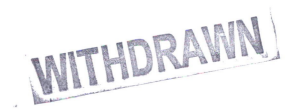

Exploring Evidence-based Practice

Despite sustained debate and progress, the evolving thing that is evidence-based nursing or practice (EBP) continues to dangle a variety of conceptual and practical loose threads. Moreover, when we think about what is being asked of students and registered or licensed practitioners in terms of EBP, it is difficult not to concede that this 'ask' is in many instances quite large and, occasionally, it may be unachievable. EBP has and continues to improve patient, client and user care, yet significant questions concerning its most basic elements remain unresolved. If nurses are to contribute to the resolution or reconfiguration of these questions then, as a first step, we must acknowledge their existence.

From a range of international standpoints and perspectives, contributors to this book focus on aspects of EBP that require development. This focus is always robust and, at times, it is unashamedly provocative. Contributors challenge readers to engage with anomalies that surround the subject and readers are asked to consider the often precarious assumptions that underpin key aspects of EBP. While both conflict and concord are evident among the various offerings presented here, the book nonetheless creates and sustains a narrative that is bigger or more substantial than the sum of individual parts. And, across contributions, a self-assuredly critical stance towards EBP as currently practiced, conceptualized and taught coexists alongside respectful admiration for all who make it happen.

Exploring Evidence-based Practice: Debates and Challenges in Nursing should be considered essential reading for academics and postgraduate students with an interest in evidence-based practice and nursing research.

Martin Lipscomb PhD RN is a senior lecturer at the University of the West of England and Secretary to the International Philosophy of Nursing Society. He is author of *A Hospice in Change: Applied Social Realist Theory*.

Routledge Key Themes in Health and Society

Exploring Evidence-based Practice

Debates and Challenges in Nursing

Edited by Martin Lipscomb

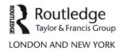

Routledge
Taylor & Francis Group

LONDON AND NEW YORK

First published 2016
by Routledge
2 Park Square, Milton Park, Abingdon, Oxon OX14 4RN

and by Routledge
711 Third Avenue, New York, NY 10017

Routledge is an imprint of the Taylor and Francis Group, an informa business

British Library Cataloguing-in-Publication Data
A catalogue record for this book is available from the British Library

Library of Congress Cataloging-in-Publication Data
Exploring evidence-based practice : debates and challenges in nursing / edited by Martin Lipscomb.
p. ; cm. — (Routledge key themes in health and society)
Includes bibliographical references and index.
ISBN 978-1-138-78990-6 (hbk.) — ISBN 978-1-315-76455-9 (ebk.)
I. Lipscomb, Martin, editor. II. Series: Routledge key themes in health and society.
[DNLM: 1. Evidence-Based Nursing. WY 100.7]
RT51
610.73—dc23
2015007302

ISBN: 978-1-138-78990-6 (hbk)
ISBN: 978-1-315-76455-9 (ebk)

Typeset in Times New Roman
by FiSH Books Ltd, Enfield

Contents

Figures and tables

Figures

Tables

Contributors

Peter Allmark PhD is Principal Research Fellow at Sheffield Hallam University. His doctorate used Aristotelian philosophy to investigate autonomy and informed consent. He has written extensively on topics in healthcare ethics and philosophy. He has also done empirical research in related areas such as parental consent to neonatal research.

Davina Banner RN PhD is an Associate Professor in the School of Nursing at the University of Northern British Columbia, Canada. Davina's clinical background is in the cardiothoracic intensive care field and her research programme focuses upon cardiovascular care and rural health service delivery. Through her research to date, Davina has worked collaboratively with a wide range of knowledge users, including healthcare providers, decision makers and patient experts. She is currently engaged in a broad range of studies, including qualitative studies of patient experiences and randomized controlled trials.

Robyn Bluhm is an Associate Professor in the Department of Philosophy and Religious Studies, and Co-Director of the Institute for Ethics and Public Affairs at Old Dominion University in Norfolk, Virginia, USA. Her research examines philosophical issues in science and medicine, with a particular focus on the relationship between ethical and epistemological questions arising in medical research or clinical practice.

Melody Carter PhD RGN is Associate Professor of Nursing at the School of Nursing and Midwifery at la Trobe University, in Australia. She has worked as a nurse, a researcher, a manager and a teacher in health and social care in London and Bristol. Her research and scholarly interests include nurse education and careers, applied social science, interprofessional practice, compassion, dignity, humanising health care and the philosophy of Pierre Bourdieu.

Bernie Garrett is an Associate Professor at the University of British Columbia School of Nursing, Canada. His work focuses on professional education, scientific philosophy, evidence-based practice and educational technologies. He is author of the textbook *Science and Modern Thought in Nursing* and over fifty journal papers on subjects including educational technology innovation, scientific philosophy and nursing policy and practice.

Rachael Grey MSc, Dip HE, RN is a Consultant Nurse in Infection Control and Tissue Viability, Yeovil District Hospital, NHS Foundation Trust. Her clinical interest is in remodelling and influencing the investigation process, resulting in a reduction of trust-apportioned infections and pressure ulcers, focusing on effective team management to promote trust-wide awareness and success.

Fred Janke MD, MSc, is an Associate Professor in the Department of Family Medicine at the University of Alberta, Canada, and the Director of Rural and Regional Health in the Division of Community Engagement. In this position he is the first 'geographic full time equivalent' member in the Faculty of Medicine to have his home base and clinical practice outside of Edmonton. In 2000, he was named as Outstanding Clinician of the Year for the David Thompson Health Region and in 2002 he was honoured for his contributions to Family Medicine through a Canadian College of Family Physician Fellowship Award.

Kathryn King-Shier RN PhD is a Professor and Guru Nanak Dev Ji DIL (Heart) Research Chair, jointly appointed to the Faculty of Nursing and Department of Community Health Sciences at the University of Calgary, Alberta, Canada. Dr. King-Shier is well known for her multi-methods programme of research, which focuses on cardiac recovery and determinants of heart health decisions, particularly focused on ethnicity and gender.

Martin Lipscomb PhD RN is a senior lecturer at the University of the West of England and Secretary to the International Philosophy of Nursing Society. He is author of *A Hospice in Change: Applied Social Realist Theory*.

Margaret Miers PhD RN retired from her role as Professor of Nursing and Social Science at the University of the West of England, Bristol, in 2010. Her publications include authored and edited texts *Gender Issues and Nursing Practice* (2000, Palgrave) and *Class, Inequalities and Nursing Practice* (2003, Palgrave). Her research interests include the evaluation of interprofessional learning and she is co-editor of Palgrave's 2010 text *Understanding Interprofessional Working in Health and Social Care: Theory and Practice*.

Deborah Neal is Consultant Physiotherapist, Yeovil District Hospital NHS Foundation Trust and Bournemouth University. Her research, clinical and service development interests are in neurology, stroke and self-management of multiple long-term conditions.

John Paley was formerly a senior lecturer in the School of Nursing, Midwifery and Health, University of Stirling, Scotland, and is currently a visiting fellow at the Centre for Health and Social Care Research, Sheffield Hallam University.

Julie Reeve is Consultant Nurse Emergency Medicine, Yeovil District Hospital NHS Foundation Trust. Her clinical focus is on developing transformational change in care delivery with specific interests in ambulatory emergency care and the development of advanced practice roles.

Mark Risjord is Professor of Philosophy at Emory University and affiliated faculty at the University of Hradec Králové, Czech Republic. His publications include *Philosophy of Social Science: A Contemporary Introduction*, *Nursing Knowledge: Science, Practice, and Philosophy* and *Woodcutters and Witchcraft: Rationality and Interpretive Change in the Social Sciences*.

Gary Rolfe is Professor of Practice Innovation and Development at Swansea University, Honorary Professor of Innovation and Development with his local health care trust and Visiting Professor at Trinity College Dublin and Canterbury Christ Church College. Gary has published ten books and over one hundred journal papers on subjects including reflective practice, practice innovation, action research, philosophy of nursing, education and scholarship.

Elizabeth Rosser DPhil, MN, Dip NEd, Dip RM, RNT is Deputy Dean, Education and Professional Practice and Professor of Nursing at Bournemouth University. She has a particular research interest in developing the health and social care workforce.

Derek Sellman RN PhD is Associate Professor in the Faculty of Nursing at the University of Alberta, Canada. Derek is the editor of the journal *Nursing Philosophy* and the author of *What Makes a Good Nurse: Why the Virtues are Important for Nurses*.

Paul Snelling is Senior Lecturer in Adult Nursing at the University of Worcester. His research interests are public health ethics and the ethics of professional regulation.

Sally Thorne, RN PhD FAAN FCAHS is Professor in the School of Nursing and Associate Dean in the Faculty of Applied Science at the University of British Columbia in Vancouver, Canada. Her substantive research is in the fields of chronic illness and cancer experience, with a particular emphasis on aspects at the intersection between system ideology and the human interface of care delivery. She is Editor-in-Chief of the journal *Nursing Inquiry* and Section Editor for *Qualitative Health Research*. She maintains a programme of scholarly activity and writing in the area of advancing applied qualitative methodology.

Janine Valentine is a Consultant Nurse for Dementia and Older People, Yeovil District Hospital NHS Foundation Trust, leading development and innovation in the care for people with dementia. Her clinical focus is specifically on evidencing therapeutic and clinical improvement through creative non-pharmacological interventions.

1   Introduction

Martin Lipscomb

Despite sustained debate and progress, the evolving and somewhat protean thing that is evidence-based nursing or practice (EBP) continues to dangle a variety of conceptual and practical loose threads. Moreover, when we think about what is being asked of students and registered or licensed practitioners regards EBP, it is difficult not to concede that this 'ask' is in many instances quite large and, occasionally, it may be unachievable. EBP has and continues to improve patient, client and user care. Yet significant questions concerning its most basic elements remain unresolved and, if nurses are to contribute to the resolution or reconfiguration of these questions then, as a first step, we must acknowledge their existence.

From a range of international standpoints and perspectives, contributors to this book focus on aspects of EBP that require development. This focus is always robust. Sometimes it is unashamedly provocative. Nonetheless, importantly, it must be stressed that this book and the arguments it contains are *not* hostile to EBP. The work does not assault or denigrate EBP and the abilities of students and nurses are not unfairly castigated. Nurses do a fantastic job in making EBP a reality and, while we need to recognise problems where they exist, and we should concede that easy answers to those problems may be unavailable (at least for now), recognising difficulties and acknowledging problems does not mean or imply that one is 'against' EBP. (Reasoned critique differs from, though it may include, pejorative denunciation.) Rather, along with the other contributors, when I am ill I want the team who care for me to incorporate evidence into decision making whenever sensible and feasible and, I trust, this incorporation will be both frequent and enabling.

A self-assuredly critical stance towards EBP as currently practised, conceptualised and taught thus merges with respectful admiration for those who make this thing happen. Contributors challenge readers to contest the mantras, platitudes and anomalies that permeate the subject and readers are asked to think about the often precarious assumptions that underpin key aspects of EBP. This is not then an introduction to EBP. Library shelves already groan beneath the weight of increasing numbers of these. Instead, while EBP's objectives, methods and conventions are outlined and explained, it will be assumed that readers are familiar with the basic concepts and activities that make up EBP. Mindful of this presumption, contributors burrow down into the messy reality of EBP's ideas and practices. Each chapter considers a vital part of what constitutes EBP and, through this process, we anticipate that understanding and perhaps even performance may improve.

Chapter 2, by Davina Banner, Fred Janke and Kathryn King-Shier begins the work. Banner and colleagues argue that, while past behaviours and attitudes are changing for the better, it must also be admitted that nurse engagement 'in the development and translation of evidence [into practice] has been somewhat lacking'. It is recognised that, despite longstanding recognition, a formidable and diverse range of overlapping barriers to EBP continue to persist. These barriers include but are not limited to, nurses' preferences for intuitive knowing over scientific and empirical knowledge, lack of confidence and competence in research finding appraisal, lack of support and influence to affect change, a dearth of facilitative mentorship and leadership and cultural and organisational obstacles. To surmount these daunting blocks upon EBP's implementation, Banner, Janke and King-Shier highlight the importance of collaborative partnership working on patient centred, clinically focused problems and, concentrating on a worked example of good practice – the management of atrial fibrillation in rural northern Canada – they illustrate how nurses and nursing can, in concert with others, foster EBP. Developing and nurturing teams that cut across traditional disciplinary, administrative and other boundaries is presented as key to successful 'real world' EBP practice. Yet shared multi-agency and interprofessional working and the benefits and difficulties that accompany such activity are noticeably underplayed or absent from student nurse education. Indeed, nurse education frequently and unrealistically anticipates a purely unidisciplinary (nursing) arena of action, whereas, if EBP is to fulfil its promise, more realistic models are needed.

Margaret Miers explores kindred themes in Chapter 3 when she speaks to the promise and potential pitfalls that accompany intra- and interprofessional working based upon or incorporating comparative effectiveness research and EBP. The importance of cross-disciplinary collaboration and working is stressed and the vital role of evidence in decision making is emphasised. Margaret notes that nursing's voice in interprofessional EBP remains fractured and muted. Moreover, reflecting continuing educational flux, nursing's competence in and commitment to EBP has historically been weak, irresolute or questionable. Indeed, while recognising the oversimplification inherent in generalising claims, Margaret nonetheless notes that an 'anti-intellectual streak' runs through elements of nursing and, in consequence, the value of research and EBP remains, for some, deeply contested. Strong nursing leadership is therefore needed. Yet, although there is much to applaud in recent developments, looking at the growth in UK nurse professor numbers as a tangential measure of leadership, only a minority of appointees have a substantive publishing history linked to healthcare practice and even fewer are obviously involved in cross-disciplinary research. Further, organisational and political barriers to nurse-initiated evidence-based change remain largely untouched despite longstanding and widespread acknowledgement of their existence (again indicating a failure in leadership). Margaret explores disputes concerning the acceptability or otherwise of different forms of evidence and, integral to these disputes, developments in decision-making theory and the roles played by differentially placed healthcare professionals in decision resolution, as well as shared decision making, are examined. As per Chapter 2, Chapter 3 nails the topics discussed to concrete problems and dilemmas. Similarly, it also highlights a host of recognised, troubling, but frequently sidestepped issues.

Picking up on issues introduced in Chapter 3, Elizabeth Rosser and colleagues (Deborah Neal, Julie Reeve, Janine Valentine and Rachael Grey) explore, in Chapter 4, the relationship between student education and practice. Like Margaret, Elizabeth and colleagues note that, while hopeful progress has and continues to be made, stubborn opposition to EBP among sections of nursing persist. For these authors, education is key to overcoming resistance. However, the standard or quality of education regarding EBP varies dramatically between institutions and, while some organisations require that lecturers have or are working towards doctorates – in contrast to more established or traditional university disciplines – many institutions employ nurse educators who have neither higher degrees nor meaningful research experience. By implication, students who are not taught by 'experts' (and this descriptor is clearly difficult to define) may fail to inculcate requisite abilities and attitudes towards EBP and research and, further, practice placements that situate students among nurses educated before EBP reached its current prominence might (assuming that lack of awareness and education may be associated with the devaluation of EBP and research) reinforce forms of enculturation that are antipathetic or even hostile towards EBP. Moreover, even institutions that place a premium on EBP and research education must cram this education into tightly packed syllabi. Collapsing important topics into circumscribed and perhaps inadequate timeslots cannot but suggest to students that EBP and research are of marginal consequence. Pointing towards the continued persistence of an 'anti-research culture' among nurses, Elizabeth and her colleagues (like others) note that students and practitioners often lack crucial resources to pursue evidence-based care improvement (including resources of confidence and cultural capital). The potentially beneficial role that nursing's professoriate might play in remedying these problems is highlighted but, again, it is stressed that professorial appointments must be clinically and patient orientated if benefits are to be garnered.

Sticking with the theme of multidisciplinary and interprofessional working, in Chapter 5, Melody Carter explores EBP from an Australian perspective. In this process, she challenges traditional ideas concerning how nurses should learn about and approach practice and, indeed, the 'principle argument [offered] is that in order to make effective contributions to interprofessional care, professionals (including nurses) need to work from a knowledge base that unifies or harmonises their practice with other disciplines'. This claim could be interpreted as undercutting professionalising agendas that promote the distinct uniqueness of nursing knowledge. However, Melody metaphorically positions nurses as 'hinge-points' through or around which interprofessional practice operates and, in this way, nursing's contribution to EBP is, or could be, facilitated and made concrete.

Illustrative stories concerning encounters with an 'early' patient with AIDS in 1985 and, later, personal loss involving the untimely death of Melody's brother to AIDS-complicated bronchial carcinoma in 2006 are used to clarify meaning. Specifically, advances in knowledge and developments in thinking about EBP 'then' and 'now' and also the comparative openness with which previously taboo topics can be discussed are sketched. It is proposed that progress in EBP implementation has occurred but that improvements need to be viewed from within 'the challenges and opportunities that face each unique country and its particular cultures, languages, political outlook and health care economy' (so EBP takes place in and is effected by forms of specific and local political, social and cultural influence). Melody introduces the ideas of French sociologist, anthropologist and philosopher Pierre Bourdieu to make sense of these influences and situations and his concept of habitus is employed to unpack factors associated with behavioural change. Chapter 5 thus explores how 'the knowledge that informs the decisions we make and the actions we take, arises from text, talk and experience'.

Chapter 6, by Mark Risjord, signals a change in direction. Using examples from everyday nursing activities (tracheal and endotracheal suctioning), Mark asks us to think about what we mean by knowledge and, further, its relation to evidence and EBP. Distinguishing between practical and propositional knowledge in clinical judgement, it is argued that 'practical activity is not the sort of thing that calls for justification' and, while evidence justifies certain forms of or rationales for action, EBP is nonetheless 'something of an oxymoron'. Acknowledging that practice guidelines should be based upon the sorts of propositional knowledge that research evidence provides, Mark notes that, problematically, instrumental action (that is, the type of action supported by practice guidelines) 'is not know-how' since know-how involves more than acting in accordance with guideline-generated rules. Indeed, the 'problem with treating evidence-based guidelines as justifying instrumental beliefs [i.e. beliefs capable of supporting acts/behaviours] is that it turns expert nursing into novice rule following'. Mark focuses on the relationship between propositional knowledge (knowledge from evidence) and practical know-how (knowledge concerning action in the world) and he suggests that, insofar as rules inevitably require interpretation (potentially an infinite regress of interpretation), propositional knowledge of the sort found in rule-forming guidelines cannot direct embodied action in any straightforward sense. Indeed, experienced nurses can and often do disregard (act outside of) evidence-based guidelines and this may be correct or appropriate. Responses to Mark's argument will depend upon one's ontological standpoint regarding agents and agency, self-knowledge and intentionality, mind and embodiment and, pivotally, the relationship of each of these concepts to environmentally situated action. While practical examples demonstrate the points being made, Chapter 6 is theoretical in tone and content. Nursing's uncertain and occasionally hostile attitude towards theory is well documented (and noted by several contributors to this book). Nevertheless, Mark's chapter successfully presses home the significance and importance of the denotation and application of evidence in decision making and, further, he challenges readers to engage with arguments and ideas that, although discussed outside of nursing, rarely receive sustained attention in 'our' literature.

In Chapter 7, Robyn Bluhm ties longstanding arguments regarding the disputed nature of generalisation to EBP. Robyn and Mark's chapters are quite dissimilar. Yet, insofar as Robyn is interested in unpicking what might colloquially be termed the 'use value' of research, both contributors focus upon common problems, albeit from radically contrasting perspectives. For Robyn, while EBP's emphasis on enabling practitioners to grasp critical appraisal skills is 'extremely valuable', EBP as traditionally presented and interpreted 'is much weaker when it comes to teaching nurses how to use the results of their critical appraisal in clinical practice'. Here, links back to previous chapters focused on interprofessional and multi-agency working can be made, since earlier contributions likewise explored (albeit from different vantages) the problematic nature of the application of EBP. Robyn notes that EBP's proponents value studies that combine participant randomisation with 'allocation concealment, and follow-up' (that is, 'good' randomised controlled trials or RCTs). This ensures internal validity. Yet too close a focus on internal validity and the concomitant devaluing of external validity limits the ability of 'nurses to use the results of research to inform patient care'. Problematically, since clinical settings rarely, if ever, mirror study settings, practitioners cannot accurately assess generalizability. Further, randomisation and allocation concealment may compound difficulties with generalizability, since unknown and known confounders (factors which may bias or skew results) cannot be known to be balanced between intervention and control arms of a study. Instead, what is required are studies that take external validity seriously. Thus, whereas RCTs actively seek to remove or limit the influence of extraneous variables (such has patient comorbidities), study results need – if they are to be useful – to beneficially inform decision making in relation to patient or client groups that almost always have multiple comorbidities and/or may differ in notable ways from research study subjects. In Robyn's words, 'while RCTs with high internal validity and narrow confidence intervals … provide clear evidence about whether the experimental intervention is better than the control, they are the *least* generalisable source of evidence when what is required is to determine whether the intervention will be effective outside of that context'. And, as a part of this problem or issue, determining the extent to which 'a' patient will or will not benefit from an intervention or treatment that has been proven to possess 'average' benefits is one of the central problems for EBP. Clearly, if accepted, Robyn's well-reasoned argument destabilises a great deal of current thinking about EBP. In particular, by highlighting problems with quantitative generalisation, Robyn undercuts the supposed value of aspects of the hierarchy of evidence.

Gary Rolfe begins Chapter 8 by outlining something of the history of EBP. This history emphasises that evidence-based nursing's progenitor, evidence-based medicine (EBM), originated as a medical educational initiative which deployed the descriptor 'evidence' solely in relation to published research reports. These published sources (ideally RCTs) were to be assessed on methodological, not practice relevant criteria, and assessment took place to facilitate students in effectively challenging otherwise omniscient clinical authority (that is, EBM was to be a counterweight to untrammelled consultant power or expert opinion). In response to criticism, EBP's proponents softened their tone and, mindful of the need to better connect research findings with clinical practice, it was recognised that evidence (still tightly limited in scope) had to be used 'judiciously' and 'conscientiously' so that it could be 'integrated' with 'expertise'. Understandably and perhaps inevitably – although also somewhat problematically – this now left it 'to the judgement of individual practitioners to decide whether and how to incorporate research findings into their clinical decisions'. Transposed into nursing, EBP began to open up the meaning and remit of evidence as, it was asserted, the goals and 'ways' of nursing differed from those of medicine. This opening up allowed qualitative researchers to claim that their studies were also evidence (of a sort). However, an allied but potentially even more profound conceptual shift occurred when nurses began to elide evidence with expertise. In some respects, this attempted conflation merely emulates and extends EBM's acknowledgement that individual clinical judgment is required when decisions about the suitability and relevance of research evidence to practice are made. Nonetheless, this was and remains a difficult move and arguments about the uncertain role of expert opinion in EBP continue unabated. Or, put another way, the disputed relationship between evidence (hierarchically organised) and expertise (opinion) – which may or may not be accorded a place in a hierarchy – still resonates. Further, when we factor in desires to meet expressed patient preferences and resource availability, it becomes clear that EBP is indeed 'a deceptively simple term for a difficult, contested and multi-faceted concept'. Engaging with this complexity, Gary suggests that two distinct approaches to best nursing practice are located within the literature (that is, best practice as 'a planned and methodical intervention' vs. 'professional artistry') and, intriguingly, each approach can be linked with separate notions of 'best evidence'. Exploration of these alternatives permits Gary to argue that 'best practice should dictate what counts as best evidence rather than vice versa'. This claim is appealing and intuitively reasonable. However, plausibility should not mask the subtle challenge that is presented here. The generality of current thinking and educational instruction regarding EBP begins with a consideration of methods and methodologies. It does not start from considerations of or from practice. This thought-provoking contribution displays commonalities in 'orientation' if not substance with chapters by Robyn Bluhm, Mark Risjord, Peter Allmark and others.

Bernie Garrett, in Chapter 9, picks up on and develops a variety of themes explored elsewhere in this volume. It is, for example, noted that undergraduate textbooks and education 'almost entirely focus on research methods and the hierarchy of evidence, presenting EBP in a manner that largely ignores non-research forms of evidence' (and indeed, all other relevant concerns). Moreover, like Gary (Chapter 8), Bernie situates EBP within an historical frame and this enables him to emphasise and explore the often overlooked dimensions of clinical expertise and patient autonomy or choice in EBP. Working through how these elements of EBP are integrated into nursing practice forms, together with an examination of non-research 'evidence', the central concern of this chapter. And, interestingly, positioning these debates within nursing's cultural history enables Bernie to identify an 'anti-science trend that is well established ... in Canada and beyond'. From this perspective, EBP is presented in certain North American nursing curricula both 'as a straw-man confection of positivist thinking ... [and as] the evidence-based tyranny of medicine'. Indeed, viewing EBP as just another of the 'ways of knowing' allows the forceful logic of its claims to be seen as 'hegemonic and oppressive'. Anti-science advocates permit unconscionable nonsense such as therapeutic touch, homoeopathy and mysticism to find a home within some nursing curricula and those who embrace postmodernist 'multiple truths' in this manner shape EBP as an 'irrelevancy'. Moreover, since the profession cannot easily embrace both stridently relativist epistemologies *and* nuanced albeit traditional empiricism, nurse education finds itself at something of a 'crossroads'.

In Chapter 10, John Paley describes the disputed and contentious place of qualitative research in the hierarchy of evidence, nurse education and, by implication, EBP. Like Bernie in Chapter 9, John recognises that EBP is seen by some as privileging quantitative ways of knowing and, again, this privileging has been considered 'an arbitrary imposition'. John further notes that powerful voices in nursing have and are seeking to raise the status of qualitative research to match that accorded to quantitative work and, in this process, weaknesses (real and imagined) in quantitative experimental design are identified and emphasised. John, on the other hand, persuasively argues that, regardless of the stridency of calls favouring qualitative inquiry, it is unclear whether 'qualitative evidence should be "on an equal footing" with evidence derived from quantitative and experimental designs'. Furthermore, insofar as statistical tests and experimental quantitative designs strive to limit the risk of inferential error, the absence of similar procedures and protocols in qualitative studies cannot but subvert claims regarding the status and use value of those findings. Indeed, unwelcome though the observation may be, it remains the case that, without such procedures and protocols, 'there is no way of discriminating between legitimate inference in qualitative research and various forms of cognitive bias: observer expectancy effects, belief bias, illusory correlation, availability cascade, selective perception, congruence bias, motivated reasoning, or outright wishful thinking'. To understand how and why nursing has become attached to qualitative inquiry, John notes that for 'the past thirty years, methodological discussion in qualitative health research ... has been subordinated to the requirements of postgraduate study'. This subordination is important. It has imposed constraints on the methodologies and methods that are available to students and, thus, in order that studies can be completed by individuals with minimal resources in short time periods, postgraduate nursing researchers have found it expedient to undertake small sample interview-based studies, which limit themselves to retrospective descriptions of the participants' experience and the 'meaning' they attach to experience. The philosophical justifications of this approach are, however, weak. And, in addition, the social psychology literature undermines the way in which 'meaning' is interpreted in most nursing qualitative studies. John's argument raises serious and awkward questions that should, if given the attention they deserve, prompt fresh thinking among educators, researchers and the consumers (readers) of research.

Continuing and developing ideas introduced in preceding contributions, in Chapter 11, Sally Thorne explores the definition, purpose and constitution of evidence, nursing's perhaps ill-advised creative expansion of the meaning of evidence and the contested status and problematic use value of qualitative research findings. It is argued that nurses have not always scrutinised their own practices as thoroughly as they do the practices of others and, moreover, misguided beliefs about EBP decision making have led some nurses to uncritically and indulgently license or embrace 'multiple ways of knowing ... [and] such attributes as pattern recognition clinical wisdom'. Broadening the range of activities and forms of understanding that are labelled evidence to include, for example, qualitative scholarship, may, however, contribute to 'the confusion and ideological posturing' that surrounds EBP. This is not an attack upon qualitative research. Sally grants that qualitative scholarship has a role to play in developing and nuancing understanding and questioning the evidential credentials of qualitative research does not mean or imply that this form of inquiry lacks merit. However, if the definitional scope or properties of evidence are carelessly blurred so that we recognise as evidence 'all forms of knowledge from which a nurse might legitimately build a good decision, we lose track of what differentiates the various knowledge forms, creating a circularity of logic within which everything is evidence and nothing remains as a corrective for false logic'. Thus not '*all* scholarly products constitute evidence' and while, in rare instances, a few qualitative products might be considered evidence, the overwhelming majority of qualitative nursing reports are simply not this thing. Again, Sally's argument is (to repeat) not hostile to qualitative inquiry and, paradoxically, the chapter supports qualitative scholarship insofar as the re-evaluation that is argued for repositions this large and non-homogenous body of scholarship on a firmer footing – that is, as a valuable non-evidential form of disciplinary focused knowledge. The chapter outlines a variety of intriguing questions and challenges and, for example, qualitative researchers are tasked with engaging more thoughtfully with often overlooked aspects of their activities. Thus, since confusion is apparent in the way qualitative findings are employed, Sally calls upon scholars to temper or finesse generalising claims and 'anticipate the implications of their findings in the hands of a practice audience'. It is difficult to argue against the logic of the arguments presented, whether those arguments will be met is of course another matter.

In Chapter 12, I argue that students and nurses generally lack the ability to appraise research findings at a level or depth commensurate with altering or informing practice on the basis of understandings gained. This argument is not antagonistic to student or nurse capabilities. It simply rests on the idea that *if* appraisal requires that appraisers are substantively able to 'follow through' how conclusions or findings are derived – if substantive understanding is necessary for practice changes to be defensible – *then* in almost all instances students and nurses who are not themselves researchers or statisticians are underprepared and thus unable to do this thing. Quantitative researchers, for example, use statistical tests that non-statisticians are unlikely to understand (non-statisticians cannot therefore know whether findings are warranted). While qualitative research reports rarely provide readers with sufficient detail to determine how findings emerged (and it may in principle be impossible for qualitative researchers to provide this detail). In consequence, I suggest that individual practitioners should not be held accountable for accessing, interpreting and implementing primary research findings. Instead, students and nurses should pay less attention to methods, methodologies and report critiques and, in contrast to other contributors to this volume, I propose that educators should emphasise to students the importance of implementing reputable guidelines. This option runs risks (see Mark Risjord, Chapter 6, and Derek Sellman, Chapter 14). However, redirecting the focus of EBP education to finding implementation and, in this process, seeking ways of overcoming political and organisational barriers to EBP might, for example, meet calls for greater intra- and interprofessional collaboration and, also, re-establish the centrality and problematic of decision making in practice.

Peter Allmark explores, in Chapter 13, ethics and EBP from an Aristotelian perspective. More specifically, Peter focuses on 'the epistemology of practice; in other words, what type of evidence or knowledge is needed in deciding how to act?'. Echoing themes raised by Mark Risjord and Gary Rolfe (among others), a distinction is made between 'practical and scientific knowledge [and] it is suggested that evidence in the form of scientific knowledge, no matter how widely defined, cannot form the basis of practice because it cannot provide the goals that action requires'. Peter argues that ethical practice or right action demands 'more than good evidence; it requires also the right ends' – and these ends or goals, the aims of action, while coming in the first instance from practice, ultimately find their origins in deeper and wider personal and social influences. To structure the work, ethical concerns or difficulties with current conceptualisations of EBP are identified. It is proposed that the common response to ethical concerns is to turn to epistemology as the source of the problem. Yet this response is inadequate. It overlooks the complexity of purposeful or intentional human motivation and action, and it ignores the practical wisdom which is embodied in craft like activities such as nursing. It also privileges executive knowledge over skill-type knowledge. Peter's critique is not anti-scientific or anti-EBP. Indeed, he argues that Aristotelian concepts provide 'tools for practitioners and researchers to note the difference between epistemic wisdom and practical wisdom' and, through the use of these tools, the 'practice of EBP is largely exonerated'. The chapter melds together ethical theory and practical insights to present a fresh perspective on issues explored by other contributors to this volume.

Picking up on themes introduced by Sally Thorne, Peter Allmark and Mark Risjord, in Chapter 14, Derek Sellman explores ethical competence from the perspective or vantage of an evidence user (that is, a nurse in practice). It is argued that, while nurses legitimately and rightly expect researchers to meet high ethical standards in establishing evidence (that is, in generating research findings), analogous ethical responsibilities rest upon nurses who are not researchers. Explicitly, when seeking to determine the use value of study findings, nurses should engage as critically and with as much integrity as researchers do when they produce findings. Specifically, nurses should 'seek answers to questions' in a manner that gives 'confidence in the value of the evidence' and significant ethical epistemic responsibilities therefore accompany or are integral to EBP. However, problematically, it is probably the case that nurses are more 'receptive to evidence that supports rather than that which refutes firmly held beliefs' and, while this unfortunate tendency is not restricted to nurses or nursing, failure to meticulously evaluate evidence for and against current practices may and perhaps should be viewed as a serious ethical lapse. Derek explores the barriers and difficulties faced by nurses in meeting their epistemic obligations and, while much stands in the way of accomplishing ideal or desirable practice, it is argued that this should not dissuade efforts to surmount obstacles whenever possible. The chapter takes an original line through ethics and EBP and, for both educationalists and practitioners alike, it details a landscape of important problems and issues that are underexplored in nursing's current literature.

Paul Snelling, in the final chapter, examines the problem, conundrum or 'myth' of evidence based (nursing) policy. Paul's argument is accessible, nuanced and, in its implications, shocking. The chapter critiques real world policy initiatives concerning intentional rounding and smoking bans. It is claimed that rounding 'has been widely implemented in the interest of a political need for action, supported by appeasing managers [including nurse managers] in the absence of any credible evidence … [while] Authoritarian and paternalistic smoking policies are given evidential gloss by NICE [National Institute for Health and Care Excellence] guidelines but are driven by imposed values'. If the arguments presented in this chapter hold – and they certainly appear reasonable – senior nurses and healthcare managers are complicit in compromising nurse regulatory requirements regards evidence use, they have undermined the concept of autonomous professional practice, and they have abused common logic. Paul's work raises difficult questions for nurse leaders and the profession more generally. Evidence's role in policy formation and labour force direction is another aspect of EBP that has yet to receive the attention it merits and, as Paul's chapter makes clear, this lacuna is of concrete importance to nurses, nursing and patient care delivery.

To conclude, EBP describes an important set of activities and ideas. Dispute surrounds significant aspects of the topic and, yet, the quality of nursing care ultimately depends upon our ability to successfully accomplish EBP. A single book or publication cannot but scratch the surface of so large a subject. Nonetheless, we would like to think that this work, by engaging with under-explored problems, contributes positively to the literature. As will by now be clear, this volume does not lay out a unified or simple set of messages. It does not provide ready answers. Instead it seeks to stimulate discussion and debate. Contributors agree and disagree with each other in their writing and conflict and concord are both present among the various offerings. Each chapter stands alone, yet collectively the work creates and sustains a narrative that is bigger or more substantial than the sum of individual parts. We hope you find the book interesting.

2 Making evidence-based practice happen in 'real world' contexts

The importance of collaborative partnerships

Davina Banner, Fred Janke and Kathryn King-Shier

Healthcare organizations around the world are striving to develop services that are evidence-based in order to improve patient care and health service outcomes (Gifford *et al.*, 2013). Evidence-based practice (EBP) has its roots in medicine through groups such as the Evidence-based Medicine Working Group and emerged in response to gaps between research and practice, as well as large variations in healthcare delivery (McGlynn *et al.*, 2003; Wennberg, 2011). The EBP movement highlights the need for decision making that is based on the best available evidence, typically randomized controlled trials and systematic reviews. This movement has permeated all healthcare disciplines and is an expectation and requirement for most healthcare providers (Canadian Nurses Association, 2010; Fineout-Overholt *et al.*, 2005; Rolfe *et al.*, 2008; Zwarenstein and Reeves, 2006). In nursing, this has included a growing focus on EBP across the administration, education, and practice settings.

Since its advent, EBP has been the topic of many publications and it is associated with improved patient and health service outcomes (Brown, 1992; Devine and Westlake, 1995; Heater *et al.*, 1988). However, it has not been without controversy. Many concerns have been raised around what constitutes evidence, causes of delay in integrating evidence into practice and the challenges of assessing evidence within the context of complex and 'real world' clinical environments (Fineout-Overholt *et al.*, 2005; Fineout-Overholt and Melnyk, 2005; French, 2002; Gifford *et al.*, 2013; Grimshaw *et al.*, 1995, 2005; Harlos *et al.*, 2012; Sackett, 2000).

Despite the widespread acceptance of EBP, nurses' interest and involvement in the development and integration of evidence has been lacking (Cutcliff and Bassett, 1997; Funk *et al.*, 1995; Pravikoff *et al.*, 2005). This has been in part due to the limited exposure of nurses to research and EBP initiatives. Likewise, research has traditionally been the domain of those in academia and, until recent years, was largely based in the university setting, with limited attention given to the clinical context and implementation of the findings. These critical disconnects have led to new fields and mechanisms of inquiry, such as implementation science and knowledge translation, that focuses not only on the development of high-quality evidence but also the integration of this evidence into practice (Zwarenstein and Reeves, 2006; Davis *et al.*, 2003; Davies *et al.*, 2010). At the heart of this is the need for meaningful collaboration between researchers and knowledge users (including community representatives, decision makers, health-care providers and policy makers). Through these partnerships, evidence can be created that is responsive to healthcare needs, is grounded in the 'real world' context and is developed in a manner that optimizes its integration into clinical practice (Davis *et al.*, 2003; Gifford *et al.*, 2013; Harlos *et al.*, 2012). It is in the context of these partnerships that the research and practice worlds become bridged and the potential of EBP can be realized. Nurses have a critical role to play in this process.

Here, we examine the role of partnerships in EBP with a particular focus upon collaborative research teams. We address how partnerships are initiated and developed and examine some of the practical considerations associated with these partnerships. We draw upon our experiences of developing a collaborative research team exploring the management of atrial fibrillation in rural and northern Canada. Atrial fibrillation is a type of irregular heartbeat that is associated with very high increases in death and disability, including a 500% increase in stroke risk (Heart and Stroke Foundation of Canada, 2014). The management of atrial fibrillation and its associated risks requires input from a wide range of healthcare providers across many community and specialist settings. There is very little literature that has examined the management of atrial fibrillation in rural settings and our team has been working to undertake exploratory studies to examine patient, provider and health service issues. Our research team comprises a broad range of researchers and knowledge users, including decision makers, interdisciplinary healthcare providers from a range of community and specialty contexts, policy makers and a patient expert. The team has developed over the past three years, initially for a qualitative study to explore the experiences of healthcare providers managing atrial fibrillation in rural communities but, more recently, has expanded into a tri-provincial Canadian partnership to collaborate on a wider range of research and clinical initiatives. In this chapter, we present some examples of our 'living partnership' and will reflect on some of the lessons learned to date.

Evidence-based practice: making it happen in the 'real world'

The need to close the gap between research and practice is an age-old issue. For decades, administrators, healthcare providers, policy makers and researchers have worked to develop strategies to optimize the integration of evidence to improve health outcomes (Brown, 1992; Devine and Westlake, 1995; French, 2000; Gifford *et al.*, 2013; Grimshaw *et al.*, 2005; Rolfe *et al.*, 2008). This EBP movement emerged largely from medicine but has pervaded most healthcare disciplines. Healthcare providers, including nurses, are required to base their practice upon the best available evidence (Canadian Nurses Association, 2010; Fineout-Overholt and Melnyk, 2005; Rolfe *et al.*, 2008; Zwarenstein and Reeves, 2006).

Great efforts have been made globally to develop and synthesize the best quality evidence, typically randomized controlled trials and systematic reviews. However, the implementation of evidence into clinical practice can be haphazard and inconsistent (Graham *et al.*, 2006). One explanation for this is that many healthcare providers are overburdened with information and have limited capacity or opportunities to critically evaluate the evidence and its application within the 'real world' clinical settings (Bero *et al.*, 1998; Graham and Tetroe, 2007; Harrison *et al.*, 2010; Zwarenstein *et al.*, 2009). For example, it can be challenging for some healthcare providers in more isolated settings to adopt best practices for the management of complex conditions, such as atrial fibrillation, in the absence of specialist assessment and monitoring facilities. Clinical practice guidelines can help to overcome some of these issues by presenting summaries of the evidence and providing important benchmarks and decision-making support for healthcare providers at the front line (Nutley *et al.*, 2003). Further, researchers also face barriers that impact the development and implementation of evidence. Since research has been traditionally grounded in the academic setting, there has been little focus on the contextual realities of clinical practice or consideration of how evidence would be integrated and used in practice.

These disparities between the research and practice settings have resulted in barriers in the creation and translation of evidence. As a result, the integration of evidence into practice is frequently delayed and can lead to poorer patient outcomes and losses in health service effectiveness (Fineout-Overholt *et al.*, 2005; Fineout-Overholt and Melnyk, 2005; French, 2002; Gifford *et al.*, 2013; Grimshaw *et al.*, 1995, 2005; Heater *et al.*, 1988; Sackett, 2000). This includes risks resulting from the overuse, underuse or misuse of pharmaceutical agents or clinical interventions, as well as greater healthcare costs related to losses in efficiency and productivity (Davis *et al.*, 2003; Harlos *et al.*, 2012; McGlynn *et al.*, 2003; Ramanujam and Rousseau, 2006).

A renewed focus upon collaborative partnerships is helping to bridge these gaps and is leading to innovative ways of undertaking research while maximizing its uptake into practice (Pope and Mays, 1995; Rapport *et al.*, 2013). This has included a diversification in research approaches, such as the integration of qualitative research into randomized controlled trials and collaborative knowledge synthesis activities, that have rendered evidence that is more attuned to the healthcare context and can be more readily integrated into clinical practice (Gibson *et al.*, 2004).

For the most part, the application of evidence requires a coordinated effort of a range of knowledge users, in addition to resources and support at the practice and organizational level. Practitioners can be overwhelmed with available evidence or faced with the need to develop solutions to highly complex clinical problems across a range of healthcare environments (Straus *et al.*, 2011). They may also face a range of barriers, including lack of knowledge, resources, skills and support, that may impact upon their ability to engage in research or other EBP initiatives. Understanding these barriers at the onset of any research or EBP activities can be helpful in developing effective processes that optimize the creation and integration of knowledge into practice (Baker *et al.*, 2010; Bosch *et al.*, 2007; Gifford *et al.*, 2013). In addition, providing support to overcome these, including mentorship, can help practitioners navigate this process (Fineholt-Overholt *et al.*, 2005). Such supports can be particularly helpful for professionals, such as nurses, who may experience many barriers to engagement in EBP activities and processes.

Evidence based practice: the emerging role of nurses

EBP is not new to nursing and strong historical and theoretical roots exist, most notably through the work of Florence Nightingale during the Crimean war, which led to significant advancements in public health and sanitation, as well as the professionalization of nursing (McDonald, 2001). However, while the virtues of EBP are well accepted, the engagement of nurses in the development and trans-lation of evidence has been somewhat lacking (Cutcliff and Bassett, 1997; Funk *et al.*, 1995; Pravikoff *et al.*, 2005). As Bluhm and Rolfe argue in Chapters 7 and 8, respectively, part of these difficulties has resulted from the perceived discon-nect between the evidence and the practice of nursing. Through such disconnects, nurses face challenges in marrying the uniqueness of the patient interaction, context of practice and the varied epistemological foundations of knowledge, with the rigidity of typical forms of higher level evidence, such as the random-ized controlled trial or systematic review. As a result of these challenges and uncertainties, many nurses have been cautious of research and EBP initiatives. Subsequently, the vital perspectives that nurses bring, including frontline insights into healthcare delivery and patient perspectives, have been largely absent (Flodgren *et al.*, 2012; Gifford *et al.*, 2013).

The level of engagement of nurses in research and EBP initiatives is gradually changing and more nurses are participating in and leading collaborative EBP initiatives (Hicks, 1995; Kitson *et al.*, 1998; Olade, 2004; Woodward *et al.*, 2007). This is likely due to educational shifts in nursing, resulting from the wide-spread introduction of baccalaureate and higher degrees, as well as greater exposure to interdisciplinary education and practice. However, numerous barriers to EBP still exist in nursing. These include:

- more limited reliance upon scientific or empirical knowledge in favour of other forms of disciplinary knowledge, such as intuitive knowing (DiCenso *et al.*, 1998; Estabrooks, 1998);
- lack of confidence and knowledge when appraising or participating in research (Gerrish *et al.*, 2003; Gifford *et al.*, 2013; Melnyk *et al.*, 2004; Rycroft-Malone *et al.*, 2004);
- lack of opportunity as a result of chronic workforce shortages and limited time release;
- lack of perceived power to generate change (Flodgren *et al.*, 2012); and
- less access to mentorship or dedicated research support and funding (Brown *et al.*, 2009; Loke *et al.*, 2014; Rosswurm and Larrabee, 1999).

For many nurses, research activities are not rewarded and many provide contributions 'off the side of their desk'. This can make sustained engagement and change challenging (Hutchinson and Johnston, 2006).

Over recent years, great efforts have been made to overcome these barriers. One mechanism to address this has been the increasing exposure of nurses to research theory and critical appraisal techniques during their nursing education (Koehn and Lehman, 2008; Fineout-Overholt *et al.*, 2005). Greater 'on the ground' support has also become more common in many healthcare organizations, typically in the form of research support roles. In addition, the growing numbers of advanced practice and healthcare leadership roles offers real potential for a cultural shift that will create space for nurses to effectively contribute and lead EBP initiatives and research (Bryant-Lukosius *et al.*, 2004; Hicks, 1995; Kitson *et al.*, 1998; Olade, 2004; Woodward *et al.*, 2007). Nurses have a critical role to play in the EBP movement and further investment is needed to provide the development and support needed to enable nurses to become active collaborators and leaders. This may include providing access to academic and practice mentors, and support for frontline nurses to champion and participate in EBP activities, such as journal clubs and educational rounds (Fineout-Overholt *et al.*, 2005).

Collaborative research partnerships

In healthcare setting across the world, there has been increasing enthusiasm for collaborative research partnerships. Such partnerships are seen as a mechanism for bringing together the critical expertise, knowledge and resources needed to improve health outcomes and build research capacity (Canadian Coalition for Global Health Research, 2014; Evans *et al.*, 2011; Mullen, 1998; Tetroe *et al.*, 2008). Through these partnerships, there is an opportunity to examine issues within the context of 'real world' health services and explore nuances that might otherwise be overlooked (Kirby, 2004). This is particularly important in the light of increasing healthcare costs and demands resulting from escalating levels of chronic disease, worsening health outcomes and growing health disparities (Alamian and Paradis, 2012; Frohlich *et al.*, 2006; McPherson *et al.*, 2001; Reeves *et al.*, 2008). There has never been a greater need for the development of high-quality evidence and its effective translation into practice.

Collaborative research partnerships are frequently created in response to a given healthcare challenge or a gap in knowledge. Through this, researchers and knowledge users work together, each contributing specific insights relevant to the research process or community and healthcare context. Activities can include primary research, quality improvement initiatives or knowledge synthesis activities, all of which contribute richly to the development of evidence-based practices and healthcare delivery. The drivers for collaborative partnerships are not just isolated to the clinical context but also reflect emerging expectations of many academic institutions, funding organizations and networks. For example, the Canadian Institutes of Health Research, the major funder of health research in Canada, requires collaborations in many of their funding competitions, including the Knowledge Synthesis and Partnerships for Health Systems Improvement grant competitions (Canadian Institutes of Health Research, 2015). In many of these competitions, it is expected that research teams are co-led by a researcher and a knowledge user, to harness the critical perspectives of the related healthcare communities, including frontline clinicians, healthcare administrators and policy makers (McLaughlin, 2006).

While collaborative research partnerships are powerful, they are also inherently complex and require a coordinated effort of a diverse range of community and healthcare partners, often over long periods of time (Bronstein, 2003). However, as these relationships mature, the partnerships can become more formalized and can result in greater alignment and synergies across different communities and organizations (Venuta and Graham, 2010). This could include the development of formalized structures and processes, such as a memorandum of understanding or collaborative research institute, to support more successive and sustained contributions to EBP and to influence the way in which services are organized and delivered. To optimize collaboration, a number of factors must be considered including team building, collaborative working, leadership and translating evidence in practice.

Team building

As previously identified, the genesis of many collaborative research partnerships arises in response to specific healthcare challenges or need. As a result, the teambuilding activities must also reflect these needs and should aim to capture a group of knowledge users from a range of disciplines, settings or populations with relevant experiences and insights (Helfrich *et al.*, 2007). As teams are initially coming together, team building may occur in a manner akin to a snowball sampling technique, whereby initial partners recommend potential team members and identify their potential contributions. For example, researchers from a range of health or related disciplines may be brought together to provide methodological or practical research expertise related to the phenomenon of interest. Likewise, a diverse range of knowledge users, including healthcare providers, administrators and policy makers, may be brought together to identify key healthcare challenges, potential barriers and enablers for EBP, to provide insight into the contextual realities for patients and healthcare providers, and to champion change with the clinical setting. Furthermore, community representatives or patient experts may also be engaged to capture key experiential insights (Chelimsky, 1995; Canadian Institutes of Health Research, 2008; Secret *et al.*, 2011; Venuta and Graham, 2010). In larger teams, members with experience in other fields, such as health informatics and management, can also be helpful (Harlos *et al.*, 2012; Walter *et al.*, 2003). As the team develops, the recruitment of new members is likely to become more strategic in nature and often involves a more deliberate process of engagement. This could, for example, include identifying and collaborating with key policy makers to scale up initiatives.

At each stage, team building must involve conscious and explicit processes for optimizing the potential contribution of the team. This includes providing opportunities to establish mutual goals, to clearly articulate expectations and to ensure that the different types of knowledge from the partners are heard and valued. As Miers highlights in Chapter 3, this includes recognizing the diverse contributions and epistemologies of the interdisciplinary audiences but could also include other forms of knowledge from community representatives (including those from Aboriginal communities) and patient groups that may be expressed in different forms and language. For our group, the initial process of team building took place over two years and is still considered to be a continuing process. In the early stages, core team members connected to gather insights into the management of atrial fibrillation in rural communities and to identify key knowledge users and informants. As a group, we then worked to build these connections, with members assisting in introductions, networking and engagement processes.

In our team's research activities to date, all of the team members have been instrumental in supporting the research activities, including identifying new sources of literature, supporting access and recruitment in clinical sites, promoting knowledge exchange and transfer, and participating in consultative activities. As part of these activities, academic and practice partners have co-presented research findings and processes to a variety of audiences, including conference presentations and webinars. In addition, the team obtained funding and undertook stakeholder consultations in three Canadian provinces to share research findings and to explore issues related to the different practice settings, including variations in practice and barriers to guideline-based care. These consultations brought together a broader range of knowledge users and stakeholders, including provincial and national policy makers, decision makers from many health authorities, and healthcare providers from a range of disciplines and settings, including family doctors and interdisciplinary specialists. The consultation meetings provided essential contextual insights that have informed the research agenda and provided critical opportunities for targeted knowledge translation activities to practice champions and policy makers. Additionally, these consultations led to the expansion of the research team to include members from across the three provinces, as well as new collaborations with other teams and networks, including a national clinical trials network. This has provided opportunities for broadening the scope of the team's activities. More recently, members of the team have begun to work with a patient expert. The patient expert not only provides critical experiential insights but is also engaged as a contributing team member to assist in the identification and prioritization of patient-orientated outcomes and research. As a team, we are cognizant of the need to promote inclusiveness for all our members through team working and minimizing any potential barriers. Overall, key elements of this process have been a continuing commitment to collaborative working and the shared goal of improving the health of Canadians with atrial fibrillation. While we may have a fair way to go on this journey, our learning as a team has provided a solid foundation for positive change.

Collaborative working

To optimize collaboration, continuing attention to the development and maintenance of team processes is required and a number of issues need to be considered.
Firstly, it is essential that trusting relationships are established; this includes
having open lines of communication so that all partners are aware of the expectations and needs of each partner (Harlos *et al.*, 2012). This includes clearly
articulating the roles of team members, as well as delineating team expectations
and processes, including the frequency of meetings, important timelines and
contributions to grants and publications (Smith *et al.*, 2002; Soydan, 2002; Roper,
2002). Secondly, regular opportunities for team members to connect and share
insights are vital if the team is to function effectively. Thirdly, ensuring and
promoting diversity in team membership is essential. This includes ensuring that
key groups are appropriately represented (Beresford, 2007; Evans *et al.*, 2011).
For example, McLaughlin (2009) argues that, often, health and social services
teams engage the 'usual suspects' and, as a result, fail to obtain adequate representation from key groups and stakeholders. This can often mean that the views
of members from vital communities or practice settings may not be heard. Finally,
it is important to recognize the unique contributions of all partners and to create
space for members to contribute fully to the development and implementation of
the research project or initiative (Mullen, 1998). This may include challenging
typical leadership and power structures, promoting openness to new approaches
and ideas, and valuing these perspectives and the wisdom brought by individual
members (Secret *et al.*, 2011).

The process of developing teams and establishing collaborative working relationships takes significant time and energy, not only to form core goals and values
but also to cultivate ways of working that are achievable within given resources
and acceptable to the team members. This may include ensuring that meetings are
accessible to participants and that training and support is available where needed
to enable members to contribute in a meaningful way (McLaughlin, 2006). Being
conscious of the needs of all team members is essential to the success of these
partnerships. Teams must therefore be receptive to news ways of working and
open to the contributions of all members so that all partners can be heard and that
conflicts or challenges can be resolved amicably and swiftly.

From our group's experiences, the initial teambuilding activities occurred best
during in-person meetings, where members were able to get to know each other
face-to-face and share their experiences and insights. These meetings allowed for
members to exchange views and seek clarification, while providing the space to
allow synergies to emerge. For our team, geographical dispersion and funding
limitations place significant limits on face-to-face activities and an amalgam of
in-person and virtual meetings are used. Most commonly, face-to-face meetings
are scheduled in alignment with key conferences or events to minimize costs and
capitalize on networking opportunities. Virtual meetings are equally important for
sustaining engagement.

Leadership

There has been great attention in the contemporary literature regarding the importance of leadership in collaborative research teams (Downey *et al.*, 2008; Nowell and Harrison, 2010; Weiss *et al.*, 2010). Effective leadership can be critical to the overall success of the team and provides the support needed to help bring the goals of the group to fruition, to promote and sustain collaborative working, to oversee team supports (such as appointed administrative or research assistants) and to resolve conflicts or challenges (Alexander *et al.*, 2001; De Dreu and Weingout, 2003; Edmonson, 1999; Van Knippenberg *et al.*, 2004). Team leaders may be appointed to represent each of the key organizations or groups, such as academic, community and practice co-leads, or may emerge naturally in the process.

As collaborative teams are becoming more diverse, there is a need for team leaders to be cognizant of power imbalances that may impair a member's ability to effectively contribute to the team. Diligence is required to ensure that different perspectives are acknowledged and respected (Dennis *et al.*, 2000; Joubert, 2006; Nembhard and Edmonson, 2006; Secret *et al.*, 2011). In healthcare teams, leadership has typically been the domain of the physician. Nurses and other allied health professionals have lacked opportunities to participate and lead in EBP initiatives. Additionally, many nurses lack confidence when faced with opportunities, owing a perceived lack of ability, autonomy and authority (Koehn and Lehman, 2008). Teams may need to overcome professional, cultural, organizational or regulatory barriers and work to establish mutual respect and equity. While this has been changing over recent years, nurses or other healthcare providers may need support to navigate this process (Pollard *et al.*, 2006). For our team, leadership emerged from an existing mentorship relationship (DB and KKS) and from connections with key healthcare providers. It was during one of the early stakeholder consultations that a new relationship was formed (FJ). This naturally emerging synergistic relationship has continued to grow and has, in itself, positively influenced the direction and focus of research activities to date, including three qualitative studies and a scoping review.

Translating evidence in practice

As discussed, collaborative teams bring together a diverse range of knowledge users and stakeholders. Subsequently, the contributions of team members can be equally varied and can span multiple disciplines, organizations and settings. This diversity can flavour the development of EBP initiatives and research and can directly impact the design, implementation and translation of EBP initiatives. For example, these differing contributions can enhance the effectiveness of knowledge translation through the development of tailored products that are appropriate and meaningful for the varied audiences. They can also facilitate connections with relevant communities and networks to optimize the sharing of the outcomes and integration into practice (Baker *et al.*, 2010; Bosch *et al.*, 2007; Gifford *et al.*,

2013; Hutchinson and Johnston, 2006; McLaughlin, 2006; Pope *et al.*, 2006). Consequently, academic partners may choose to take the lead on producing technical reports and peer-reviewed publications, while practice partners and community representatives may lead the development of presentations, briefing notes and other translation products (such as blogs and leaflets) that are aimed at community and healthcare audiences. For our team, the knowledge-user partners have been central to the development of presentations to both academic and healthcare audiences. This has led to a bigger focus on barriers to atrial fibrillation management in the rural community and upon the identification of strategies to optimize the enactment of clinical guidelines in the clinical setting.

Collaborative research partnerships: common challenges

While the benefits of collaborative research teams are widely recognized, the process itself can be complex and can give rise to a number of challenges. Such challenges can be related to engagement, group membership, sharing information and resources.

Engagement in collaborative research partnerships

Partnerships are diverse and levels of engagement between researchers and knowledge users can vary considerably between partners and over time. It can take a significant amount of time to establish partnerships and comfortable patterns of working. Equally, it can be challenging for team members to navigate this engagement within the context of their own workload and organizational responsibilities. Team leaders must also be cautious not to overburden team members, particularly healthcare providers, amid high healthcare demands, and should be flexible where possible to appropriately pace activities to facilitate sustained contributions. This can sometimes create challenges in balancing the needs of team members alongside inflexible research funding opportunities and changing organizational demands (Galinsky *et al.*, 1993). For example, INVOLVE (2004) explored community engagement in participatory research and identified a 'ladder of participation' with participation that ranges on a continuum from consultation to full engagement. During consultation, members may contribute to the direction of research activities without a clearly defined role, whereas full engagement would assume delineated contributions or team leadership (Arnstein, 1971; INVOLVE, 2004; McLaughlin, 2006). Advisory groups or steering committees would provide a middle ground of engagement. In such cases, members would assist in the development, implementation and translation of research and provide strategic guidance or financial or procedural surveillance of research activities, including the integration of findings into practice. Collaborative teams may consist of members whose participation spans the whole continuum of engagement. Each can be essential, particularly in research in areas where there may be fewer resources (such as rural and remote settings) or with special or vulnerable populations.

For our team, the process of deciphering how and when to engage team members was something that emerged from trial and error. This was in part because one of the team leads (DB) was an early career investigator and also because of the diverse range of knowledge users engaged. During the initial research activities, it became apparent that engaging a diverse range of team members in each and every decision was neither feasible nor helpful. This was addressed as a team and we delineated informal guidelines to assist in decision making. This process included identifying areas where team members were happy to delegate the responsibility for decision making to the team leads and identifying other areas where consultation would be expected. As our team has continued to develop, this has become considerably easier to navigate. As such, members may experience ebbs and flows in participation, while knowing that the group as a whole remains committed. Our collaborative team is relatively small compared with many and these interactions can be more readily achieved. Further, we consider our collaborative team to be a work in progress and strive to remain open to new directions and strategies to help us strengthen our partnerships and achieve our goals. In larger teams, it can be more difficult to foster these collaborative relationships and careful and effective communication within the team becomes critically important.

Group membership

Members of any collaborative team may change throughout the duration of a research study or EBP initiative or research study, either because of the changing needs of the research or through attrition, conflicts or delays experienced by group members. For example, when working with a broad range of partners, changes in personal circumstances or organizational structures may occur and individuals may move out of positions or may be unable to participate due to workload demands. As this occurs, new relationships may need to be formed and new members will require additional time or supports to orientate themselves with group processes or projects (McLaughlin, 2006). Similarly, team membership may expand as an EBP initiative or research activity unfolds. For our team, a research plan has been a helpful mechanism to communicate overarching team goals and processes as team changes occur or new projects are explored. Revisiting team processes on a regular basis can be helpful in ensuring that lines of communication remain open.

Sharing information

The storage and transfer of research data can present logistical challenges for many research teams, particularly for large collaborative teams that span a wide range of healthcare organizations or regions. Teams working on EBP initiatives or research may collect or use data that may be confidential. Having robust processes for data handling, in addition to confidentiality agreements, can be helpful. These agreements could include the identification of those with whom data can be shared, how data can be transferred between group members and documenting any organizational or regional legislation or policy. Team leaders may be allocated the responsibility for the storing and providing access to the data. The sharing of data should be carefully planned. In most cases, data sharing occurs only if there is a justified need and there is a secure mechanism in place, such as a password-encrypted online data storage repository. Other study data, such as meeting minutes, should also be made available to partners.

Similarly, teams need to be cognizant of the sensitivity of data, particularly data related to specific healthcare organizations. In our study of healthcare providers' experiences of managing atrial fibrillation in the rural and northern settings, a number of issues were highlighted related to the organization and delivery of healthcare services, including distrust of new clinical therapies and challenges related to the exchange of information across community and special-ist settings. These were discussed with knowledge-user partners to ensure that the communication of issues and messaging was appropriate and sensitive.

Resources

Collaborative teams require commitment and resources, including financial resources (McLaughlin, 2006; Evans *et al.*, 2011). For teams to function well, provisions must be made to cover both the research and team expenses. Research costs include expenses related to undertaking the research itself and can include salaries for research support staff, such as research assistants and project coordi-nators, as well as other costs related to the collection and analysis of data. Team expenses are likely to include financial support for meetings (including travel and venue costs), as well as any staffing costs (such as an administrative and research assistants or project managers) or resources (office space, information technology and supplies). In many cases, this financial support comes from research grants, as well as in-kind support from partnering healthcare organizations, such as health authorities.

For our team, funding has come from a variety of sources, including the Canadian Institutes for Health Research, health networks and health authority partners, and has been used to support a range of research and team activities. One example of this was our tri-provincial stakeholder consultations. The team funding was used to support the meeting costs but the majority of travel costs were covered by in-kind support from the partnering healthcare organizations. This enabled us to bring together a full complement of stakeholders. However, while this funding has been sufficient to cover the costs of most of our consulta-tive and knowledge translation activities, as well as some support for a graduate research assistant, it has been inadequate to sustain a permanent research coordi-nator position. This has been a key barrier for our team and has resulted in difficulties in coordinating schedules for regular meeting and supporting team travel for face-to-face meetings. As a team, we are striving to secure more substantial funding to address some of these barriers and assist us in achieving our goal to improve the health outcomes of Canadians with atrial fibrillation.

Conclusion

The integration of best evidence into practice has been widely shown to improve patient outcomes and optimize the use of clinical interventions and healthcare resources (Heater *et al.*, 1988; Devine and Westlake, 1995; Brown, 1992). Despite the increasing range of clinical practice guidelines and literature supporting the benefits of EBP, large variations in care exist and much evidence fails to reach the bedside (McGlynn *et al.*, 2003; Wennberg, 2011). Collaborative partnerships are inherently complex but harnessing the power of these relationships across multiple settings and organizational levels offers the opportunity to maximize the development and implementation of responsive evidence to improve patient and health outcomes. To optimize this collaborative process, attention to team building, collaborative working, leadership and translation strategies are important. Through these collaborative processes, a solid foundation can be developed to support the creation and translation of evidence that can bring about positive change.

References

Alamian, A. and Paradis, G. (2012) Individual and social determinants of multiple chronic disease behavioral risk factors among youth. *BioMed Central Public Health*, 12, 224.

Alexander, J. A., Comfort, M. E., Weiner, B. J. and Bogue, R. (2001) Leadership in collaborative community health partnerships. *Nonprofit Management and Leadership*, 12(2), 159–75.

Arnstein, S. (1971) A ladder of citizen participation. *Journal of the Royal Planning Institute*, 35(4), 216–24.

Baker, R., Camosso-Stefinovic, J., Gillies, C., Shaw, E. J., Cheater, F., Flottorp, S. and Robertson, N. (2010) Tailored interventions to overcome identified barriers to change: effects on professional practice and health care outcomes. *Cochrane Database Systematic Review*, 17(3). doi:10.1002/14651858.CD005470.pub2.

Beresford, P. (2007) User involvement, research and health inequalities: developing new directions. *Health and Social Care in the Community*, 15(4), 306–12.

Bero, L. A., Grilli, R., Grimshaw, J. M., Harvey, E., Oxman, A. D. and Thomson, M. A. (1998) Closing the gap between research and practice: an overview of systematic reviews of interventions to promote the implementation of research findings. *British Medical Journal*, 317(7156), 465–8.

Bosch, M., Van Der Weijden, T., Wensing, M. and Grol, R. (2007) Tailoring quality improvement interventions to identified barriers: a multiple case analysis. *Journal of Evaluation in Clinical Practice*, 13(2), 161–8.

Bronstein, L. R. (2003) A model for interdisciplinary collaboration. *Social Work*, 48, 297–306.

Brown, S. A. (1992) Meta-analysis of diabetes patient education research: variations in intervention effects across studies. *Research in Nursing and Health*, 15(6), 409–19.

Brown, C. E., Wickline, M. A., Ecoff, L., and Glaser, D. (2009) Nursing practice, knowledge, attitudes and perceived barriers to evidence-based practice at an academic medical center. *Journal of Advanced Nursing*, 65(2), 371–81.

Bryant-Lukosius, D., DiCenso, A., Browne, G., and Pinelli, J. (2004) Advanced practice nursing roles: development, implementation and evaluation. *Journal of Advanced Nursing*, 48(5), 519–29.

Canadian Coalition for Global Health Research (2014) Building respectful and collaborative partnerships for global health research. Available online at: www.ccghr.ca/resources/partnerships-and-networking/building-respectful-and-collaborative-partnerships-for-global-health-research (accessed 9 March 2015).

Canadian Institutes for Health Research (2008) *Framework for Citizen Engagement.* Participation and Citizen Engagement Branch. Ottawa: CIHR. Available online at: www.cihr-irsc.gc.ca/e/41270.html (accessed 9 March 2015).

Canadian Institutes of Health Research (2012) Guidelines for health research involving aboriginal people. Available online at: www.cihr-irsc.gc.ca/e/29134.html (archived site; accessed 9 March 2015).

Canadian Institutes of Health Research (2015) Funding overview. Available online at: www.cihr-irsc.gc.ca/e/37788.html (accessed 9 March 2015).

Canadian Nurses Association (2010) *Evidence-informed Decision-making and Nursing Practice*, Position Statement 113. Ottawa: CNA. Available online at: www.cna-aiic.ca/~/media/cna/page-content/pdf-en/ps113_evidence_informed_2010_e.pdf?la=en (accessed 9 March 2015).

Chelimsky, E. (1995) Where we stand today in the practice of evaluation. *Knowledge and Policy*, 8, 8–19.

Cutcliffe, J. R. and Bassett, C. (1997) Introducing change in nursing: the case of research. *Journal of Nursing Management*, 5(4): 241–7.

Davies, P., Walker, A. E., and Grimshaw, J. M. (2010) A systematic review of the use of theory in the design of guideline dissemination and implementation strategies and interpretation of the results of rigorous evaluations. *Implement Science*, 5(14), 5908–5.

Davis, D., Davis, M. E., Jadad, A., Perrier, L., Rath, D., Ryan, D., Sibbald, G., Straus, S., Rappolt, S., Wowk, M. and Zwarenstein, M. (2003) The case for knowledge translation: shortening the journey from evidence to effect. *BMJ*, 327(7405), 33–5.

De Dreu, C. K. and Weingart, L. R. (2003) Task versus relationship conflict, team performance, and team member satisfaction: a meta-analysis. *Journal of Applied Psychology*, 88(4), 741–9.

Dennis, M. L., Perl. H. I., Huebner, R. B. and McLellan, A. T. (2000) Twenty-five strategies for improving the design, implementation and analysis of health services research related to alcohol and other drug abuse treatment. *Addiction*, 95, 281–308.

Devine, E. C. and Westlake, S. K. (1995) The effects of psychoeducational care provided to adults with cancer: meta-analysis of 116 studies. *Oncology Nursing Forum*, 22(9), 1369–81.

DiCenso, A., Cullum, N. and Ciliska, D. (1998) Implementing evidence-based nursing: some misconceptions. *Evidence Based Nursing*, 1(2), 38–9.

Downey, L. M., Ireson, C. L., Slavova, S., and McKee, G. (2008) Defining elements of success: a critical pathway of coalition development. *Health Promotion Practice*, 9(2), 130–9.

Edmondson, A. (1999) Psychological safety and learning behavior in work teams. *Administrative Science Quarterly*, 44(2), 350–83.

Estabrooks, C. A. (1998) Will evidence-based nursing practice make practice perfect? *Canadian Journal of Nursing Research*, 30, 15–36.

Evans, S., Corley, M., Corrie, M., Costley, K. and Donald, C. (2011) Evaluating services in partnership with older people: exploring the role of community researchers. *Working with Older People*, 15(1), 26–33.

Fineout-Overholt, E. and Melnyk, B. (2005) Building a culture of best practice. *Nurse Leader*, 3(6), 26–30.

Fineout-Overholt, E., Melnyk, B. M. and Schultz, A. (2005) Transforming health care from the inside out: advancing evidence-based practice in the 21st century. *Journal of Professional Nursing*, 21(6), 335–44.

Flodgren, G., Rojas-Reyes, M. X., Cole, N. and Foxcroft, D. R. (2012) Effectiveness of organisational infrastructures to promote evidence-based nursing practice. *Cochrane Database Systematic Review*, 15(2), CD002212. doi: 10.1002/14651858. CD002212.pub2.

French, P. (2002) What is the evidence on evidence-based nursing? An epistemological concern. *Journal of Advanced Nursing*, 37(3), 250–7.

Frohlich, K. L., Ross, N. and Richmond, C. (2006) Health disparities in Canada today: some evidence and a theoretical framework. *Health Policy*, 79(2), 132–43.

Funk, S. G., Tornquist, E. M. and Champagne, M. T. (1995) Barriers and facilitators of research utilization. An integrative review. *Nursing Clinics of North America*, 30(3), 395–407.

Galinsky, M. J., Turnbull, J. E. Meglin, D. E. and Wilner, M. E. (1993) Confronting the reality of collaborative practice research: issues of practice, design, measurement, and team development. *Social Work*, 38, 440–9.

Gerrish, K., McManus, M. and Ashworth, P. (2003) Creating what sort of professional? Master's level nurse education as a professionalising strategy. *Nursing Inquiry*, 10(2), 103–12.

Gibson, G., Timlin, A., Curran, S. and Wattis, J. (2004) The scope for qualitative methods in research and clinical trials in dementia. *Age and Ageing*, 33(4), 422–6.

Gifford, W. A., Graham, I. D. and Davies, B. L. (2013) Multi-level barriers analysis to promote guideline based nursing care: a leadership strategy from home health care. *Journal of Nursing Management*, 21(5), 762–70.

Graham, I. D. and Tetroe, J. (2007) How to translate health research knowledge into effective healthcare action. *Healthcare Quarterly*, 10(3), 20–2.

Graham, I. D., Logan, J., Harrison, M. B., Straus, S. E., Tetroe, J., Caswell, W. and Robinson, N. (2006) Lost in knowledge translation: time for a map? *Journal of Continuing Education in the Health Professions*, 26(1), 13–24.

Grimshaw, J., Freemantle, N., Wallace, S., Russell, I., Hurwitz, B., Watt, I. and Sheldon, T. (1995) Developing and implementing clinical practice guidelines. *Quality in Health Care*, 4(1), 55–64.

Grimshaw, J. M., Thomas, R. E., MacLennan, G., Fraser, C., Ramsay, C. R., Vale, L., Whitty, P., Eccles, M. P., Matowe, L., Shirran, L., Wensing, M., Dijkstra, R. and Donaldson, C. (2005) Effectiveness and efficiency of guideline dissemination and implementation strategies. *International Journal of Technology Assessment in Health Care*, 21(1), 149.

Grimshaw, J. M., Eccles, M. P., Lavis, J. N., Hill, S. J. and Squires, J. E. (2012) Knowledge translation of research findings. *Implementation Science*, 7(1), 50. doi:10.1186/1748-5908-7-50.

Harlos, K., Tetroe, J., Graham, I. D., Bird, M. and Robinson, N. (2012) Mining the management literature for insights into implementing evidence-based change in healthcare. *Healthcare Policy*, 8(1), 33–48.

Harrison, M. B., Légaré, F., Graham, I. D. and Fervers, B. (2010) Adapting clinical practice guidelines to local context and assessing barriers to their use. *Canadian Medical Association Journal*, 182(2), 78–84.

Heart and Stroke Foundation of Canada (2014) Statistics. Atrial Fibrillation. Available online at: www.heartandstroke.com/site/c.ikIQLcMWJtE/b.3483991/k.34A8/Statistics.htm#atrialfib (accessed 9 March 2015).

Heater, B. S., Becker, A. M. and Olson, R. K. (1988) Nursing interventions and patient outcomes: a meta-analysis of studies. *Nursing Research*, 37(5), 303–7.

Helfrich, C. D., Weiner, B. J., McKinney, M. M. and Minasian, L. (2007) Determinants of implementation effectiveness adapting a framework for complex innovations. *Medical Care Research and Review*, 64(3), 279–303.

Hicks, C. (1995) The shortfall in published research: a study of nurses' research and publication activities. *Journal of Advanced Nursing*, 21(3), 594–604.

Hutchinson, A. M. and Johnston, L. (2006) Beyond the BARRIERS Scale: commonly reported barriers to research use. *Journal of Nursing Administration*, 36(4), 189–99.

INVOLVE (2004) *Involving the Public in NHS, Public Health and Social Care: Briefing Notes for Researchers*. Eastleigh: INVOLVE. Available online at www.invo.org.uk/posttypepublication/involve-briefing-notes-for-researchers (accessed 9 March 2015).

Joubert, L. (2006) Academic-practice partnerships in practice research: a cultural shift for health social workers. In G, Rosenberg and A, Weissman (eds), *International Social Health Care: Policy, Programs and Studies* (pp. 151–61). Binghamton, NY: Haworth Press.

Kirby, P. (2004) *A Guide to Actively Involving Young People in Research: For Researchers, Research Commissioners and Managers*. Eastleigh: INVOLVE.

Kitson, A., Harvey, G. and McCormack, B. (1998) Enabling the implementation of evidence based practice: a conceptual framework. *Quality in Health Care*, 7(3), 149–58.

Koehn, M. L. and Lehman, K. (2008) Nurses' perceptions of evidence-based nursing practice. *Journal of Advanced Nursing*, 62(2), 209–15.

Loke, J. C., Laurenson, M. C. and Lee, K. W. (2014) Embracing a culture in conducting research requires more than nurses' enthusiasm. *Nurse Education Today*, 34(1), 132–7.

McDonald, L. (2001) Florence Nightingale and the early origins of evidence-based nursing. *Evidence Based Nursing*, 4(3), 68–9.

McGlynn, E. A., Asch, S. M., Adams, J., Keesey, J., Hicks, J., DeCristofaro, A. and Kerr, E. A. (2003) The quality of health care delivered to adults in the United States. *New England Journal of Medicine*, 348(26), 2635–45.

McLaughlin, H. (2006) Involving young service users as co-researchers: possibilities, benefits and costs. *British Journal of Social Work*, 36(8), 1395–410.

McLaughlin, H. (2009) What's in a name: 'client', 'patient', 'customer', 'consumer', 'expert by experience', 'service user' – What's next? *British Journal of Social Work*, 39(6), 1101–17.

McPherson, K., Headrick, L. and Moss, F. (2001) Working and learning together: good quality care depends on it, but how can we achieve it? *Quality in Health Care*, 10(2), 46–53.

Melnyk, B. M., Fineout-Overholt, E., Fischbeck Feinstein, N., Li, H., Small, L., Wilcox, L. and Kraus, R. (2004) Nurses' perceived knowledge, beliefs, skills, and needs regarding evidence-based practice: implications for accelerating the paradigm shift. *Worldviews on Evidence-Based Nursing*, 1(3), 185–93.

Mullen, E. J. (1998) Linking the university and the social agency in collaborative evaluation research: principles and examples. *Scandinavian Journal of Social Welfare*, 7, 152–8.

Nembhard, I. M. and Edmondson, A. C. (2006) Making it safe: the effects of leader inclusiveness and professional status on psychological safety and improvement efforts in health care teams. *Journal of Organizational Behavior*, 27(7), 941–66.

Nowell, B. and Harrison, L. M. (2010) Leading change through collaborative partnerships: a profile of leadership and capacity among local public health leaders. *Journal of Prevention and Intervention in the Community*, 39(1), 19–34.

Nutley, S., Walter, I. and Davies, H. T. (2003) From knowing to doing a framework for understanding the evidence-into-practice agenda. *Evaluation*, 9(2), 125–48.

Olade, R. A. (2004) Evidence-based practice and research utilization activities among rural nurses. *Journal of Nursing Scholarship*, 36(3), 220–5.

Pollard, K. C., Miers, M. E., Gilchrist, M. and Sayers, A. (2006) A comparison of inter-professional perceptions and working relationships among health and social care students: the results of a 3-year intervention. *Health and Social Care in the Community*, 14(6), 541–52.

Pope, C. and Mays, N. (1995) Qualitative research: reaching the parts other methods cannot reach: an introduction to qualitative methods in health and health services research. *British Medical Journal*, 311(6996), 42–5.

Pope, C., Robert, G., Bate, P., Le May, A. and Gabbay, J. (2006) Lost in translation: a multi-level case study of the metamorphosis of meanings and action in public sector organizational innovation. *Public Administration*, 84(1), 59–79.

Pravikoff, D. S., Tanner, A. B. and Pierce, S. T. (2005) Readiness of US nurses for evidence-based practice: many don't understand or value research and have had little or no training to help them find evidence on which to base their practice. *American Journal of Nursing*, 105(9), 40–51.

Ramanujam, R. and Rousseau, D. M. (2006) The challenges are organizational not just clinical. *Journal of Organizational Behavior*, 27(7), 811–27.

Reeves, S., Zwarenstein, M., Goldman, J., Barr, H., Freeth, D., Hammick, M. and Koppel, I. (2008) Interprofessional education: effects on professional practice and health care outcomes. *Cochrane Database of Systematic Reviews*, 23(1): CD002213. doi: 10.1002/14651858.CD002213.pub2.

Rolfe, G., Segrott, J. and Jordan, S. (2008) Tensions and contradictions in nurses' perspectives of evidence-based practice. *Journal of Nursing Management*, 16(4), 440–51.

Roper, L. (2002) Achieving successful academic–practitioner research collaborations. *Development in Practice*, 12, 338–45.

Rapport, F., Storey, M., Porter, A., Snooks, H., Jones, K., Peconi, J., Sánchez, A., Siebert, S., Thorne, K., Clement, C. and Russell, I. (2013) Qualitative research within trials: developing a standard operating procedure for a clinical trials unit. *Trials*, 14(1), 54. doi:10.1186/1745-6215-14-54.

Rosswurm, M. A. and Larrabee, J. H. (1999) A model for change to evidence-based practice. *Journal of Nursing Scholarship*, 31(4), 317–22.

Rycroft-Malone, J., Harvey, G., Seers, K., Kitson, A., McCormack, B. and Titchen, A. (2004) An exploration of the factors that influence the implementation of evidence into practice. *Journal of Clinical Nursing*, 13(8), 913–24.

Sackett, D. L. (2000) Evidence-based medicine. In Armitage, P. and Colton, T. (eds), *Encyclopedia of Biostatistics*, 3. Chichester: Wiley.

Secret, M., Abell, M. L. and Berlin, T. (2011) The promise and challenge of practice–research collaborations: guiding principles and strategies for initiating, designing, and implementing program evaluation research. *Social Work*, 56(1), 9–20.

Smith, R., Monaghan, M. and Broad, B. (2002) Involving young people as co-researchers: facing up to the methodological issues. *Qualitative Social Work*, 1, 191–207.

Soydan, H. (2002) Formulating research problems in practitioner–researcher partnerships. *Social Work Education*, 21, 297–304.

Straus, S. E., Tetroe, J. M. and Graham, I. D. (2011) Knowledge translation is the use of knowledge in health care decision making. *Journal of Clinical Epidemiology*, 64(1), 6–10.

Tetroe, J. M., Graham, I. D., Foy, R., Robinson, N., Eccles, M. P., Wensing, M., Durieux, P., Légaré, F., Palmhøj Nielson, C., Adily, A., Ward, J. E., Porter, C., Shea, B. and Grimshaw, J. M. (2008) Health research funding agencies' support and promotion of knowledge translation: an international study. *Milbank Quarterly*, 86(1), 125–55.

Van Knippenberg, D., De Dreu, C. K. and Homan, A. C. (2004) Work group diversity and group performance: an integrative model and research agenda. *Journal of Applied Psychology*, 89(6), 1008–22.

Venuta, R. and Graham, I. D. (2010) Involving citizens and patients in health research. *Journal of Ambulatory Care Management*, 33(3), 215–22.

Walter, I., Davies, H. and Nutley, S. (2003) Increasing research impact through partnerships: evidence from outside health care. *Journal of Health Services Research and Policy*, 8(2), 58–61.

Weiss, E. S., Taber, S. K., Breslau, E. S., Lillie, S. E. and Li, Y. (2010) The role of leadership and management in six southern public health partnerships: a study of member involvement and satisfaction. *Health Education and Behavior*, 37(5), 737–52.

Wennberg, J. E. (2011) Time to tackle unwarranted variations in practice. *BMJ*, 342, d1513. doi: http://dx.doi.org/10.1136/bmj.d1513.

Woodward, V., Webb, C. and Prowse, M. (2007) The perceptions and experiences of nurses undertaking research in the clinical setting. *Journal of Research in Nursing*, 12(3), 227–44.

Zwarenstein, M. and Reeves, S. (2006) Knowledge translation and interprofessional collaboration: Where the rubber of evidence-based care hits the road of teamwork. *Journal of Continuing Education in the Health Professions*, 26(1), 46–54.

Zwarenstein, M., Goldman, J. and Reeves, S. (2009) Interprofessional collaboration: effects of practice-based interventions on professional practice and healthcare outcomes. Cochrane Database Systematic Reviews, 8(3), CD000072. doi: 10.1002/14651858.CD000072.pub2.

3 Intra- and interprofessional working

Pitfalls and potential

Margaret Miers

The importance of evidence-based practice (EBP) is now widely accepted across the range of professions involved in health and social care. A shared zeal for evidence-informed practice has the potential to enhance collaborative intra- and interprofessional working and to enhance provision of effective care. This chapter considers the potential for EBP to unite nurses and other professionals in efforts to improve care, as well as the difficulties in fulfilling such potential.

International collaborations, such as the Cochrane Collaboration (www.cochrane.org) and the Campbell Collaboration (www.campbellcollaboration.org), as well as national and international professional organisations have promoted shared understanding and acceptance of models of accessing, appraising and synthesising evidence. In addition, these shared approaches to gathering and assessing evidence have been used, in some instances, to develop evidence-based guidance for practice. In the United States, for example, as early as 1998, the American Psychology Association listed sixteen 'empirically supported treatments' (such as cognitive behavioural therapy for panic disorders) for dissemination to training programmes (Chambless *et al.*, 1998). In the UK, the National Institute for Health and Care Excellence (NICE) has provided the National Health Service with advice on effective and good-value health care since 1999. In April 2013, NICE gained new responsibilities for providing guidance for those working in social care. More recently, the United States government has provided a significant boost to EBP through legislation supporting 'comparative effectiveness research' (AHRQ, 2015). This more specific term refers to research designed to determine the benefits and harms of treatments, tests, public health strategies and other healthcare services for the population and for different groups within the population. The American Recovery and Reinvestment Act 2009, passed to facilitate measures to ensure economic recovery, authorised an additional US$1.1 billion to be spent on comparative effectiveness research. The effectiveness of treatment has become important within debates about US health reform.

The US health reform legislation (the Patient Protection and Affordable Care Act 2010) established a new non-governmental entity, the Patient-Centred Outcomes Research Institute (PCORI) to oversee and set guidelines for the research. The law has also established funding streams for the research, including through a tax paid into a trust fund by Medicare and private health insurance companies (Donnelly 2010). Unlike NICE, the US legislation bans the use of quality of life years and other cost-effectiveness measures in determining comparative effectiveness. Although these US developments remain topics of active debate, the US 'push' for research into effective practice is likely to shift the discursive landscape around EBP, not least through growing use of the term 'comparative effectiveness research' and through the emphasis on patient-centred outcomes. As in the UK, the US organisations established to oversee research and guidance for practice (the National Institutes of Health, the Agency for Healthcare Research and Quality and the Office of the Secretary of Health and Human Services) involve a range of professionals, researchers and patient and patient advocacy groups. The board of governors of PCORI includes a nurse and a chiropractor, as well as medical practitioners, researchers, policy makers and administrators. Non-professionals are members of key advisory groups. Such developments suggest that EBP has a growing potential to promote shared under-standings and shared competencies in producing and using evidence in clinical practice across medical and non-medical professions. Nurses and allied health professionals have opportunities to play an active role in developing effective care.

The role of nursing in EBP, both as 'consumers' and 'producers' of evidence, however, remains unclear. Medicine's leadership in health care may be enhanced rather than reduced by the EBP movement and comparative effectiveness research, not least through the nursing profession's inexperience in conducting and using research. Although the PCORI Methodology Committee includes a nurse member, and patients and patient advocates are well represented on the advisory panels, medicine dominates the Methodology Committee. Nursing's role in research leadership is still limited. It is worth noting that, when, in 2012, The International Council of Nurses (ICN) produced a toolkit, *Closing the Gap: from Evidence to Action*, an editorial in the *Lancet* (2012) expressed surprise at the ICN's tardy promotion of EBP. The *Lancet* editorial was critical of the toolkit's content as well as its late arrival, suggesting doubts about nursing's EBP competence and commitment. A defensive letter in response by leading nurse researchers did little to allay the Lancet's doubts (Clark *et al.*, 2012). Whilst asserting the importance of collaboration in medicine and nursing, the letter iden-tifies nursing's challenges as relating to identity and confidence and a 'strong anti-intellectual streak … which is hostile to research'. Far from being a collabo-rative profession, nursing is revealed as being divided and divisive, with scepticism about EBP rife amongst many practitioners. Intra-professional differ-ences about EBP require some exploration and explanation.

Intra-professional differences in nursing: why do nurses resist EBP?

One obvious reason for intra-professional differences lies in different educational preparation for practice. Many nurses (and other health and social care profes-sionals) initially gained qualifications before the advent of the EBP movement.

Nursing teams will often comprise qualified staff who have experienced different educational programmes prior to registration. For nursing in the UK, the rapidity of educational change has been particularly acute. Until the 1990s, most student nurses were part of the workforce, learning while working; study time was limited and training programmes of different duration (two or three years) led to qualification as an enrolled or registered nurse. The abolition of enrolled nurse status in the 1990s and the introduction of diploma-level education as the minimum academic qualification for new entrants to the profession brought some uniformity. Degree-level entry programmes, offered in some universities for some branches of nursing since the 1970s, however, maintained differences in educational experience amongst nurses until the recent movement towards all graduate level entry. The EBP movement, begun in the 1990s, has emerged during decades of change and reorganisation in nurse education across the world. Nurses entering the workforce after completing degree-level preparation programmes that include courses on EBP work alongside nurse colleagues educated through different systems. Education level has consistently been found to influence attitudes towards EBP, with degree-level education being associated with more positive views. In a US study of nurses' perceptions of evidence-based nursing practice, for example, Kochn and Lehman (2008) found statistical differences for attitudes between those with baccalaureate qualifications and higher education experience compared with those with associate qualifications and diploma-level education. Frequent educational change has meant that, for decades, experienced staff may have felt devalued by progressive change in role and expectations and by new entrants to the profession. Educational change itself provides the opportunity for the development of workforce subcultures that are capable of promoting mutual distrust and denigration, particularly around an unhelpful clever/caring dichotomy. Such conflict of cultures (and scepticism about EBP) is exacerbated by public discourse about nursing. When newsworthy stories about poor standards of care receive widespread public attention it is commonplace in the UK for journalists, patients and medical staff to attribute poor care to educational change. Nurses, therefore, can feel justified in sharing such views. Online comments on a *Nursing Times* editorial (Middleton, 2013) illustrate the support of some practising nurses for the view that the problem of non-caring nurses 'lies with the training which now focuses on academia rather than caring'. As Clark *et al.*'s letter to the *Lancet* notes, some nurses do seek a 'return to a supposed halcyon era opposed to the use of research in health care' (Clark *et al.*, 2012).

Whereas public discourse about nursing may be particularly unhelpful in legitimising nursing's 'anti-intellectual streak' in clinical settings, scepticism about EBP is common amongst many professions. Nursing is not alone. There have been considerable changes in the education and training of practitioners over recent decades across all health and social care professions. In the United States, Lilienfeld *et al.* (2013) have documented the scepticism and resistance towards EBP of clinical psychologists and have argued that dismissing resistance as 'reflections of ignorance and anti-intellectualism' and neglecting the causes of such resistance hinders efforts to disseminate effective evidence-based therapy.

Lilienfeld *et al.* (2013) advocate looking at the reasons for resistance. These include the fact that relying on clinical experience rather than research evidence was commonplace in training programmes prior to the EBP movement and hence older psychologists (and nurses) understandably have difficulty changing their way of thinking. Reviewing surveys of clinical psychologists' attitudes towards EBP, Lilienfeld *et al.* (2013) report that past clinical experiences are considered more influential in practice than 'current research on treatment outcome'. Social work, similarly, has developed as a profession around clinical experience and, hence, many practitioners have resisted EBP, seeing it as dismissing an 'essential part of their professional identity and expertise' (Drisko and Grady, 2012: 245). Diverse views amongst professionals are understandable but may nevertheless inhibit nurses and other professionals from working together effectively.

A positive view of the tardiness of the ICN in developing and promoting an EBP tool kit, is that this reflects the ICN's sensitivity towards the diversity of nursing across the globe. The ICN emphasises the pivotal role of national nurses' associations in leadership to ensure patients receive effective care. Nursing organ-isations in Africa, for example, face different challenges from nursing organisations in the United States, Canada, Australia, the UK and other countries, where graduate-level preparation, electronic resources and research funding are an accepted part of the nursing landscape. The Collaboration for Evidence Based Healthcare in Africa (cebha.org), founded in 2011, makes it clear that imple-menting findings relevant to Africa involves taking into account later disease presentation, co-infections, malnutrition, high levels of self-medication, use of traditional remedies, reduced level of resources, including human resources, and political instability. Shaibu (2006) emphasises the importance of cultural sensi-tivity in introducing evidence-based nursing practice in Botswana. She concurs with the ICN in emphasising the importance of national organisations creating role models and reward systems for nurses and midwives that are successful in using an evidence base for decision making. Cultural sensitivity is also important in better resourced countries to avoid an unhelpful 'us versus them', 'pro EBP versus anti-intellectual' mentality.

Cultural sensitivity can help professionals to work together through finding shared points of understanding and addressing barriers to EBP. Lilienfeld *et al.* (2013) note that psychotherapists are routinely taught that repeated client resist-ance should not be ignored or dismissed. They argue that, by analogy, reasons for resistance to EBP should be explored and understood. They identify important sources of resistance to EBP that need to be addressed. Although their list applies to psychotherapy, it is equally relevant to nursing. The sources of resistance include 'naïve realism' (that is, a belief in the need to see 'with their own eyes'); myths and misconceptions about human nature (in nursing this can include the beliefs that nurses are born not made and that caring cannot be taught); the chal-lenge of applying group probabilities to individuals; reversal of the onus of proof (that is, expecting proof for the effectiveness of new practices but ignoring the need to prove the effectiveness of current routines); mischaracterisation of what EBP is; and, finally, pragmatic, educational and attitudinal obstacles. This final source of resistance includes the 'gap' between researchers and academics, who are generally the 'producers' of evidence, and the practitioners who are expected to use such evidence in their practice. Suggested ways of addressing sources of resistance include ensuring that student education emphasises the rationale for a scientific approach to practice and not just a 'protocol-based' (or 'cook book') approach to EBP, avoiding an 'ivory tower' approach to disseminating evidence by forging close alliances between research orientated and practice-oriented professionals and hence avoiding supporting the appearance, if not the reality, of separate cultures. This book aims to help nursing move forward by avoiding a 'cook book' approach to EBP, exploring what is meant by 'science or evidence based' more thoroughly, and, in this chapter as well as others, forging a closer link between research and practice through examining practice-based decision making in more depth.

It is worth noting that the emphasis in comparative effectiveness research on comparing the outcomes of treatment options, including current routines, may help nurses to understand the relevance of EBP. A 2013 online forum discussion about comparative effectiveness research amongst American nurses involves suggestions from nurses for further effectiveness research. These include comparative effectiveness research on turning for pressure ulcer prevention (for example, a randomised controlled trial on two- versus three-hour turning intervals in acute care) and an examination of the evidence base for nursing physical assessments for hospitalised people. Frequent assessments are time consuming and disruptive to patients but are often ordered as routine. Although these topic suggestions may be prompted partly by nurses' concern for their own workload, there is little evidence about the effectiveness of such commonplace nursing actions for patient outcomes (AHRQ 2013).The discussion forum suggests interest in improving the evidence base for nursing practice and willingness to question the effectiveness of current practice.

Nursing leadership in EBP: meeting the challenge

The *Lancet's* criticisms of the ICN and lead nurse researchers' criticisms of the profession suggest that the nursing profession's response to its responsibility to provide leadership and role models in EBP warrants critical examination. Leadership approaches to promoting EBP vary across the world. In some countries, programmes have been developed to build the research and leadership skills of nurses. In the UK, as Rosser *et al.* explain in Chapter 4, the United Kingdom Clinical Research Collaboration has introduced a Clinical Academic Career pathway to help build research capability amongst nursing, midwifery and allied health professions. Without such a career pathway, it is difficult for nursing to provide role models for practice-based research leadership. In Canada, research funding and awards support nurses to build research skills, as well as experience in research partnerships and research leadership. Davina Banner, Fred Janke and Kathryn King-Shier explore, in Chapter 2, the challenges in such partnerships. In the United States the National Institute for Nursing Research provides funding support for research leadership. In Australia, the Joanna Briggs Institute provides, *inter alia*, a library of resources, training in systematic reviews, a database of best practice information sheets and international support for collaborating centres across the world.

Nurse leadership in research teams producing evidence relevant to practice is still developing. The skills for research leadership involve more than skills in research. They include the ability to gain research funding, the ability to support and develop junior researchers through doctoral and postdoctoral programmes, the ability to build collaborative relationships with practice-based professionals and with patient research partners as well as research participants. The skills required include liaison with multiple research settings and management of multi-centred studies, following the highest standards of research governance. Skills and experience in publishing and disseminating research findings are further role requirements. In the UK, the Royal College of Nursing awards Fellowships to acknowledge the significant contributions of individual nurses to the profession. In 2011, a Fellowship was awarded to Professor Sarah Hewlett for her significant contribution to rheumatology through her research leadership and clinical practice (Hewlett *et al.*, 2011a). Her work is an exemplar of research leadership and of research centred on patient interests, needs and priorities. Her work developing understanding of the personal impact of rheumatoid arthritis and her collaboration with patients as research partners has seen medical communities internationally call into question how outcome measures are devised. Hewlett's research incorporating the patient perspective into outcome measures has strongly influenced the international body for the development of outcomes measurement in rheumatology clinical trials (OMERACT; omeract.org), which established an international patient perspectives group (Kirwan *et al.*, 2011). Hewlett's research team of doctoral students, research assistants and postdoctoral fellows, comprising nurses, podiatrist, physiotherapists, psychologists and patient partners, is funded by a range of national and international organisations. She currently leads a study exploring rheumatoid arthritis flare and self-management across five countries and the team's research includes studies of foot care, physical activity and stiffness symptoms (Dures *et al.*, 2012). Such achievements have been celebrated as an example of nurse leadership in research. They are also, importantly, grounded in effective interprofessional collaboration, including collaboration between nurses and doctors.

The Royal College of Nursing conducts regular surveys to monitor the development of research leadership in the UK. The number of professors of nursing in the UK increased from 132 in 2003 to 262 in 2013. However, of those 262, only 29 were joint appointments between universities and healthcare organisations. Details of the inaugural lectures presented by the professoriate suggest that the expertise and interests of many of the professors concern workforce issues, the nature and history of nursing and midwifery, health services research, nurse education and issues concerning the nature of research and research development within the profession. Few focus on healthcare practice. Nevertheless, practice-relevant research includes growing expertise in researching the patient experience and biopsychosocial aspects of the illness experience. Research into wound care, ageing, dementia and palliative care suggest a growth in nurse leadership in those areas.

Despite these significant examples of leadership, research studies indicate that at a local level nurse leaders and managers can be significant barriers to implementing EBP (Melnyk *et al.*, 2012). In a US survey, Melnyk *et al.* found that lack of time and an unsupportive organisational culture were seen by nurse respondents as the two most significant barriers to EBP. Lack of support from mentors, ward managers and more senior managers contributes to perceptions of organisational barriers. Brown *et al.* (2009), in a study of nurses' perceptions, found that nurses' lack of autonomy and lack of authority to change practice were significant barriers to their EBP. Carrying out medical orders and medicine's view of nursing as a subordinate profession meant that nurses' engagement with EBP was not facilitated. The need for an organisational approach to EBP, led by senior staff, is now widely recognised. In the United States, Magnet accreditation has been a significant driver towards EBN. Magnet accreditation is awarded to organisations providing good evidence-based care and supportive work environments. As Wise (2009) reports, after initial accreditation, to maintain Magnet status, hospitals must show improved outcomes and clinical practice based on current evidence. Developing EBP committees is one way of fulfilling Magnet expectations. Such committees provide an organisational approach to improving practice decisions based on current research. Leadership at an organisational level can avoid the limitations of relying on leadership and mentorship at ward level. Access to internet and other resources and ensuring the availability of evidence in a manner concordant with normal workflow are all facilitators of EBP that need to be addressed at organisational level.

Interprofessional working: transdisciplinary models of evidence based practice

Although successful leadership of research teams by nurses is increasing, medical scepticism about nursing's commitment to EBP remains. Conditions for effective collaboration include 'willingness to trust, respect and value the contributions of all involved in the delivery of care' (Pollard and Harris 2010: 147). Barriers to effective interprofessional working can include different professional priorities, lack of understanding of the roles and obligations of others, hierarchical structures and poor communication methods and interpersonal skills (Barrett and Keeping, 2005).

A barrier to effective collaboration across professions in research teams lies in differing views about 'legitimate' research approaches and methods. The *Lancet*'s 2012 editorial is critical of the ICN toolkit's ambivalent approach to EBP, noting that the content is 'uncritical of an egalitarian attitude to research findings and reluctant to distinguish between evidence and experience'. Reasons for nursing's reluctance to accept medicine's hierarchical view of evidence are ably explored in this book, with some chapters arguing for an inclusive view of evidence and

John Paley (Chapter 10) challenging nurses to make greater use of social psychology when considering the strengths and weaknesses of qualitative research. It is important to recognise that nursing is not alone in accepting a broader range of evidence as relevant to practice than medicine. As Satterfield *et al.* (2009) make clear in their review of professional models of EBP, nursing, public health and social work have all expanded the scope of what is perceived as evidence. All these professions accept qualitative data as 'best available' research evidence, not least because evidence from randomised controlled trials is rarely available for community or society based interventions. Public health policies draw on evidence from cross-sectional studies, quasi-experimental designs and time series analyses. Social work and nursing both value evidence from qualitative research for its insights into client experiences and the influence of social context. Research teams incorporate qualitative data into patient-centred outcomes research. Hewlett and colleagues, for example, have demonstrated effectively how qualitative data about patient experiences of rheumatoid arthritis symptoms can provide the basis for developing research tools that can be used to explore the impact of treatments on outcomes relevant to patients. Qualitative research into the experience of rheumatoid arthritis fatigue, alongside a Cochrane systematic review (Cramp *et al.*, 2013), for example, has led to the development of the Bristol Rheumatoid Arthritis Fatigue Scales (University of the West of England, 2010), now widely used as outcome measure in effectiveness studies (Hewlett *et al.*, 2011b).

It is important to recognise that there is growing and considerable interest in promoting the integration of diverse information and methodologies into health research and, hence, in building interdisciplinary research teams comprising, for example, biological, health and social scientists. This interest is fuelled in part by the recognised importance of translational research, linking laboratory-based biomedical research to patient and client outcomes but also by the recognition of the significance of patient and user involvement. In the United States, the National Institute of Nursing Research (2014) issued a call for proposals in January 2014 entitled Centers of Excellence for Self Management Research: Building Research Teams for the Future. The aim of the research funding stream is to expand the number of research investigators involved in interdisciplinary nursing science research intended to promote integration of diverse information for molecular and biological processes with patient-reported outcomes (symptoms, financial status, health-related quality of life). An earlier (2012) call for proposals for interdisciplinary work in symptom science has led, for example, to Duke University School of Nursing's Center of Excellence for Adaptive Leadership for Cognitive/Affective Symptom Science and the John Hopkins School of Nursing Center for Sleep-Related Symptom Science. These centres support nursing leadership and experience in interdisciplinary research. Recognition of the importance of behavioural science research in health care has increasingly established qualitative methods as integral to research involving patient priorities and perspectives. The place of qualitative research in treatment trials is becoming well established. Rapport *et al.* (2013) have developed and publicised a standard operating procedure for the use of qualitative research within trials for one clinical trial centre. These developments suggest that nurses' qualitative research expertise can contribute to building an evidence base about effective care.

Nursing is also not alone in seeing qualitative research as relevant to decisions about care of individual patients. Psychology is also more accepting of a range of research designs than medicine and, importantly, places strong emphasis on the importance of patients' characteristics, context and values in determining appropriate professional practice. Social work also emphasises the importance of clients' characteristics when considering interventions and both nursing and psychology recognise the importance of patient preferences to decisions regarding care.

Satterfield *et al.* (2009) confirm the importance of the patient/client perspective and characteristics in EBP by proposing a transdisciplinary EBP model that places decision making in its centre. They propose a model of EBP in which decision making is based on: i) best available research evidence; ii) client/population characteristics, state, needs, values and preferences; and iii) resources (including the practitioner's expertise). The model also acknowledges that all decisions take place within an organisational context and wider environment. The legal framework, for example, constrains healthcare decision making.

The significance of this transdisciplinary model lies in both the emphasis on the patient/client perspective and in placing decision making at the centre of the EBP model. The gap between the producers and users of evidence is exacerbated by the evidence producers' lack of concern about the theory and practice of practice-based decision making. Effective EBP relies as much on understanding decision making as it does on understanding the nature of evidence. It is the dominant role of medical practitioners in decision making that amplifies their dominance in EBP. Satterfield *et al.*'s transdisciplinary model, however, does little to clarify how information about effectiveness, client and resources, including the practitioner's own expertise, can or should be used. Practitioners are left on their own to analyse and reflect on their own decision making. As such, the model is unlikely to contribute to shared decision making across professions (nor shared use of any relevant evidence base). Similar decision-making models offered within EBP literature are also unlikely to enable shared decision making with patients, as is now widely recommended with health care (and supported by, for example, the US PCORI). Whereas it is beyond the scope of this chapter to explore fully the terrain of the study of decision making, failure to recognise and acknowledge that evidence becomes relevant to practice through the process of decision making and at the point of decision leads to scepticism about EBP amongst practitioners. Thompson *et al.* (2005) have argued for a greater focus on decision making in EBP but their call has not been widely taken up. Focusing on decisions as a way of drawing attention to comparative effectiveness research, as well as clients' values and preferences, would require a shared approach to how to think about and understand decisions.

Decision making and EBP

The problem with recognising the importance of analysing the process of decision making, as well as the nature of evidence, is the breadth of literature and perspectives involved. During their education, nurses are generally introduced to normative models of rational decision making reliant on expected utility theory of human behaviour (Chapman and Sonnenberg, 2000). Nurses may also be introduced to descriptive models for how people actually behave using intuitive, heuristic or analytical processing. Descriptive models reveal the poor quality of judgment and decision making. The challenge in focusing more on the point of decision is that the study of decision making evolves as rapidly as healthcare research. Modes of making decisions such as intuition, ill-defined deliberative processes such as 'taking into account and bearing in mind' (Dowie and Kaltoft, 2011); decision analysis, with or without decision aids, are now commonly termed 'decision technologies' and recognised simple models of expected utility (such as simple decision trees) are now seen as masking real-life complexity. Dowie *et al.* (2013) have termed ward-based argumentation considering, *inter alia*, the best available research evidence concerning outcomes, the client's preferences and values, the available clinical and other resources 'verbal multicriteria decision deliberation' (MCDD). The alternative to this approach is an analytical numerical approach multi-criteria decision analysis (MDCA), which recognises that options have multiple attributes that are assessed through multiple criteria, accorded different weightings according to the values and preferences of the parties involved. A further growing area in the study of decision making is techniques and aids used to improve the quality of decision making, often involving use of information technologies. Different aids support MCDD or MDCA. A proliferation of academic disciplines and sub-disciplines are involved in this endeavour, notably informatics, ethics and cognitive psychology. It can be argued that the search for transdisciplinary understanding of EBP and of decision making is seriously impeded by the proliferation of academic disciplines and sub-disciplines (and accompanying journal titles) involved in both research and in analysing decision making.

Kaltoft (2013) has identified the disconnect between disciplines and sub-disciplines as a significant difficulty in making effective progress towards effective decision making in nursing. She discussed the disconnect between nursing informatics and nursing ethics, noting that nursing informatics literature and nursing ethics literature support separate communities, both seeing their role as providing decision support, by way of information inputs and ethical insights, respectively. Kaltoft identified information about comparative effectiveness research as decision information inputs that can be supplied through informatics. Informatics can also supply web-based decision support tools that can assist the process of identifying options, information supporting beliefs about likelihoods of outcomes and their multiple attributes, as well as providing templates for considering preferences and values. Nursing ethics supports decisions by articulating and clarifying values and principles and the importance of diverse parties to the decision. Kaltoft identifies Annalisa (http://maldaba.co.uk/products/annalisa) as an example of a support tool that facilitates the inclusion of value-based preferences into a decision-making process alongside beliefs about the likelihood of diverse outcomes occurring (see café Annalisa: cafeannalisa.org.uk). Kaltoft's arguments and the structure of and rationale for decision aids such as Annalisa warrant closer attention than space allows here. Kaltoft's conclusion is that the disconnect between informatics and ethics illuminates the opportunity and need to develop 'nursing decisionics' as a discipline, complementary to nursing informatics and nursing ethics. 'Nursing decisionics' would be a discipline that focuses specifically on the point of decision. The curriculum for such a discipline would be three main 'decision technologies', identified as: i) 'clinical judgment'; ii) MCDD; iii) MCDA. She argues that 'decisionics' would help make the decision-making process much more transparent. In a separate paper, Kaltoft *et al.* (2013) have also argued that the decision-making process should include deciding how to decide.

The disconnect between the communities that Kaltoft identifies is only one of many. The disconnect between EBP and health informatics is equally significant, as is the disconnect between EBP and the study of decision making and of decision analysis. Nursing's growing (yet separate) communities focused on EBP, on informatics and on ethics exemplify the profession's ability to sustain and retain diverse and separate sub-groups, as well as academic tribalism. The complexity and unfamiliarity of the proposed 'decisionics', however, is unlikely to help to bridge the barriers between nurses educated through different systems or nurses working in education and research settings and nurses working in community and clinical practice. Nevertheless, any brief foray into decision making literature raises important points for serious consideration by any professionals interested in integrating evidence into practice. Hitherto, nursing research into decision making has focused on the use of cues in judgments (Manias *et al.*, 2004) and on nursing autonomy (McCarthy 2003). Lack of autonomy and lack of authority have been shown to be barriers to EBP. It is likely that, if nurses lack autonomy to make decisions and have limited understanding of the cues they use in making judgments, in-depth study of decision making may well seem irrelevant to practice-based nurses. Nevertheless, in-depth study of the nature of evidence without study of decision making will also alienate nurses, who will increasingly work in a climate of shared decision making.

Shared decision making: potential and challenges for nurses

Recent years have seen the development of nursing roles with an increased level of autonomy. In the UK, these include consultant nurses, advanced practice nurses, clinical nurse specialists, nurse practitioners and nurse prescribers. The contribution of such nurses to EBP and to informed decision making is still developing, as is the evidence base about the contribution of such roles. Whereas many early questionnaire-based descriptive studies of such nurses have hitherto demonstrated self-reported continuing educational needs, more recent observational studies and case studies of advanced practice nurses have shown the positive impact of such roles. Gerrish *et al.* (2011) found that advanced practice nurses acted as knowledge brokers in promoting EBP among clinical nurses, accumulating, synthesising and disseminating evidence in varied ways and developing skills through role modelling and problem solving. Williamson *et al.* (2012), in an ethnographic study of advanced nurse practitioners in an acute medical setting, found that they acted as a 'lynchpin', using expertise, networks and insider knowledge to facilitate care and nursing and medical practice. The lynchpin concept suggests that nurses with higher levels of autonomy can play a positive role in facilitating informed decision making.

One of the key developments in both research and in decision analysis is the recognition of the importance of patient-centred practice. Patient-centred outcome research and patient ownership of decisions and modes of decision making are changing ways of thinking. Shared decision making is becoming a healthcare aim. NHS England's Shared Decision Making programme, part of its Improving Patient Experience strategy, has developed tools for shared decision making. Current decision aids available are 18 option grids, 10 brief decision aids and 36 patient decision aids (NHS England, 2015). It is possible that nurses' role in EBP can evolve through a facilitative role in supporting patients to make their own informed decisions about health and health care. Senior nurses' ability to play a lynchpin role suggests this is the case but, as yet, there is limited evidence about nurses' effectiveness in shared decision making. Upton *et al.* (2011), in a study of primary care nurses' views on sharing decisions regarding asthma treatment, found that, despite holding positive views about sharing decision making with patients, nurses only offered opportunity for shared decisions based on their pre-selected recommendations. Shared decision making was used in a paternalist rather than an egalitarian approach. This study reflects the complexity of shared decision making and the need for nurses to reflect on the attitudes, emotions and values, as well as the knowledge base they bring to their practice. Nurses' paternalism, however, may not be surprising, given the long and established tradition of professionals taking control within health care. Some patients and clients may prefer to rely on trusting the professionals to make decisions or may base their decisions on accepted approaches to decision making within the family or community. Preferred decision technologies may be faith or chance based rather than deliberative or analytical. Kaltoft *et al.* (2013) are right to note that decision making first involves deciding how to decide. The more the complexity of shared approaches is considered, the more challenging it appears. Nevertheless, shared decision making, as Friesen-Storms *et al.* (2015) discuss, will be increasingly important in the management of long term conditions.

It is understandable that the complexity of decision making has led to a proliferation of specialist knowledge areas, all relevant to the delivery of care. There is a danger that such specialisation will lead to knowledge silos similar to the professional silos that can inhibit collaborative working and shared understanding amongst those involved in delivering effective care. The concept of EBP has provided unifying potential, offering an approach to practice that all professions support (despite debates about hierarchical or inclusive views on evidence and differing levels of skills and experience amongst practitioners). Amongst nurses, sceptical views about EBP persist not least because the nature of evidence readily available to practising nurses can seem to have little relevance to the daily experience of client-focused care. Although limited educational preparation and lack of supportive leadership contributes to such scepticism, it is important to recognise that EBP has serious limitations as an overarching framework for practice. Practice-based decisions are not based solely on evidence and information. Practice is also based on, *inter alia*, preferences, values, ethical principles and available resources. The focus on a shared decision process makes this particularly clear. Involving patients/clients in the process makes it harder for professionals to mask their own professional and self-interests, emotions and values by concentrating on information and evidence. Decision making becomes more open to scrutiny.

Acknowledging EBP's inadequacy as an overarching framework for practice involves creating more complex, or at least different, models to guide education and practice. Educators face the challenge of shaping curricula to support an understanding of shared decision making at all levels of experience, even though many nurses will practise with limited levels of authority and autonomy. Nursing is now making progress in building skills and experience in producing and using evidence through research leadership and more autonomous senior roles. Nurses in autonomous roles have 'lynchpin' opportunities to promote shared evidence-informed decision making. Their practice will be constrained by their capacity for effective collaborative working and by their own educational preparation. This chapter and this book aim to support such nurses by broadening perspectives and deepening enquiry into EBP.

References

AHRQ (2013) Comparative effectiveness research in nursing care. *Allnurses*, 27 June. Available online at http://allnurses.com/ahrq-effective-health/comparative-effectiveness-research-841227.html (accessed 9 March 2015).

AHRQ (2015) Agency for Healthcare Research and Quality Effective Health Care Program: Helping You Make Better Healthcare Choices. Available at www.effectivehealthcare.ahrq.gov (accessed 9 March 2015).

Barrett, G. and Keeping, C. (2005) The processes required for effective interprofessional working. In Barrett, G., Sellman, D. and Thomas, J. (eds) *Interprofessional Working in Health and Social Care: Professional Perspectives*. Basingstoke: Palgrave Macmillan, 18–31.

Brown, C. E., Wickline, M., Ecoff, L. and Glaser, D. (2009) Nursing practice, knowledge, attitudes and perceived barriers to evidence-based practice at an academic medical centre. *Journal of Advanced Nursing*, 65(2): 371–81.

Chambless, D. L., Baker, M. J., Baucom, D. H., Beutler, L. E., Calhoun, K. S., Crits-Chrisoph, P., Daiuto, A., *et al.* (1998) Update on empirically validated therapies, II. *Clinical Psychologist*, 51(1): 3–16.

Chapman, G. B. and Sonnenberg, F. A. (eds) (2000) *Decision Making in Health Care, Theory, Psychology and Applications*. Cambridge: Cambridge University Press.

Clark, A. M., Thompson, D. R., Walson, R. and Norman, I. (2012) The state of nursing and evidence-based practice, *Lancet*, 380: 472.

Cramp, F. A., Hewlett, S., Almeida, C., Kirwan, J. R., Chpoy, E., Chalder, T., Pollock, J. and Christensen, R. (2013) Non-pharmacological interventions for fatigue in rheumatoid arthritis. *Cochrane Database of Systematic Reviews*, 8, CD008322. doi: 10.1002/14651858.CD008322.pub2.

Donnelly, J. (2010) Comparative Effectiveness Research. *Health Policy Brief: Health Affairs*, October 5. Available online at www.healthaffairs.org/healthpolicybriefs/brief.php?brief_id=27 (accessed March 24, 2015).

Dowie, J. and Kaltoft, M. K. (2011) Deciding how to decide – and how to support decisions. Nuffield Webinar, 21 November. Available online at www.nuffieldtrust.org.uk/sites/files/nuffield/jack_dowie_21.11.11_for_pdf.pdf (accessed 9 March 2015).

Dowie, J., Kaltoft, M. K., Salkeld, G. and Cunich, M. (2013) Towards generic online multicriteria decision support in patient-centred health care. *Health Expectations*, first published online 2 August, doi: 10.1111/hex.12111.

Drisko, J. W. and Grady, M. D. (2012) *Evidence-Based Practice in Clinical Social Work*. New York: Springer Science and Business Media.

Dures, E., Kitchen, K., Almeida, C., Ambler, N., Cliss, A., Hammond, A., Knops, B., Morris, M., Swinkels, A. and Hewlett, S. (2012) 'They didn't tell us, they made us work it out ourselves': patient perspectives of a cognitive-behavioural programme for rheumatoid arthritis fatigue. *Arthritis Care and Research*, 64(4): 494–501.

Editorial (2012) Science for action-based nursing. *Lancet*, 379: 1763.

Friesen-Storms, J. H. H. M., Bours, G. J. J. W., van der Weijden, T., Beurskens, A. J. H. M. (2015) Shared decision making in chronic care in the context of evidence based practice in nursing. *International Journal of Nursing Studies*, 52(1): 69–76.

Gerrish, K., McDonnell, A., Nolan, M., Guillaume, L., Kirshbaum, M. and Tod, A. (2011) The role of advanced practice nurses in knowledge brokering as a means of promoting evidence-based practice among clinical nurses. *Journal of Advanced Nursing*, 67(9): 2004–14.

Hewlett, S., Chalder, T., Choy, E., Cramp, F. A., Davis, B., Dures, E., Nicholls, C. and Kirwan, J. R. (2011a) Fatigue in rheumatoid arthritis: time for a conceptual model [editorial]. *Rheumatology*, 50(6): 1004–6.

Hewlett, S., Sanderson, T., May, J., Alten, R., Bingham, C. O. 3rd, Cross, M., March, L., Pohl, C., Woodworth, T. and Bartlett, S. J. (2011b) I'm hurting, I want to kill myself: rheumatoid arthritis flare is more than a high joint count – an international patient perspective on flare where medical help is sought. *Rheumatology*, 51(1): 69–76.

International Council of Nurses (2012) *Closing the Gap: from Evidence to Action*. Geneva: ICS. Available online at www.icn.ch/publications/2012-closing-the-gap-from-evidence-to-action (accessed 9 March 2015).

Kaltoft, M. K. (2013) Nursing informatics and nursing ethics: addressing their disconnect through and enhanced TIGER-vision. *Studies in Health Technology and Informatics*, 192: 879–83.

Kaltoft, M. K., Cunich M., Salkend, G. and Dowie, J. (2013) Assessing decision quality in patient-centred care requires a preference-sensitive measure. *Journal of Health Services Research and Policy*, 19(2):110–17.

Kirwan, J. R., Boonen, A. and Hewlett S. (2011) OMERACT 10 patient perspective virtual campus: valuing health: measuring outcomes in RA fatigue, sleep, arthroplasty, systemic sclerosis; and the clinical significance of changes in health. *Journal of Rheumatology*, 38(8): 1728–34.

Kochn, M. L. and Lehman, K. (2008) Nurses' perceptions of evidence based nursing practice. *Journal of Advanced Nursing*, 62: 2009–15.

Lilienfeld, S. O., Ritschel, L. R., Lynn, S. J., Cautin R. L. and Latzman, R. D. (2013) Why many clinical psychologists are resistant to evidence-based practice: root causes and constructive remedies. *Clinical Psychology Review*, 33: 883–900.

Manias, E., Atkins, R. and Dunning, T. (2004) Decision-making models used by 'graduate nurses' managing patients' medications. *Journal of Advanced Nursing*, 47(3): 270–8.

McCarthy, M. C. (2003) Detecting acute confusion in older adults: comparing clinical reasoning of nurses working in acute, long-term and community health care environments. *Research in Nursing and Health*, 26(3): 202–13.

Melnyk, B. M., Fineout-Overholt, E., Gallagher Ford, L. and Kaplan, L. (2012) The state of evidence based practice in U.S. nurses: critical implications for nurse leaders and educators. *Journal of Nursing Administration*, 42(9): 410–17.

Middleton, J. (2013) Nurse education is not to blame for care failings [editorial]. *Nursing Times* 109(13): 1.

National Institute of Nursing Research (2014) FOAs: Centers of Excellence for Self-Management Research. Available online at www.ninr.nih.gov/newsandinformation/newsandnotes/foa-selfmanagementcenters-2014#.VP3NoUKyQQ4 (accessed 9 March 2015).

NHS England (2015) Tools for shared decision making. Available online at www.england.nhs.uk/ourwork/pe/sdm/tools-sdm (accessed 9 March 2015).

Pollard, K. and Harris, F. (2010) Interprofessional working. In Sellman, D. and Snelling, P. *Becoming a Nurse: A Textbook for Professional Practice*. Harlow: Pearson, pp. 138–63.

Rapport, F., Storey, M., Porter, A., Snooks, H., Jones, K., Peconi, J., Sanchez, A., Siebert, S., Thorne, K., Clement, C. and Russell, I. (2013) Qualitative research within trials: developing a standard operating procedure for a clinical trials unit. *Trials*, 14(1): 54. doi:10.1186/1745-6215-14-54.

Satterfield, J. M., Spring, B., Brownson, R. C., Mullen, E. J., Newhouse, R. P., Walker, B. B. and Whitlock, E. P. (2009), Toward a transdisciplinary model of evidence-based practice. *Millbank Quarterly*, 87: 368–90.

Shaibu, S. (2006) Evidence-based nursing practice in Botswana: issues, challenges, and globalisation. *Primary Health Care Research and Development*, 7: 309–13.

Thompson, C., McCaughan, D., Cullum, N., Sheldon, T. and Raynor, P. (2005) Barriers to evidence-based practice in primary care nursing – why viewing decision-making as a context is helpful. *Journal of Advanced Nursing*, 4(52): 432–44.

University of the West of England (2010) Bristol Rheumatoid Arthritis Fatigue Scales. Available online at http://bit.ly/15DH1i9 (accessed 9 March 2015).

Upton, J., Fletcher, M., Madoc-Sutton, H., Sheikh, A., Caress, A.-L. and Walker, S. (2011) Shared decision making or paternalism in nursing consultations? A qualitative study of primary care asthma nurses' views on sharing decisions with patients regarding inhaler device selection. *Health Expectations*, 14(4): 374–82.

Williamson. S., Twelvetree, T., Thompson, J. and Beaver, K. (2012) An ethnographic study exploring the role of ward-based Advanced Nurse Practitioners in an acute medical setting. *Journal of Advanced Nursing*, 68(7): 1579–88.

Wise, N. J. (2009) Maintaining magnet status: establishing an evidence-based practice committee. *AORN Journal*, 90(2): 205–13.

4 Evidence-based practice as taught and experienced

Education, practice and context

Elizabeth Rosser, Deborah Neal, Julie Reeve,
Janine Valentine and Rachael Grey

Introduction

It is widely recognized that nursing as a profession has changed almost unrecognizably over the last 60 years, both in what nurses are expected to do in practice and in the way they are prepared. Since September 2013, in the UK, all students are required to complete a degree-level programme leading to registration/licensure and, as such, they are expected to be familiar with the research process and to understand the relevance, authority and utility of research (Christie *et al.*, 2012). This is reinforced by the current Nursing and Midwifery Council Standards (NMC, 2010, R5 6.1) which states that: 'All nurses must appreciate the value of evidence in practice, be able to understand and appraise research, apply relevant theory and research findings to their work and identify areas for further investigation' (NMC, 2010: Domain 1: 9, p. 14).

Whilst research understanding is key to achieve the higher education experience, evidence-based practice (EBP) is not merely about research. EBP has been defined in a number of ways and Sackett *et al.* (2000) refer to it as the integration of the best research evidence with clinical expertise and patient values to facilitate clinical decision making. It is a means of ensuring that effective care is delivered and embraces a combination of knowledge for the head (technical knowledge based on research evidence), knowledge for the hand (professional and life resources) and knowledge for the heart (first person accounts of patient experience) (Galvin and Todres 2012). Whilst research is only one form of evidence in the EBP approach, and although it is considered the strongest form of evidence, if it is 'de-contextualised' or separated from other forms of knowledge, it can be misleading. Forms of evidence other than research are considered in depth in Chapter 9 of this book. Education for registration, which embraces all three forms of evidence, is crucial to promoting the delivery of consistent, high-quality care (Rolfe *et al.*, 2008).

The early introduction of EBP into the pre-registration programme and its integration throughout the preparation for professional life is key to setting the culture of EBP. It follows that those involved in educating the emerging professional are central to setting the tone of its importance and encouraging a commitment by them to embracing its principles throughout their professional career. However, whilst acknowledging EBP as a major policy drive in modern healthcare systems, this chapter considers in more detail the challenges and potential solutions to its adoption from the education perspective for students in both the education and practice settings but also among clinicians in the 'real world' of practice. Particular attention will be given to:

- developing the new workforce
- culture in practice
- confidence of the individual
- resource constraints within the organization.

Developing the new workforce

Historical development of the profession

Within the UK, preparation to become a registered nurse has traditionally been based on the apprenticeship model, training in the rudiments of practice skills and procedures supported by underpinning knowledge. Then, from the first degree programme leading to registration delivered by Edinburgh University in 1960, it was almost 30 years later when nursing programmes moved wholesale into higher education, with the compulsory Diploma in Higher Education with Registration in 1989 (Project 2000). Then, a further 25 years later, in September 2013, the all-graduate intake became compulsory across the UK. Increasingly, graduate status is being required internationally for registered nurse status in order to develop nursing workforce capability (Spitzer and Perrenoud, 2006; Watson, 2006).

In the early 1990s, within the UK, removal of the student body as an integral part of the clinical nursing workforce has had far-reaching consequences. With the elimination of this 'cheap' labour, the NHS has had to reorganize its workforce by re-skilling its healthcare assistants (clinical bands 2–4) and subsequently its professional nursing workforce, with students gaining supernumerary status. Over the last 20 years, the advantages that EBP appears to have brought to professional nurses are immense. Its adoption may even be considered as justifying the existence of professional practitioners, as distinct from the informal care given by well-meaning family members (who are often eager to access the latest research themselves). More importantly, with the readily available access to the worldwide web and the increasing move towards the patient as consumer, the role of the nurse and wider healthcare professional has changed to working in partnership with their increasingly informed patients. To manage the shift in power, nurses will need to be at least as well informed as their patients so that they can support informed decision making. It is not surprising that EBP has been well received. Indeed, on the one level, its rapid and widespread acceptance was demonstrated in its first ten years of adoption, as Rolfe suggests, by the considerable rise in published papers on the topic from 1 in 1992 to 1760 in 2000 (Rolfe *et al.*, 2008: 441). However, on a second level, there continues to be widespread resistance to its continued adoption and, as Melnyk *et al.* (2012) suggests, the role of education to improve the skills of those in practice is fundamental if those on the front line are to be successful in achieving an evidence-based culture. Whilst there is no disputing that EBP is highly valued, as Miers noted in Chapter 3, given its intro-duction since the early 1990s, many registered nurses who have been employed in practice for a number of years have not been prepared using an EBP approach. This, together with the increasing volume of healthcare assistants with no formally recognized preparation, serves to dilute the student exposure to an evidence-based culture in practice. Even now, UK nursing's regulatory body, the Nursing and Midwifery Council (NMC) requires higher education institutions to employ teachers of students on programmes leading to qualified nurse registra-tion to have a basic undergraduate degree (the same level as those they are teaching), an active professional registration and an approved teaching qualifica-tion, with no requirement for higher degrees and competence in research. At the other extreme, many higher education institutions in the UK, where nursing programmes are being delivered, require their education staff to achieve doctoral status to establish leadership in research. However, research capability and research leadership within nurse education is not uniform across the sector. The importance of both research and education for the emerging professional has been reinforced very recently by Lord Willis (2012) in his report, *Quality with Compassion: The Future of Nursing Education*. Although as yet, not all higher education institutions require their staff to compulsorily undertake doctoral study, those who are less confident in teaching research and EBP may convey a less than positive attitude to research. One of the greatest criticisms, as Melnyk *et al.* (2012) suggest, is that educators spend more time teaching the skills of *doing* research rather than teaching students how to *use* research. Given that students are exposed in practice to practitioners with a range of educational backgrounds and educationalists with different perspectives on research and EBP, it is not surpris-ing that challenges to the adoption of EBP remain.

Developing capacity and capability in research and EBP

There is no doubt, as evidenced from the changing NMC requirements for nurse registration, that the curriculum preparing the next generation of qualified nurses changes regularly by statute and continues to have many demands placed upon it. Many have suggested that, with a 45-week curriculum, the programme is already 'over stuffed', yet every higher education institution delivering the programme has the freedom to interpret the NMC standards and put their unique selling point on its delivery. However, programmes leading to registered nurse status have varied so considerably in their make-up across the country, that the United Kingdom Clinical Research Collaboration (UKCRC, 2007) suggests that many leave with little knowledge of research by the time they register. With a full-to-bursting curriculum, the small-scale nature of suitable projects and the challenges of ethics approval, it is acknowledged that there are significant challenges to offering any undergraduate nursing student hands-on experience of empirical research and, for the same reasons, this is mirrored at masters level. So, without the opportunity to gain hands-on experience of empirical research, the mystique and fear of research potentially remains. Indeed, Cliska (2005) in Canada and Mattila and Eriksson (2007) in Finland suggest that most students do not envisage themselves undertaking a research project, so their motivation to learn is low, they fail to see the relevance and they find the sessions boring or even anxiety provoking. With research understanding having key importance in the implementation of EBP, it is not surprising that student nurses leave their programme feeling under confident about their grasp of EBP and an understanding of what constitutes 'evidence'. In the UK, the NMC (2010) is perfectly clear in its requirements of the new standards that approved education providers are expected to underpin their programmes with evidence-based sources. This expectation is evident in nursing programmes more widely across the globe (Winters and Echeverri, 2012; Chew, 2014; Barria, 2014; Florin *et al.*, 2011). Educators are then charged with engaging students in a meaningful way to feel excited by research and to understand the range and strength of the different types of available evidence. More importantly, educators who develop a culture that challenges existing practice, who are open to embracing new evidence and who welcome and support new ways of working based on best evidence are crucial to developing capacity and capability in EBP.

Whilst there is ample evidence to suggest that students value research methodology as important knowledge to gain from their undergraduate studies, Melnyk *et al.* (2012) found that support structures in practice are lacking. They suggest that EBP mentorship would be more appropriate than a token one- or two-day workshop and that mentors experienced in the delivery of EBP should work closely with practitioners to help them learn the skills and consistently implement EBP for the culture to begin to change. From the practice education perspective, Christie *et al.* (2012) found that educators play a key role in ensuring a commitment to research during the socialisation of students to the profession. They suggest that, if this approach is not embedded throughout the programme, students quickly learn the hidden messages of its lack of relevance for practice.

So, it appears that the educator has a key role in developing the capacity and capability of students in the nature of research evidence (authority), the type of research required in clinical practice (relevance) and the potential power of research to transform and improve practice (utility); and that this needs to be embedded throughout the curriculum. Additionally, Christie *et al.* (2012) confirm that consistent appreciation of the value of research in practice is important throughout the undergraduate nursing programme delivered by enthusiastic academics expert in research and its application to practice. Indeed, Winters and Echeverri (2012) offer a range of learning and teaching strategies that can be used to build the skills of critiquing, interpreting and using research by those knowledgeable and excited themselves about research. Girot (2013) acknowledged in her qualitative study of four higher education institutions in south-west England that, as educationalists complete their doctoral studies as required by their employing institution, they embrace the new order and move from a place of anti-intellectualism to a position where they feel responsible for changing the culture within their own organization. Participants in Girot's (2013) study confirmed their own responsibility for bridging the divide between teaching and research and the need to value both. They also recognized the importance of clinicians in practice having a sound knowledge of EBP and research methodology. There is great danger of the theory–practice divide, with research methodology being embedded within the undergraduate curriculum yet its translation into everyday practice lacking. Some organizations continue to employ lecturer practitioners who bridge the divide between higher education institutions and practice and are able to promote and actively encourage an EBP approach to practice.

New workforce developments

How can the nursing workforce embrace the sophisticated skills of research within the clinical environment? Where are the role models to support expert clinical researchers? Girot (2013) found that nurses enter the profession first and foremost to practise nursing and their first inclination when they qualify as a registered nurse is to seek employment in practice to consolidate their skills as a professional. Perhaps newly qualified nurses could be encouraged to undertake part-time doctoral study immediately following qualification to allow new registrants to develop their practice alongside higher level study to embed research and practice as the norm, right from the start. In the past, it was likely that it would be some time before any serious thought of a career in nursing research or indeed in education, became a reality. Nevertheless, there are currently over 10 000 clinical research nurses (CRNs) in England and, as Gelling (2010) admits, their work historically has varied considerably, with no recognized benchmark qualification. Many, certainly in the early days, failed to qualify to take a leadership role in research projects, often choosing such a career for its sociable work schedule. For many, their role has been quite separate from a purely clinical role and CRNs have been disadvantaged by professional isolation, with few recognized expectations for their career progression. However, in 2008, national competencies for the role were introduced to guide their development and to be used alongside a structured education programme (Gelling, 2010) in an attempt to attract new recruits and offer career development. Nevertheless, to develop a critical mass of senior researchers, able to lead major projects in clinical practice, requires recognized and sophisticated preparation for the role. Additionally, developing research leaders has been the subject of long debate and also requires flexible employment models that embrace both research and practice, with significant funding to support their career progression. With the *Developing the Best Research Professionals* report of the UKCRC (2007), the new role of clinical academic was introduced for nurses (and subsequently for allied health professionals), with a clear career trajectory in clinical research. The National Institute for Health Research (NIHR) has now taken on the administration and funding of these posts and the dedicated research training from master's degree in clinical research, through to doctorate in clinical research, before taking up a postdoctoral fellowship and then senior clinical academic fellowship, which will be joint funded with practice to drive expert clinical researchers into the heart of clinical practice. Ultimately, as Miers acknowledges in Chapter 3, joint appointments at professorial level would go some way to embed 'practice' research jointly within the world of education and clinical practice. Expert clinicians, including consultant nurses with research expertise, who hold strategic positions in both education and in practice, will help to bridge the theory–practice gap with regard to clinical research in both education and practice. This level of research leadership by individuals who are experts in practice and research and who are approachable and accessible will enhance the culture and acceptance of EBP as the accepted norm.

Culture in practice

Organisational culture does have a significant bearing on the uptake of EBP. A student nurse in placement for exactly half of their education programme, leading to registration as a qualified nurse (within the UK and Europe this equates to 2300 hours in both theory and practice), will learn through experience the value that professional practice places on EBP. Indeed, as already noted, if research-informed nursing knowledge is not consistently valued or used throughout their education programme, Christie *et al.* (2012) suggest that there is a risk of developing a 'hidden curriculum', where students unintentionally learn the lack of importance of research in practice. Several researchers argue that whilst graduate nurses do have the ability to appraise research, the main barriers to research implementation remain in practice (Christie *et al.*, 2012). However, as Rolfe argues convincingly in Chapter 6, best practice should dictate what counts as best evidence rather than vice versa. It follows that, seeing the purpose and understanding the nature of evidence and its relationship with practice as a whole needs to be embedded in the fabric of every practising nurse, to the benefit of patient care. Indeed, Wallis (2012: 15) emphasizes: 'EBP … that integrates the best evidence from well-designed studies with clinicians' expertise, patient assessments, and patients' own preferences, leads to better, safer care; better outcomes; and lower healthcare costs'.

A culture that embraces EBP as a tripartite relationship (head, hand and heart) will lead to more cost-effective practice, improved quality of care and greater satisfaction. Senior nurses on the front line confirm their experiences of colleagues who are passionate about their practice and devour research articles and who, given the right circumstances, endeavour to implement their findings in practice. The educator's belief in the strength of EBP and the practitioner's application of their knowledge and their collective ability to critique the nature of that evidence is central to its acceptance among students' learning the craft of their profession.

EBP and effective clinical decision making

Miers explores the connection between EBP and clinical decision making in Chapter 3. Additionally, Christie *et al.* (2012) confirm that EBP has been linked to clinical governance as a way of ensuring that practitioners employ safe and effective decision making; yet it appears that practitioners still lack the power and influence to make research-based changes. From their own study, Gerrish *et al.* (2008) reinforce that junior nurses, in particular, felt that they lacked the autonomy required to change practice.

At a time when education expectations have been rising for the profession, the emphasis on clinical decision making based on best evidence has become of paramount importance. One of the reasons for the widespread adoption of EBP is that it offers a foundation on which to support this (Sackett *et al.*, 1996). Indeed, its development and growth is embedded in demands by the profession and the public for quality, safety and accountability in the profession (Stevens and Staley, 2006). Students experiencing placement in organisations where clinical decision making is based on best evidence are likely to be positively influenced by their potential to impact change. However, there is little appetite for lone workers introducing unilateral change. Ultimately, the aim is to collectively promote a culture where EBP becomes the norm for all and where interprofessional teams are open to embracing change based on best evidence. It is worth considering whether lessons can be learned from allied health professions which moved to an all-graduate intake some years previously and whether nursing students across the UK will, in time, become more confident to impact change and influence the implementation of research into practice.

As already noted, nurse education across the western world has increasingly moved to a university-based programme and, as such, the nursing workforce capability in EBP is likely to improve if the curriculum supports such a preparation (Christie *et al.*, 2012). Indeed, similar challenges experienced by educators in the UK are evident in the United States and within Europe. In the United States, Krainovich-Miller *et al.* (2009) confirm the historical beginnings of teaching research and EBP within the profession, with the majority of faculty members learning about research from a traditional conduct of research perspective. In Sweden, Florin *et al.* (2011) found, in their national survey of nursing students' experiences of the education support they received for research utilization, that experiences differed depending on which university they attended. Their capability beliefs regarding EBP varied considerably affecting their potential to implement it in the 'real world'. Interestingly, this did not seem to affect the clinical element of their programme to the same extent. Nevertheless, leadership in clinical research and practice is crucial if the culture of EBP is to be encouraged and adopted. In time, the development of a critical mass of nurses who choose to progress a clinical academic career, alongside educators who also require doctoral status to teach will significantly improve the motivation and confidence to encourage its adoption.

Organisational context

If, as previously noted, EBP consists of the use not merely of research evidence but of a range of evidence from the head, hand and heart (Galvin and Todres,

2012), it seems that knowledge of the hand (professional experience) and knowledge of the heart (patients' views, which may be drawn from empirical research) are as important if not more important in decision making in practice than knowledge of the head (empirical research) (Gerrish *et al.*, 2008; Estabrooks, 1998). However, Sitzia (2002) suggests that, collectively, lack of time and incentives and a nursing culture based on custom and practice, task completion and autocratic leadership, rather than on autonomous decision making, contrive to produce a workforce which rejects a culture of EBP. Students exposed to such environments, although not the norm, are less likely to feel empowered to change or influence a change in practice, particularly when organizational context is often challenged by the increasing acuity of care and the workforce is focused on fire-fighting rather than proactive improvement. Many international studies, irrespective of country, emphasize the lack of time either on or off duty for qualified nurses to read about research (Gerrish *et al.*, 2008). Additionally, in an environment where students are learning their craft, qualified nurses believe that they lack the ability and have insufficient resources to apply research into practice (Gerrish *et al.*, 2008; Caldwell *et al.*, 2007; Ryecroft-Malone *et al.*, 2004). Meijers *et al.* (2006), in their systematic review, explore the relationship between contextual factors and the use of research in nursing. They found that, in spite of the limitation of methodological quality and recognizing the complexity of context in which nursing practice occurs, contextual factors may well influence the implementation of research in practice. In particular, they suggest that context, culture and leadership have a positive influence on research use by nurses. In an environment where EBP is perceived negatively, or urgent issues distract the committed professional towards fundamental priorities as maintaining basic patient safety, the context can have a significant negative influence on the adoption of EBP.

Gerrish *et al.* (2008), in their review of the literature, reinforce that organizational context and the constraints under which nurses work should be considered when setting out to promote EBP within the organizational culture. In spite of the considerable investment made across the western world to increase the potential for care to be delivered based on best evidence, organizations have a responsibility not only to ensure that evidence-based protocols and guidelines are in place but that students and staff are using them (Rycroft-Malone *et al.*, 2004). They should ensure that mechanisms such as the use of complete audit cycles against evidence based guidelines are in place to review and appraise them. However, as Rycroft-Malone *et al.* (2004) argue, the complexity of implementing evidence into practice reinforce that it is unlikely that the mere presence of protocols and guidelines will ensure their appropriate implementation. Students, sensitive of the need to be socially accepted within their placement will be strongly influenced by those in a position of authority with either a positive or negative view on EBP and this will subsequently have an impact on their future practice. As Rycroft-Malone *et al.* (2004: 915) suggest, 'context has been found to be a potent mediator of the successful implementation of evidence into practice'. Indeed, with the proliferation of the use of professional and social networks, Rycroft-Malone *et al.* (2004)

recognize the role these networks can play in shaping views on the impact of particular evidence, affecting different approaches to working practices and influencing change. The active use of social media among the emerging professional is probably one of the most significant positive influences on the organizational culture and students are well placed to be supported by these media.

Whilst there seems sufficient evidence to suggest that, strategically, EBP is a worthwhile pursuit, over the 25 years since its inception, there remain considerable challenges to its implementation. There are a number of studies evidencing the anti-research culture among students within their undergraduate, prequalifying programmes, as well as their exposure to a negative attitude to the acceptance of research within the practice setting (Hannes *et al.*, 2007: 163; Burke *et al.*, 2005). Within the UK, recent media portrayals have evidenced patients at risk of neglect in a range of care settings. These portrayals reinforce that there exist multiple examples of 'real world' practices which not only lack an evidence base to care but present a culture that devalues its relevance.

Confidence of the individual

There are numerous examples of students and newly qualified practitioners who lack confidence to challenge existing practice. They also lack time and confidence to read and critically appraise the evidence and disseminate good practice and these are areas which require to be addressed (Zipoli and Kennedy, 2005; Nagy *et al..*, 2001; McCaughan *et al.*, 2002). Three of the most documented barriers to the implementation of EBP affecting the confidence of the individual are:

- the lack of knowledge and skills of the practising nurse to identify and appraise research reports (Gerrish *et al.*, 2008);
- misperceptions of or negative attitudes about research and evidence-based care (Melnyk *et al.*, 2012);
- inconsistent understanding among nurse executives of the meaning of evidence-based nursing (Alspach, 2006).

Within the UK, it is well recognized that the NMC (2015) requires qualified nurses to be responsible and accountable for providing safe, person-centred, evidence-based care. This impacts directly on how the education programme to support undergraduate nursing students equips students with knowledge and skills and enables their understanding of implementing research into practice (Christie *et al.*, 2012). Yet, in Finland, the study of Mattila and Eriksson (2007) stated that undergraduate nursing students are under-committed to research as a result of having little exposure to research implementation during their clinical placements. This is reinforced by others within the UK who suggest that a lack of research knowledge during their undergraduate nursing programme impacts on the poor application of research by qualified nurses (Marsh *et al.*, 2001; Closs *et al.*, 2000). However, more recently, the rapid rise in research knowledge for nursing practice has of itself become a barrier to research use even among research active nurses (Carrion *et al.*, 2004; Adamsen *et al.*, 2003). Learning to manage the volume of appropriate and respected research evidence will become a lifelong learning competence that nurses will be required to embrace as they progress in their career (Alien *et al.*, 2008) and a skill that needs harnessing during their undergraduate preparation.

Whilst the NMC (2010) requires nursing students to be competent in delivering evidence-based care at point of registration and to maintain that competence after registration (NMC, 2015), the UKCRC (2007) has reinforced that, in spite of the move of nurse education into institutions of higher education nationally, some students leave the programme with little knowledge of research by the time that they register. With the advent of nursing becoming an all-graduate intake in the UK and advanced practice nurses requiring masters level study (Department of Health, 2010), it is likely that advanced academic study will become a requirement for more senior posts. Clinical leaders are already being called to evidence their level of critical thinking and decision making for such demanding roles, and it is likely that higher degrees for specialist and advanced practitioners will become the norm. Although most consultant nurses have master's degrees, increasingly they are undertaking doctoral study to support the four dimensions of their role (research, education, clinical practice and their leadership of service development). So, although Caldwell *et al.* (2007) suggest that nurses lack the confidence in the willingness of their organization to support EBP, with more senior nurses undertaking higher degrees, and with EBP being a required standard in pre-registration nursing programmes, this picture is likely to change.

Misperceptions or negative attitudes about research and evidence-based care

In spite of exposure to the concept of EBP during nurses' prequalifying preparation and, in some institutions, its application as a foundation to all clinical skills teaching, the culture of the organization in the practice arena will significantly influence their ability to implement such a philosophy.

Gerrish *et al.* (2008), in their own study of senior and junior nurses in the development of EBP, questioned where the educational emphasis should lie in order to maximize the development of such a culture in practice. Whilst, traditionally, the focus has been on preparing nurses in clinical practice with the skills to access, critique, interpret and apply research findings to practice, there are a number of international studies which have shown that nurses fail to implement research in practice, owing to a lack of ability to do so, lack of time and of resources (Bryar *et al.*, 2003; Glacken and Chaney, 2004; Hutchinson and Johnson, 2004; McKenna *et al.*, 2004). Additionally, there has existed an 'anti-research culture' (Hannes *et al.*, 2007: 163), with students developing a negative attitude to the use of research evidence, even early in their career (Burke *et al.*, 2005), with the public referring to nurses becoming 'too clever to care'. Nevertheless, Gerrish *et al.* (2008: 70) propose that EBP requires the critique and interpretation of a much wider range of types of evidence. They recommend that, more realistically perhaps, they should be developing the skills to critique research 'products', such as clinical protocols, within the context of their own setting. Since the publication of these studies, the landscape has been changing. As previously acknowledged, many higher education institutions require their teaching staff to achieve doctoral status as compulsory and, through their own education, nurse educators are beginning to overcome the tendency to anti-intellectualism and to promote confidence in research through their own increasing competence and credibility (Girot, 2013). Importantly, within the first decade of the 21st century, competition across UK higher education institutions with healthcare faculties has now become a reality for the Research Excellence Framework, where faculties strive to increase their reputation in research output and impact. Indeed, as already acknowledged, the requirement for a master's qualification for specialist and advanced practitioners and the introduction of clinical academic careers, where excellent practitioners can build confidence and credibility in research, is significant progress for the profession.

Inconsistent understanding among nurses of the meaning of evidence-based nursing

The concept of EBP originated with the evidence-based medicine movement in Canada (Sackett *et al.*, 2000) and, since then, the nursing profession has tackled a steep learning curve to embrace research and an evidence base as part of their professional identity. Alspac (2006) has estimated that 64 per cent of registered nurses have limited understanding of evidence-based nursing and, in particular, that nurse executives also have an inconsistent understanding of the term (Sredl, 2008). Indeed, Rolfe addresses this in some detail in Chapter 8 of this book. So, clearly, in spite of the strategic imperative to embrace the EBP movement, there seems to be considerable uncertainty about its interpretation in the 'real world' of practice, which poses a problem for students in the practice setting and for their confidence in its use (Christie *et al.*, 2012). Indeed, methodologically, there have been mixed views from those who have entered the debate from an informed perspective. With randomized controlled trials being deemed as the 'gold standard' of research in terms of their influence on EBP (authority), there have been those who have challenged their position in this hierarchy for nursing, where such approaches tend to encourage a standardization of approach rather than an individualized approach to care (Mantzoukas, 2008; Adib-Hajbaghery, 2009). Clearly, positivistic methodology has its place in the development of protocols. Naturalistic methodology and its interpretation for practice from the patient perspective is as important in assisting students and practitioners to understand the situation from the 'inside'. However, nurse educators need to equip students to appraise the 'authority' of the evidence before they can make informed decisions about its utility (Christie *et al.*, 2012).

Assisting students to be lifelong learners once they qualify is crucial, so that they can learn to access, understand and appraise research and make a clear decision as to its relevance to their practice. Indeed, Isaac and Franceschi (2008) and Christie *et al.* (2012) confirm the need for educators to have an important role in producing easily understandable versions of relevant and important research for practice by using summaries or other media to disseminate principles that could be applied in practice and to whet the appetite of novice and experienced practitioners to grasp challenging and difficult concepts. It is also important to support student understanding of the purpose, limitations and strengths of various research designs for practice-based decision making to aid their confidence in implementation.

Given that students join teams of qualified staff to learn the craft of nursing practice, these teams comprise practitioners at different stages of their career and experience. In a study of senior and junior nurses' experiences of developing EBP, Gerrish *et al.* (2008) illustrated important differences between the two. Surprisingly, junior nurses were less likely to know where to find sources of evidence, such as organizational information, and were less likely than senior nurses to know how to appraise it or implement it in their practice. Whilst it is more likely that student nurses on placement align themselves with the more junior nursing staff than the more senior nurses, learning by example is likely to hamper the sustainability of implementing EBP. A culture where junior as well as senior nurses feel confident to effect change and to become more involved in supporting EBP, through for example the use of journal clubs, will significantly influence the future workforce for students on their journey to registration.

Resource constraints in the organization

It seems clear from the literature that getting evidence into practice is to some extent dependent on organizational 'fit' and the resources that organisations invest in enabling its success (Rycroft-Malone *et al.*, 2004: 921). It has already been shown that providing funding and additional staff to enhance implementation is a key factor to success. However, the relationship between resources and the adoption of evidence into practice is highly complex and does not merely require an increase in both of these resources without the acceptance by those on the front line (Rycroft-Malone *et al.*, 2004). Students involved in placement activity and junior nurses in preceptorship preparation for their early career development quickly learn the rules of engagement and the informal and often 'unsaid' priorities for every organization they are exposed to. Caldwell *et al.* (2006) found, in their examination of four professional groups (nurses, social workers, occupational therapists and physiotherapists), that there was no significant difference across the professional groups in their proactive use of research resources with two-thirds of respondents accessing bibliographical databases only twice or less over the previous 12 months. Whilst this is further supported by Webster *et al.* (2003) for nurses and McColl *et al.* (1998) for general practitioners, it illustrates that it is not a problem solely for nurses. Given that most of the participants in Caldwell *et al.*'s (2007) study had been qualified for less than 12 months, it is likely that the change in pattern of usage in their professional lives has significantly changed from their experience as a student. Indeed, as already noted, Gerrish *et al.* (2008) found in their more recent study that senior nurses were more confident in finding, reviewing and using different sources of evidence, were more likely to use published information, and more likely to show interest in the effective use of research in their practice than junior nurses. This suggests that junior nurses lack the skills to use evidence-based guidelines and as such, this presents a considerable barrier to the implementation of EBP.

Although this study reported over six years ago, nurse education within the UK moved to a higher education qualification with registration over 25 years ago. One of the expectations of a university preparation would be that those completing such a preparation would be well skilled in the use of bibliographical databases and would have a good grounding in the importance of EBP. This suggests that there is a disconnect between their educational preparation and its acceptance in practice. Indeed, Gerrish et al. (2008) found that nurses use experiential knowledge and work-based information to inform their practice, supporting the work of Thompson et al. (2004) and Winters et al. (2007), who confirm that many qualified nurses rely on their peers to support them in keeping up to date with the evidence base for their practice. Anecdotally, practice colleagues suggest that a culture of desk-based activity is not seen as being 'proper' work. Clearly, this is unsustainable for nurses to be confident in the currency of information and suggests a thoroughly uncritical approach to practice.

Access to online resources for research has become increasingly more important, owing to the ease of access of the worldwide web, as long as practitioners and students know how to use the systems. Indeed, McNeil et al. (2003) suggest that nurse education has focused too readily on using computers for access rather than using the literature, leaving students and practitioners unable to critically appraise the literature once it has been accessed. However, time and availability of these resources are not accessible to all owing to firewall barriers and also a lack of investment by healthcare organizations (Edwards and Lockett, 2004). Nevertheless, organizations are beginning to use electronic health records, with many senior staff using tablets and other mobile devices to access the internet regularly at work. Thus, in time, access to and ability to critique the literature should become more commonplace. Additionally, investment in cyber cafes in work canteens and, perhaps for some, a quiet room or library where resources can be accessed, with expertise in building information literacy skills to support practitioners, will be a cost needing to be borne by the NHS. For NHS trusts that offer student placements, additional funding is offered by commissioners in the UK to ensure students and staff have access to the literature and other resources.

In Yeovil District Hospital NHS Foundation Trust, some professional groups, such as physiotherapy and occupational therapy, have a tradition of in-service training in which recent graduates take turns as equal members of a professional group with other highly experienced clinicians to lead a session in which they present the evidence for a specific topic. This encourages new information to be introduced by those at all levels of the hierarchy in a non-threatening way and generates healthy debates around clinical reasoning. Whilst this is not the current situation for nurses in the same NHS trust, participants in Caldwell *et al.*'s (2007) study positively responded to the effect that they were actively encouraged to read research relevant to their practice and had access, through work, to electronic databases. However, few seemed to be using them. As previously acknowledged, the constraints on time and confidence to use the computers for best evidence seem to conspire against their regular use.

Whilst the employment of clinical research nurses has been problematic in terms of stability of employment and lack of a secure career trajectory to support them, the new Clinical Academic Career structure provides the opportunity for experienced nurses and allied health professionals with an interest in a clinical research career to pursue this without penalty. Ultimately, the development of a critical mass of clinical researchers, equipped to lead the development of meaningful research will expose newly qualified nurses to live a truly EBP experience in the practice setting. Additionally, the appointment of clinical chairs, part funded by the higher education institution and the NHS trust, will encourage the voice of practice in the institution and the voice of research in practice to be heard. Such appointments will evidence a commitment from both education and practice to fund significant clinical research leaders to lead and support research for practice.

Conclusion

With the recent move of nurse education to achieve an all-graduate intake of prequalifying students, EBP has become a key requirement for qualified nurses across the UK. However, much of the literature dwells in the past, in an anti-intellectual culture, a climate based on custom and practice, task completion and autocratic leadership, where educators lack confidence to embrace the new world and to take forward a philosophy which values practice based on best evidence. Whilst fire fighting to maintain basic patient safety continues to be a focus, owing to competing priorities for resources, we are witnessing significant change going forward. Students are becoming more vocal and challenging existing practice. Consultant nurses with a remit for research and service improvement and advanced practitioners are both required to have master's level study and educators need doctoral status; so the profession continues its journey of radical change. In particular, a new workforce is emerging. Senior nurses experienced in both practice and clinical research will, in time, change the culture in practice, increase the confidence of the emerging practitioner and demand resources to support them. However, this new clinical academic career pathway is in its infancy. In time, it will have considerable impact on practice in all its guises, as well as on education. Senior nurses who have a joint appointment in both practice and education and who are skilled both clinically and in clinical research will bring EBP into the common vocabulary of practice and universities and reinforce its presence in both.

References

Adamsen, I., Larsen, K., Bjerregaard, I. and Masden, J. K. (2003) Danish research-active clinical nurses overcome barriers in research utilization. *Scandinavian Journal of Caring Sciences* 17(1), 57–65.

Adib-Hajbaghery, M. (2009) Evidence-based practice: Iranian nurses' perceptions. *Worldviews in Evidence-based Nursing* 6(2), 93–101.

Alien, P., Lauchner, K., Bridges, R.A, Francis-Johnson, P., McBride, S. G. and Olivarez, A. Jr (2008) Evaluating continuing competency: a challenge for nursing. *Journal of Continuing Education in Nursing* 39(2), 81–5.

Alspach, G. (2006) Nurses' use and understanding of evidence-based practice: some preliminary evidence. *Critical Care Nurse* 26(6), 11–12.

Barría, R. M. (2014) Implementando la Práctica basada en la evidencia: un desafío para la práctica enfermera [Implementing evidence-based practice: a challenge for the nursing practice; editorial; Spanish]. *Investigación y Educación en Enfermería* 32(2), 191–3.

Bryar, R. M., Closs, S. J., Baum, G., Cooke, J., Griffiths, J., Hostick, T., Kelly, S., Knight, S., Marshall, K. and Thompson, D. R. (2003) The Yorkshire barriers project: diagnostic analysis of barriers to research utilization. *International Journal of Nursing Studies* 40(1), 73–84.

Burke, L. E., Schlenk, E. A., Sereika, S. M., Cohen, S. M., Happ, M. B. and Dorman, J. S. (2005) Developing research competence to support evidence-based practice. *Journal of Professional Nursing* 21(6): 358–63.

Carrion, M., Woods, P. and Norman, I. (2004) Barriers to research utilization among forensic mental health nurses. *International Journal of Nursing Studies* 41(6), 613–19.

Caldwell, K., Coleman, K., Copp, G., Bell, L. and Ghazi, F. (2007) Preparing for professional practice: How well does professional training equip health and social care practitioners to engage in evidence-based practice? *Nurse Education Today* 27, 518–28.

Chew, B. W. K. (2014) Exploring factors influencing the development and Implementation of evidence-based healthcare practice in emergency care setting. *Singapore Nursing Journal* 41(2), 29–34.

Christie, J., Hamill, C. and Power, J. (2012) How can we maximize nursing students' learning about research evidence and utilization in undergraduate, preregistration programmes? *Journal of Advanced Nursing* 68(12), 2789–801.

Ciliska, D. (2005) Educating for evidence-based practice. *Journal of Professional Nursing* 21(6), 345–50.

Closs, S. J., Baum, G., Bryar, R. M., Griffiths, J. and Knight, S. (2000) Barriers to research implementation in two Yorkshire hospitals. *Clinical Effectiveness in Nursing* 4(1), 3–10.

Department of Health (2010) *Equality and Excellence: Liberating the NHS*. London: Department of Health.

Edwards, N. and Lockett, D. (2004) The prohibitive costs of accessing evidence online. *Journal of Continuing Education in Nursing* 35(2), 89–90.

Estabrooks, C. A. (1998) Will evidence-based nursing practice make practice perfect? *Canadian Journal of Nursing Research* 30(1), 15–36.

Florin, J., Ehrenberg, A., Wallin, L. and Gustavsson, P. (2011) Educational support for research utilization and capability beliefs regarding evidence-based practice skills: a national survey of senior nursing students. *Journal of Advanced Nursing* 68(4), 888–97.

Galvin, K. and Todres, L. (2012) *Caring and Well-being: a Lifeworld Approach*. Abingdon: Routledge.

Gelling, L. (2010) Clinical research nursing has a bright future. *Nurse Researcher* 17(2), 3.

Gerrish, K., Ashworth, P., Lacey, A. and Bailey, J. (2008) Developing evidence-based practice: experiences of senior and junior clinical nurses. *Journal of Advanced Nursing* 62(1), 62–73.

Girot, E. A. (2013) Shaping clinical academic careers for nurses and allied health professionals: the role of the educator. *Journal of Research in Nursing* 18(1), 51–64.

Glacken, M. and Chaney, D. (2004) Perceived barriers and facilitators to implementing research findings in the Irish practice setting. *Journal of Clinical Nursing* 13(6), 731–40.

Hutchinson, A. and Johnson, L. (2004) Bridging the divide: a survey of nurses' opinions regarding barriers to, and facilitators of, research utilization in the practice setting. *Journal of Clinical Nursing* 13, 304–15.

Hannes, K., Vandersmissen, J., De Blaeser, L., Peeters, G., Goedhuys, J. and Aertgeerts, B. (2007) Barriers to evidence-based nursing: a focus group study. *Journal of Advanced Nursing* 60(2), 162–71.

Isaac, C. A. and Franceschi, A. (2008) EBM: evidence to practice and practice to evidence. *Journal of Evaluation in Clinical Practice* 14(5), 656–9.

Krainovich-Miller, B., Haber, J., Yost, J. and Kaplan Jacobs, S. (2009) Evidence-based practice challenge: teaching critical appraisal of systematic reviews and clinical practice guidelines to graduate students. *Journal of Nursing Education* 48(4), 186–95.

Mantzoukas, S. (2008) A review of evidence-based practice, nursing research and reflection: leveling the hierarchy. *Journal of Clinical Nursing* 17(2), 214–23.

Marsh, G. W., Nolan, M. and Hopkins, S. (2001) Testing the revised barriers to research utilization scale for use in the UK. *Clinical Effectiveness in Nursing* 5(2), 66–72.

Mattila, L. R. and Eriksson, E. (2007) Nursing students learning to utilize nursing research in clinical practice. *Nurse Education Today* 27(6), 568–76.

McCaughan, D., Thompson, C., Cullum, N., Sheldon, T. and Thompson, D. (2002) Acute care nurses' perceptions of barriers to using research information in clinical decision-making. *Journal of Advanced Nursing* 39(1), 46–60.

McColl, A., Smith, H., White, P. and Field, J. (1998) General practitioners' perceptions of the route to evidence based medicine: a questionnaire survey. *British Medical Journal* 316 (7128), 361–5.

McKenna, H., Ashton, S. and Keeney, S. (2004) Barriers to evidence-based practice in primary care. *Journal of Advanced Nursing* 45, 899–914.

McNeil, B., Elfrink, V., Bickford, C., Beyea, S., Averill, C., Klappenback, C. (2003) Nursing information technology knowledge, skills and preparation of student nurses, nursing faculty, and clinicians: a US survey. *Journal of Nursing Education* 42(8), 341–9.

Meijers, J. M. M., Janssen, M. A. P., Cummings, G. G., Wallin, L., Estabrooks, C. A. and Halfens, R. Y. G. (2006) Assessing the relationship between contextual factors and research utilization in nursing: systematic literature review. *Journal of Advanced Nursing* 55(5), 622–35.

Melnyk, B. M., Fineout-Overholt, E., Gallagher-Ford, L. and Kaplan, L. (2012) The state of evidence-based practice in US nurses: critical implications for nurse leaders and educators. *Journal of Nursing Administration* 42(9), 410–17.

Nagy, S., Lumby, J., McKinley, S. and MacFarlane, C. (2001) Nurses' beliefs about the conditions that hinder or support evidence-based nursing international. *Journal of Nursing Practice* 7(5), 314–21.

NMC (2015) *The Code: Professional Standards of Practice and Behavior for Nurses and Midwives*. London: Nursing and Midwifery Council. Available online at www.nmc-uk.org/The-revised-Code (accessed 10 March 2015).

NMC (2010) *Standards of Pre-registration Nurse Education*. London: Nursing and Midwifery Council. Available online at www.nmc-uk.org/Publications/Standards (accessed 10 March 2015).

Rolfe, G., Segrott, J. and Jordan, S. (2008) Tensions and contradictions in nurses' perspectives of evidenced-based practice. *Journal of Nursing Management* 16, 440–51.

Rycroft-Malone, J., Harvey, G., Seers, K., Kitson, A., McCormack, B. and Titchen, A. (2004) An exploration of the factors that influence the implementation of evidence into practice. *Journal of Clinical Nursing* 13, 913–24.

Sackett, D., Rosenberg, W. M., Muir Gray, J. A., Haynes, R. B. and Richardson, W. (1996) Evidence based medicine: what it is and what it isn't. *British Medical Journal* 312(7023), 71.

Sackett, D. L., Srauss, S. E., Richardson, W. S., Rosenberg, W. M. C and Haynes, R. B. (2000) *Evidence-based Medicine: How to Practice and Teach EBM*. London, Churchill-Livingstone.

Sitzia, J. (2002) Barriers to research utilization: the clinical setting and nurses themselves. *Intensive Critical Care Nursing* 18(4), 230–43.

Spitzer, A. and Perrenoud, B. (2006) Reforms in nursing education across Western Europe: implementation processes and current status. *Journal of Professional Nursing* 22(3), 162–71.

Sredl, D. (2008) Evidence-based nursing practice: what US nurse executives really think. *Nurses Researcher* 15(4), 51–67.

Stevens, K. R. and Staley, J. M. (2006) The quality chasm reports, evidence-based practice and nursing's response to improve healthcare. *Nursing Outlook* 54(2), 94–101.

Thompson, C., Cullum, N., McCaughan, D., Sheldon, T. and Raynor, P. (2004) Nurses, information use and clinical decision making – the real world potential for evidence-based decisions in nursing. *Evidence-based Nursing* 7(3), 68–72.

UKCRC (2007) *Developing the Best Research Professionals: Qualified Graduate Nurses: Recommendations for Preparing and Supporting Clinical Academic Nurses of the Future*. London: United Kingdom Clinical Research Collaboration.

Wallis, L. (2012) Barriers to Implementing Evidence-Based Practice Remain High for U.S. Nurses. *American Journal of Nursing* 112(12), 15.

Watson, R. (2006) Is there a role for higher education in preparing nurses? *Nurse Education in Practice* 6(6), 314–18.

Webster, J., Davies, J., Holt, V., Stallan, G., News, K. and Yegdich, T. (2003) Australian nurses' and midwives' knowledge of computers and their attitudes to using them in practice. *Journal of Advanced Nursing* 41(2), 140–6.

Willis Commission (2012) *Quality with Compassion: The Future of Nursing Education. Report of the Willis Commission on Nursing Education*. London: Royal College of Nursing. Available online at www.will003commission.org.uk (accessed 10 March 2015).

Winters, C. and Echeverri, R. (2012) Teaching strategies to support evidence-based practice. *Critical Care Nurse* 32(3), 49–54.

Winters, C. A., Lee, H. J., Besel, J., Strand, A., Echeverri, R., Jorgensen, K. P and Dea, J. E. (2007) Access to and use of research by rural nurses. *Rural and Remote Health* 7(3), 758.

Zipoli, R. and Kennedy, M. (2005) Evidence-based practice among speech–language pathologists: attitudes, utilization and barriers. *American Journal of Speech–Language Pathology* 14(3), 208–20.

5 Critical considerations in evidence-based interprofessional practice

Melody Carter

Introduction

Effective interprofessional practice has been a key aspiration of modern health and social care services for many years. The majority of the effort to achieve these goals has been directed towards improving team structures, improving relationships, service design and in the education of professionals (Townsend *et al.* 2003, Meads and Ashcroft 2005, Pollard 2006, 2009, Miers *et al.* 2009, Quinlan 2009). I suggest that a further dimension can be added whereby we critically examine the role of professional and institutional knowledge and interprofessional practice more closely. My principle argument is that in order to make effective contributions to interprofessional care, professionals (including nurses) need to work from a knowledge base that unifies or harmonises their practice with other disciplines. They need to do this so that they can fully participate in the assessment of need, decision making and evaluation processes that are so crucial to patient care. This means that the nurse's critical thinking needs to act as the 'pivot' or 'hinge point' between their use of knowledge (the evidence base for practice) and their approach to care in an increasingly complex multidisciplinary health and social care landscape.

Evidence-based practice (EBP), like interprofessional practice, represents a 'movement' of ideas (for practice) that seeks to fundamentally change traditional approaches to discipline and service-orientated professional health care. When I write about EBP, I am following the definitions outlined for us by nurse scholars who consider evidence for nursing practice in its broadest definition (Pearson *et al.* 2005, Pearson 2013). Although stemming from different problems or challenges, both evidence-based and interprofessional healthcare practices and activities can be understood in the way that they occupy and translate into social and professional space. They challenge the implementation of traditional ideas about the way that nurses should learn and approach their practice to make a difference to healthcare outcomes and the patient's experience of care.

This essay links together EBP (the formal knowledge that informs practice) and interprofessional practice (the interprofessional and multi-dimensional forms of care delivery). It argues that, from a critical sociological point of view, these are interrelated concepts, shaped by both individuals and institutions, through social processes and actions. Effective practice is dependent on the application of more than research evidence in a traditional or western sense, for this tends to disconnect practice from the experience of health and health care. For nurses who wish to work in a way that responds to people as individuals and upholds ethical approaches to nursing, we need to give the broadest possible considerations to the conditions under which we deliver care and the way that our patients experience it.

Both evidence-based and interprofessional practice can be understood as ideas (a way of seeing the world of practice) and as practice (a way of behaving or acting) in themselves. Interprofessional approaches are expected but are not always understood or governed by the idea of an evidence-based approach to interprofessional care. Healthcare practice (interprofessional or otherwise) is difficult to evaluate systematically but there are a number of exceptions, where the body of evidence explains or directs us towards a particular model of care, that enable or encourage delivery models to change, adapt or evolve.

The approach to understanding the relationship between these two distinct and yet interrelated movements, in this discussion at least, is one that is reflective, by which I mean standing in one place and looking back and thinking critically about what and why something happens and what this means. It is a real and common-sense approach. It is one that situates these considerations within a critical sociological context. Dorothy E. Smith's (2005, 2006) work on institutional ethnography and, earlier, Pierre Bourdieu's (1977, 1989, 2001) sociology offer ideas that have been taken up in healthcare research and therefore allow others to critically consider; to ask probing questions, about the place of evidence-based and interprofessional practice in nursing and, in particular, why and how they flourish or flounder?

Critical sociological perspectives: text, talk and experience

I have said that evidence-based and interprofessional practice represents a movement (a journey from one way of doing things to another). From an institutional ethnographic perspective, we are considering text (what is written down) and talk (what is spoken) that relates to the care of individuals with a range of health and social care needs. The advice we have on EBP directs us towards a hierarchy of evidence but we know that, for some areas and dimensions of practice, we need to think beyond traditional or conventional sources to inform us of how we should be thinking and acting. When I think about EBP and interprofessional practice in health care, I am thinking in essence about the sociological processes, the rules, practices and actions that initiate and govern our actions. I am thinking about the institutional structures and the agency of individuals that create the social space where groups of people and individuals take part in these processes. Institutional ethnography asks questions about how the social relations (or regulations) of organisations or institutions develop, evolve and operate. In the case of inter-professional, multidisciplinary or interagency practices that operate within health and social care, these are represented by three dimensions, namely knowledge that is conveyed through text, talk and (I suggest) experience.

Through the texts and the talk of EBP (let us call this knowledge) and in the texts and talk of interprofessional practice (let us call this knowledge plus the work), we have the experience of patients and professionals (so let us call this knowledge plus experience). But do all texts (authoritative sources of knowledge or otherwise) that support the expectations for evidence-based and interprofessional practice get written into policy and guidance? How do other sources, including tacit knowledge (experiential or local wisdom) become translated into or begin to count in practice? Smith (2005, 2006) argues that these processes do not happen in objective isolation, but are dependent upon (and are subject to) the sociological features of a field, in this case of health and social care practice. The nurse's engagement in and impact upon healthcare experience, through the acquisition of an evidence base for their practice and the subsequent translation of this into effective articulated expression of interprofessional care should therefore be a self-conscious act of deliberate agency. Likewise Bourdieu's (1986) ideas of a field of practice, the acquisition of economic, cultural capital, understanding the rules of the game, as well as possessing the habits of practice all describe the factors that enable or disable the best intentions of practitioners to use their knowledge of all kinds to best effect.

HIV/AIDS: a case example of evidence based interprofessional practice

At the time of writing this chapter, Melbourne has just hosted the World AIDS Conference (AIDS 2014). This conference brings together research scientists and professionals from all over the world. It is in itself as good an illustration of an interprofessional, evidence-based developing practice as it is possible to find. Melbourne 2014 is more than just a conference; it is an 'event'. Participants include both established and novice, research scientists, health and social care professionals but also activists, campaigners, service users and carers; politicians and even celebrities attend. AIDS 2014 gained high-profile coverage locally and around the world and emphasised what an impact this interdisciplinary, multi-agency and global approach has had on this most devastating global pandemic.

It was widely reported in Australia and across the world, particularly because of the attendance of some high-profile people who came to urge and encourage the researchers and professionals to continue to work together. Following the coverage on television and through social media, I was struck by the way that the understanding, the care and experience of patients with HIV/AIDS had been transformed in a thirty-year period as a result of interprofessional and evidence-based approaches to the challenge of this personal and public health crisis by researchers, health and social care practitioners, humanitarian campaigners and volunteers and, of course, by those who live with the illness each day. It made me recall this past event.

In 1985, I was employed as a nurse in a London intensive therapy unit. I was working the late shift and was given the care of a young man who had been admitted as an emergency in severe respiratory distress. He had a severe pneumonia that was clearly not responding to any of the treatments he had received so far. The 'handover' I received was unremarkable; the patient required invasive mechanical ventilation, was sedated and had a high fever, although his illness was suspected to be viral in origin. I was not especially curious about the unknown illness but set about the routine of caring and planning all the therapeutic interventions scheduled for him that day. During the course of the afternoon his mother visited, she was tense and confused, she had been advised that he had not responded to the treatment that been tried so far; she sat by his bed and asked if she could hold his hand.

As the shift progressed, a series of curious events occurred. A number of medical staff visited and stood studying 'the charts' and assessed his condition. At one stage, the sister in charge brought me a full gown, mask and a box of gloves. Her words were, 'we are not sure what it is so we need to take precautions'. Without any curiosity or concern, I gowned and gloved myself and continued with my duties. I did ask what the view was about his condition; the doctor said she had not encountered the illness before but that it bore similarities to a number of cases recently seen in the United States of America.

An hour or so later, goggles and a 'larger' box full of gloves and surgical masks were brought. I noticed that I was getting fewer interruptions, the patient's mother had left the ward and it was just me and him, with just the sound of the ventilator breathing in and out for him and the sound of my breath inside my mask.

When the shift came to its end, we moved the patient to a single room, I gave my handover to the night staff and went home. The next day I heard that he had died. He was the first patient I had met with HIV/AIDS and he had died so suddenly that the professionals had very little evidence or experience to draw upon and, except for his mother and what little I contributed, there had been no help for him.

From the earliest stages, this illness was more than a medical phenomenon but, as my reflection reminds me, it came later to be viewed as a social, psychological and, of course, a deeply political one. What I recall most from this event is the lack of discussion or dialogue that occurred between myself and the other practitioners involved in his care. I was operating in a total knowledge vacuum beyond responding to the immediate practical, clinical care needs that were presented. I had no knowledge (tacit or otherwise) with which to process or analyse the events. There was very little conversation between me and his mother; I had no insights to offer except for what was obvious within the moment. For me, this illustrates the way that effective interprofessional practice is dependent on knowledge, text, talk and experience – ideally, all three, but even one of these three dimensions would have been a start. Over the next few years, we learned so much more about this condition and its relative risks to people and healthcare professionals (Searle 2007). We cared for more patients and heard about more around London. The year after, having seen several of his friends fall ill, my own brother had a blood test and found that he too was HIV positive. Both he (and we) thought he would die soon; he was ill with a series of serious episodes of illness but he always recovered. He spoke of his isolation and loneliness and economic hardship; this was an illness which set people apart. He was and felt stigmatised by it. He first was diagnosed aged twenty-five, was very sick for five years, but then lived until he was forty-three. In that short time, new therapies and under-standings of the illness emerged from a whole new area of medical research and from all parts of the world. On reflection, the development of a new language and a way to explain its impact, new discourses and narratives of illness emerged around this condition and new health and social care practices.

My own brother was fortunate to have been cared for by a team who accessed the best evidence and enabled him to cope and recover from episodes of illness and reach a degree of stability and wellness. The specialist nurse who was part of the team that cared for him was considerably better educated than I had been. His quality of life was dependent not just upon the improving application of newly emerging treatments but also on the evidenced-based and compassionate response of a range of collaborating agencies in health, housing and social care. These, and eventually the hospice where he died, deployed a model of interprofessional holistic practice that dignified his and our experience at the most difficult of times. Fast forward again to today and the link between interprofessional health and social care practice and the evidence base for the interventions and advances in treatment remain inseparable. The current work of Unicef illustrated this for me through the voice of a young teenager in Malawi, explaining the impact on her life, her education, her future. The intergenerational impact of this illness requires prevention and treatment in countries where there is little or no infrastructure for health and where the head of the household has died or is very ill. Making a difference in this one area of healthcare practice has required interprofessional and inter-agency collaboration through research, education, treatment and care on a local and a global scale.

The institutional ethnography of evidence-based and interprofessional practice

Understanding any practice requires some analysis of the intellectual and practi-cal space that it occupies and the relationships that exist with other such practice-related concepts. Both are principally intellectual ideas that are derived from western traditions of thought. They make demands of professionals (in this case, health and social care practitioners) and the institutions (that employ and manage) responsible for care organisation and delivery. The relationship between practices for evidence-based and interprofessional care should be reciprocal and mutual. Meaning that all care should be based upon the best available evidence and, in turn, EBP activities in terms of research questions, studies and dissemina-tion should respond to the complex challenges and problems of the people who depend upon interprofessional efforts to meet their health care needs.

If we are thinking ethnographically, we are paying particular attention to the cultures to which we belong and with which we interact. People who have grown up in one culture may not see anything around them as extraordinary at all. This chapter is written by someone who is seeing this issue through the eyes of someone recently arrived in a new place. For me, the things that are ordinary and everyday for everyone around me tend to look extraordinary, and things that are familiar to me (my behaviours, language, style of dress and other preoccupations, for example) look pretty strange to others (Hammersley and Atkinson 1995).

The history, institutional structures and cultures, within which academics and practitioners work, are pretty important for both evidence-based and interprofessional practice. If we start with the person in need of health and social care, we have the prospect that a number of individuals or agencies may be involved. The more complex the person's healthcare needs, the more likely that numerous professionals representing a particular speciality or subspecialty will be represented in their care experience. The individual practitioner will work sometimes within one organisation but often across many. These services, in turn, will have a number of possible funding, charging or commissioning arrangements, with different routes for access and eligibility criteria. Equally, the more people involved in a person's care, the more fragmented it is likely to be. These arrangements are not of the individual's making and probably not of the professional's either but, rather, they stem from a set of policy and procedural arrangements instigated by healthcare organisations to manage demand and delivery. They tend to evolve and to be implemented according to a set of (politically driven) principles or imperatives set down in text and actioned, for better or worse, through the process of professional talk.

An exploration of progress of the EBP movement cannot take place without due acknowledgement and recognition of the challenges and opportunities that face each unique country and its particular cultures, languages, political outlook and healthcare economy. The education and careers of health professionals, moreover, play an essential part in the way that institutions operate. Rather than making spontaneous progression and improvement, institutional cultures tend to reproduce themselves through the behaviour and language of individuals (Bourdieu 1989, 1993, Bourdieu and Passeron 1990). French sociologist Pierre Bourdieu (1930–2002) writes that individuals behave and act according to individual dispositions that he terms the 'habitus'. They tend to follow rules according to their individual dispositions and to make use of the capital (that is, economic, cultural and social, for example) they have at their disposal. This has the potential to undermine the aspirations of organisations to change practice through policy that is only text based. In order to adopt an evidence-based approach to practice and to be a successful contributor to interprofessional practice, the practitioner needs to be able to recognise, desire and act on this capital. Bourdieu's ideas also suggest that individuals will only make a change to their practices when crises arise. This suggests that, for improvements in healthcare practices to become accessible and properly translated for all who might benefit, it is necessary to think about the way that new evidence (the models and rules for the way that care should be provided) is translated for and by practitioners within a particular field. This is more than just an act of dissemination but needs to include a close examination of what existing rules, understandings and habits of nursing practices must be first 'unpicked' for this new rule to become established or translated to a new practice (Carter 2014).

An example of this can be seen in the development of the Australian nursing service. In the nineteenth and twentieth centuries, the health and welfare of aboriginal people was catastrophically damaged by the effects of colonisation and settlement. The response to this at the time was simply to superimpose a Eurocentric model of health care and nursing that completely failed to recognise either the causes of poor health in aboriginal people or to provide an appropriate (culturally safe) and effective response (Best and Fredericks 2014). This text highlights the interest of Florence Nightingale in indigenous health. Best and Fredericks describe the way that Nightingale published results of a 'survey' in 1865. The survey identified that some of the health problems that indigenous people were experiencing were due to attempts by incomers to 'civilise' them. Nightingale's nineteenth-century model of nursing, based upon a western perspective about what nursing was (and was not), failed to take into account what was really at stake for indigenous people and what would really help to reverse or slow what was happening. It has taken another 150 years for nursing in Australia to begin to respond appropriately, for example, through a change in the Australian Registered Nurse Accreditation Standards in 2012 (Australian Nursing and Midwifery Accreditation Council 2012).

When I consider my local field of practice, I would conclude that a twenty-first-century western-style healthcare system has developed and dominates. It takes effort to visualise Indigenous Australia and to see where its healthcare traditions and practices are celebrated and valued (Best and Fredericks 2014). Australia's health and social care systems and approach cannot be explained without acknowledgement of the continuing struggle towards reconciliation and inclusion of a range of peoples, cultures, traditions, belief systems, languages and towards an equitable provision of service to meet healthcare needs. The inequities in health are well documented and evaluated (Thompson 2003) and for the Aboriginal and Torres Strait Islander population, healthcare outcomes are said to be enduringly poor (Rosenstock *et al.* 2013). This is reflected both in the epidemiological healthcare data and in the experience of those who work in the healthcare services that support these communities (Australian Indigenous HealthInfoNet 2014, Australian Institute of Health and Welfare 2014).

Because of the need to move ideas from text into talk, the struggle for dominance in healthcare ideas (including evidence-based and interprofessional practice) cannot be separated from the struggle for sociopolitical or economic ideas. This is true on the macro (public health) level and on the micro (personal) level. In a country that is both very old in one way and very young in others, this makes for a unique set of challenges, including the work towards reconciliation (of indigenous peoples, European settlers and contemporary migrants from all over the globe). For nurses and for those they work alongside, this must inevitably mean the inclusion or recognition of the ideas (or rules that govern thinking) of a range of peoples, cultures, traditions and belief systems. The argument therefore is that EBP should stem from a broad definition of what constitutes evidence and this necessarily includes patient's experiences and preferences.

The way in which the rule of an evidence-based approach to nursing practice is moving across the profession is global. Australia's media and political class is also very much exercised about its changing relationship with the region and within its own borders and the relationships between different cultural and national groups are subject to a lively and critical discourse in the media and in the everyday concerns of its public institutions, including nursing. However, the extent to which this will be taken up in all areas of healthcare practice is not dependent on whether it is just a 'good' or 'right' thing but will be determined by the relationships that institutions have/create with the knowledge that is available and how it is translated and shared.

EBP is both, in the first place and in itself, an idea circulated within institutions in text. This does not in itself make it a practice; for this to happen, text must become knowledge and then it must translate into talk and then into practice. Similarly, the idea of interprofessional practice in health care is an idea that is only widely available as text. Translation into practice is far from universal and it is adopted in a way that obeys local rules and aspirations and these are subject as much to personal and cultural conditions as they are to professional and political ones.

Reflexive considerations

If we are going to get further into this topic we need to ask what interprofessional or evidence-based practice means to me and to you. What experiences have you had; what comes to mind? Shortly after I arrived as a newcomer to an Australian university, I attended a seminar where some excellent 'work in progress' was presented to those with an interest in Indigenous health. As a guest and a newcomer, I absorbed it all, paying great attention to the questions being asked, the different methods of research and the fascinating findings. The topics included infant and maternal health, epidemiological studies and community health studies. It was all following a conventional format and we had reached the plenary; the researchers were responding to questions. A member of the audience asked a question; 'What is your epistemology?' He was a senior academic who identified himself as Indigenous. He was asking a 'Who do you think you are?' or 'Where are you coming from?' question. He said (I paraphrase) 'that Aboriginal people get sick and tired of non-Indigenous researchers coming out to their place to look at their (wrist) watch to tell them what time it is'. This was an important lesson for me, the outsider. Those in the room who did not declare what their interest was in what they were doing had risked giving the appearance of taking an uncritical approach to their activities and thus compounding the inequalities that Indigenous people experience. The question was apposite and one that could be asked of all researchers, especially those working with groups who are under-represented in institutions or the establishment. The commentator was making a point about the nature of this field of research but, in fact, it applies to all fields of research with human subjects and those who wish to take an evidence base approach to their practice; we should all be asking ourselves: 'Who am I and why am I doing this?'.

Research practice should be reflexive and undertaken in a partnerships, beyond interprofessional partnerships, to one which includes the perspective and experience of its vulnerable subject, which takes us all a bit beyond the general expectations of obtaining informed consent as understood in most fields of medical research. Even valid and reliable research will often not be translated or applied; it will sit there and make little impact to changing practice. It may be read by others with an interest (it will have some impact) but it will not make people's health better or change the ways in which we work. These thoughts started with my drifting into a setting because I was 'curious' and ended up with me rethinking all my understandings of the role that epistemology and power play in research and evidence based interprofessional practice.

Person centeredness and interprofessional practices

I have described the way that I see interprofessional and evidence-based practice as stemming from different sources but they have not necessarily been explored as interrelated concepts governed by similar social and institutional rules and practices. However, I offer a further example here to illustrate this point. We have already looked at an interprofessional response to a public health phenomenon (HIV/AIDS). The second example offered is one where the approach is generally focused on individual experiences of care when old.

The development and approach to interprofessional practice appears to depend on many factors, including the personal and professional culture, the local population's health needs, the kind of evidence available and the organisational features of healthcare institutions and services. In the context of the first example, I made the individual the starting point and, in the second, I am approaching the issue the other way around; that is, thinking about the way that the institution, service or professional approaches or organises care for some of its most vulnerable people and how this in turn impacts on individual experience. Whether we are thinking of a newly emerging complex healthcare condition for young people or the well-known predicament of growing old, successful care depends on the way that professionals respond to human need, down to the point of what they think a human being is and how the experience of illness (in all its variations) should be understood and responded to.

In my second case example, I want to consider the relationship between the concept of person-centred care (Parse 2004, McCormack and McCance 2006, Slater 2006) and interprofessional practice or multidisciplinary or inter-agency care. I want to begin by asking why do people with health and social care needs have to depend on a set of practices and processes that involve so many participants? Why does it have to be so complicated? This change to the experience of care is an institutionally driven one and increasingly dehumanises the experience of care. Increasingly, these changes are seen to relate to political imperatives to increase efficiency and cost containment. This can be observed as pattern of successive health and social care reforms across the UK the United States and Australia (Arbuckle 2013). It has been observed that, where the knowledge about and the motive for providing care becomes separated from the governance of institutions and their reforms becomes detached, the patient and the staff experience will deteriorate.

There are real concerns for professionals to consider in this, too. As we specialise, we seem to separate but, if my needs are complex or extend beyond the scope of one professional role, that separation can compromise my care. So, having specialised ourselves apart, crucial partnerships need to be rebuilt around specific practices. For example, physician and pharmacist, nurse and physician, anaesthetist and surgeon, social worker and psychiatrist, general practitioner and community nurse. These partnerships are mutually beneficial and, where they operate within the same model of care and the same institutional setting and are not in competition for any capital goods, they can work to my good. However, where structural or institutional divides exist and where a different model (including the source and degree of EBP) underpins the approach to care, the partnerships are less obvious and, as a patient, I will feel the gaps opening around me and obstacles to what I think I need rising up before me.

Where the agreements and understanding about the ways of working (social actions and processes) are not clear to professionals and patients, my care will fragment. By which I mean it will become an issue for dispute, rationing, decisions, unmet needs and confusion. Some of these separations are resolved by re-consolidation through commissioning specialised services to work together: stroke care services, palliative care and the hospice movement and children's services are obvious examples in some contexts, but what if I am a person whose situation does not specifically align to one specialty or area of interest?

The care and discharge from hospital of frail, older adults is a topic that gets to the heart of what hospital care is for and is the ultimate test (in my view) of where the practice of person-centred care gets properly put to the test across health systems (Bauer *et al.* 2009, Carter 2010, Dilworth *et al.* 2012, Parliamentary Health Service Ombudsman 2011). One of the most interesting dynamics here arises from the institutional and organisational operations that centre on the use and control of inpatient beds. Worth a closer look is the way that organisations seek to govern and direct this and the way that such texts (this can include state legislation, policies, guidelines, charters and operating rules) become translated into practice, through staff talk, interactions and patient and carer experiences. The clinical, commercial and political imperatives of organisations and institutions providing emergency and elective care often fail to protect the interests of those who recover slowly, whose future is uncertain and whose care needs are complex and need many different interventions, across a range of institutional boundaries and services to meet them. A nurse working in a field of practice where the pathway for patients is uncertain or subject to collaboration with external agencies will inevitably find themselves at a point of tension between the organisational imperatives of the employer and the person at the centre of care. Where there is disconnect between that organisational expectation and the central needs of the person at that juncture, there is a risk to the dignity and continued wellbeing of the person and sometimes the wellbeing of staff. This was starkly highlighted in the UK and elsewhere in the published investigations of a number of infamous healthcare failures over the years (Garling 2008, Flynn 2012, Mid-Staffordshire NHS Foundation Trust Inquiry 2013, Arbuckle 2013).

As nurses, we are encouraged to think of care in terms of a process or processes rather than as a series of isolated tasks. Interprofessional practices can be considered at each stage in the same way as assessment (diagnosis), planning, implementation and evaluation. There are different levels and sources of evidence to support each stage of a process for a patient's care and, under most regulatory standards, an expectation that nurses will seek out and evaluate knowledge and apply the best available evidence to all aspects of their practice.

Australia: nexus of past and present

In understanding the development of evidence-based and interprofessional practice in Australia, it is important to consider the history of ideas about science, scientific tradition and models of health care from a wider or global perspective. The EBP tradition in the UK (particularly in nursing) increasingly makes a strong case for a broader evidence base for practice. Australia (if not as 'country' but as an institution) is fairly young. Until fairly recently, its public, political and philosophical face has been orientated towards Europe, the UK, the United States and now towards China. However, there is 'another country'. Australian Indigenous population has a culture that is more than 60,000 years old and contains numerous cultures and subcultures that co-exist, including a health practice tradition that stretches back, beyond living memory (Best and Fredericks 2013). In a world of competing ideas, values and traditions, we need to consider these perspectives as we make sense of how knowledge in text and in talk is used and applied in practice.

So how could we theorise about this? We have political, ethnographic (cultural) sociological, anthropological and multiple health dimensions, just for starters. My argument draws upon Smith's (2005) ideas about institutional ethnography as a way of conceptualising the interface between the complex notions of improving nursing care through an evidence-based approach to nursing in an interprofessional context. We are not all clear about the direction or barriers to improving health care of complex populations and diverse peoples. However, if we understand the way that policy shapes practice, we can at least begin to move beyond reading and hearing about barriers that exist and begin to think about how we are part of the institution that needs to make a difference.

Practices adopted by the institutions that are inhabited and dependent upon historically tried and tested practices will tend to lean towards the 'unidisciplinary' rather than the 'interprofessional', because this is where medical and allied healthcare 'specialisms' and professional ambition will lead it. Both evidence-based and interprofessional practices are social practices and ideologies that will to a greater or lesser extent govern the practice habits of its players. The success of the operation of both evidence-based and interprofessional practice is dependent upon the individual habitus of its players and upon the particular features and dynamics of that field of practice. These practice habits are subject to individual operations, which may or may not recognise the mission of others in the field to move toward or by an interprofessional and/or evidence-based approach to practice. They might operate and organise themselves quite separately and even to be resistant to that hegemonic top-down directive, bottom up entreaty or sideways obligation, that says to approach our work in this way is a 'good thing'.

Conclusion

In so many areas of practice, aspirations to work for the good of patients and to improve patient care get thwarted. Understanding the way that the knowledge which informs the decisions we make and the actions we take arises from text, talk and experience is one way of making sense of our practice, both in relation to the patients we meet and in our relationships with health and social care colleagues.

The importance of reflexivity cannot be underplayed in understanding my argument about what it is to nurse effectively and with kindness. Reflecting on practice is important but we need to go beyond this to ask ourselves the 'Who am I?', 'What am I doing here?' and the 'What don't I know?' questions. Evidence for practice is not a simple given but relies on our active curiosity, reflexive interactions and receptiveness to listen and to process the range of information available to us.

Effective care is said to be largely dependent on effective decision making. The reliability and validity of our decision making will be hugely dependent not only on the quality of the evidence available but how much of this is part of the nurse's working knowledge and how good are we at sharing it. Even finely honed clinical skills cannot compensate for an absence of appropriate knowledge with which to work.

In interprofessional practice, all participants in care must work together in decision-making activities; they coordinate care and are expected to work towards a set of shared goals and milestones, but the ways that they share their knowledge and understanding through talk and text is a key critical concern. If they do not do this, care will be incoherent, confused and even dangerous.

Regardless of where in the world we are, the nurse who thinks about what they have learned from text, from talk and from their own study of the evidence for practice and the experiences of others, has the potential to be an effective practitioner. Therefore, it is more than just what we think, believe or learn about our own individual behaviours and practices. It is also about what we understand and take from the experience of peers and from the people we care for, as illustrated by the context of culturally safe practices in Australia and elsewhere. Effective interprofessional practice needs an evidence base that moves from the page and from talk into the practice of the nurse and the organisational process that frame their activities. Moreover, if the organisations and professional and economic structures (local and national) support an interdisciplinary multi-agency approach then interprofessional practice will flourish. That is not to say that individual champions are not important but little is achieved without the context and the culture being right. The interplay between the institutional and the individual actions is of critical concern and needs to be scrutinised and reflected upon.

Nurses are often at the centre of those healthcare processes and practices where dignity is compromised or threatened. These concepts and experiences are at the centre of patient wellbeing and these are small examples of where structures, organisational cultures, groups and individual practice need to respond to the widest range of evidence and its application. As nurses, we live in the centre of the social world of practice. We do not stand outside of this world; therefore, we need to own and share all kinds of evidence for practice and the relational, inter-professional practices that spring from it.

Acknowledgements

As I write and share these ideas, I would like to acknowledge the traditional owners of this land; the Wurundjeri people, and to pay my respects to elders past and present. You can read more about their history online (Yarra City Council 2013) and I recommend Best and Frederick (2014) too.

I would also like to acknowledge the advice of my colleague Dr Louise Ward, Senior Lecturer Mental Health Nursing, School of Nursing and Midwifery at La Trobe University, in the preparation of this chapter.

BBC News (2014) reported that, on 17 July 2014, the Malaysian Airlines flight MH17 crashed in Eastern Ukraine killing all passengers and crew on board. A number of the passengers were travelling from Northern Europe to contribute to the AIDS 2014 conference in Melbourne, Australia. In writing this, I am offering a personal acknowledgement of the consequences of this act. I acknowledge its impact on all people affected by this event and to pay my personal respects to those conference delegates and to all the others who died.

Finally, I pay my respects to my brother Michael (1962–2007) and to those who cared for him. I hope my retelling of part of his story is helpful; the experiences of others always teach us something.

References

AIDS (2014) AIDS 2014: 20th International AIDS Conference, Melbourne, Australia, July 20–25. See http://aids2014.org/Default.aspx?pageId=689 (accessed 10 March 2015).

Arbuckle, G. A. (2013) *Humanising Health Care Reforms*. London: Jessica Kingsley.

Australian Indigenous HealthInfoNet (2014) Overview of Australian Indigenous health status 2013. Edith Cowan University. Available online at www.healthinfonet.ecu.edu.au/health-facts/overviews (accessed 10 March 2015).

Australian Institute of Health and Welfare (2014) Australia's Health 2014. Available online at http://aihw.gov.au/australias-health/2014/how-healthy (accessed 10 March 2015).

Australian Nursing and Midwifery Accreditation Council (2012) *Registered Nurse Accreditation Standards*. Canberra: ANMAC.

BBC News (2014) MH17 Crash Dutch Investigator's first findings available. *BBC News Europe*, 9 September. Available online at www.bbc.co.uk/news/world-europe-29122816 (accessed 10 March 2015).

Best, O. and Fredericks, B. (2014) *Yatdjuligin: Aboriginal and Torres Strait Islander Nursing and Midwifery Care*. Melbourne: Cambridge University Press.

Bauer, M., Fitzgerald, L., Haesler, E. and Manforn, M. (2009) Hospital discharge planning for frail older people and their family, are we delivering best practice? A review of the evidence. *Journal of Clinical Nursing* 18(18), 2539–46.

Bourdieu, P. (1977) *Outline of a Theory of Practice*. Cambridge: Cambridge University Press.

Bourdieu, P. (1986) *Distinction: A Social Critique of the Judgment of Taste*, trans. Richard Nice. London: Routledge.

Bourdieu, P. (1989) Symbolic space and symbolic power. *Sociological Theory* 7(1), 14–25.

Bourdieu, P. (2001) *Practical Reason: On the Theory of Practice*. Cambridge: Polity.

Bourdieu, P. and Passeron, J. C. (1970) *Reproduction in Education, Society and Culture*. London: Sage.

Carter, M. (2010) Telling tales: 'atrocity' stories and the patient experience. *Nursing Management* 16(9), 28–31.

Carter, M. (2014) Vocation and altruism in nursing: the habits of practice. *Nursing Ethics* 21(6), 695–706.

Dilworth, S., Higgins, I. and Parker, V. (2012) Feeling let down: an exploratory study of the experience of older people who were readmitted to hospital following a recent discharge. *Contemporary Nurse* 42(2), 280–8.

Garling, P. (2008) *Final Report of the Special Commission Inquiry: Acute Care Services in NSW Public Hospitals: Overview*. Sydney, NSW: NSW Department of Premier and Cabinet.

Flynn, M. (2012) *Winterbourne View Hospital: A Serious Case Review*. Bristol: south Gloucestershire Council for South Gloucestershire Safeguarding Adults Board.

Hammersley, M. and Atkinson, P. (1995) *Ethnography: Principles in Practice*, 3rd edn. London: Routledge.

McCormack, B. and McCance, Tanya V. (2006) Development of a framework for person-centred nursing. *Journal of Advanced Nursing* 56(5), 472–9.

Meads, G. and Ashcroft, J. (2005) *The Case for Interprofessional Collaboration in Health and Social Care*. Oxford: Wiley-Blackwell.

Mid Staffordshire NHS Foundation Trust Inquiry (2013) *Report of the Mid Staffordshire NHS Foundation Trust Public Inquiry*, Chaired by Sir Robert Francis QC. Presented to Parliament pursuant to Section 26 of the Inquiries Act 2005. HC947. 3 vols. London: TSO.

Miers, M. E., Rickaby, C. E. and Clarke, B. A. (2009) Learning to work together: health and social care students' learning from interprofessional modules. *Assessment and Evaluation in Higher Education* 34(6), 673–91.

Quinlan, E. (2009) The 'actualities' of knowledge work: an institutional ethnography of multi-disciplinary primary health care teams. *Sociology of Health and Illness*. 31(5), 625–41.

Parliamentary Health Services Ombudsman (2011) Care and Compassion? Report of the Health Service Ombudsman on ten investigations in NHS care of older people. Available online at www.ombudsman.org.uk/reports-and-consultations/reports/health/home (accessed 25 March 2015).

Parse, R. R. (2004) Person-centred care. *Nursing Science Quarterly* 17(3), 193.

Pearson, A. (2013) Translation science: transforming everything changing nothing? *International Journal of Evidence-Based Healthcare* 11(3), 147. doi: 10.1111/1744-1609.12036.

Pearson, A., Wiechula, R., Court, A. and Lockwood, C. (2005) The JBI model of evidence-based healthcare. *International Journal of Evidenced Based Healthcare* 3(8), 207–15.

Pollard, K. (2009) Student engagement in interprofessional working in practice placement settings. *Journal of Clinical Nursing* 18, 2846–56.

Pollard, K. C., Miers, M. E., Gilchrist, M. and Sayers, A. (2006) Comparison of interprofessional perceptions and working relationships among health and social care students: the results of a 3-year intervention. *Health and Social Care in the Community* 14(6), 541–52.

Rosenstock, A., Mukandi, B., Zwi, A. B. and Hill, P. S. (2013) Closing the gaps: competing estimates of Indigenous Australian life expectancy in the scientific literature. *Australian and New Zealand Journal of Public Health* 37(4), 356–64.

Thompson, N. (2003) *The Health of Indigenous Australians.* Oxford: Oxford University Press.

Townsend, E., Langille, L. and Ripley, D. (2003) Professional tensions in client-centered practice: using institutional ethnography to generate understanding and transformation. *American Journal of Occupational Therapy* 57(1), 17–28.

Searle, S. E. (1987) Knowledge, attitudes and behaviour of health professionals in relation to AIDS. *Lancet*, 329(8523), 26–8.

Slater, L. (2006) Person-centeredness: a concept analysis. *Contemporary Nurse* 23, 135–44.

Smith, D. E. (2005) *Institutional Ethnography: A Sociology for People.* Oxford: Rowman and Littlefield.

Smith, D. E. (2006) *Institutional Ethnography as Practice.* Oxford: Rowman and Littlefield.

Yarra City Council (2013) The Aboriginal History of Yarra. Available online at http://aboriginalhistoryofyarra.com.au (accessed 10 March 2015).

6   Evidence and practical knowledge

Mark Risjord

The puzzle of evidence-based practice

The phrase "evidence-based practice" is something of an oxymoron. Evidence provides justification, yet practical activity is not the sort of thing that calls for justification. Clinical practice requires a suite of abilities, instruments, tools, and materials, not to mention patients. People, objects, and activities are simply not the sort of thing that can be justified by evidence. Justification is appropriate for what philosophers call "propositional knowledge" or "knowledge-that." In these cases, the knowledge can be expressed in a sentence (hence, *propositional* knowledge). Something is evidence only insofar as it gives us confidence that a proposition (expressed as a sentence, judgment, or belief) is true. To have practical knowledge, by contrast, is to have knowledge-how: it is the ability to do something. Questions of justification cannot arise for know-how. Strictly speaking, then, "evidence-based practice" is a logical impossibility.

The ambivalence about names – are we talking about evidence based "medicine", "nursing," "policy", "guidelines", "practice" or what? – is a symptom of the tensions within the project. Evidence-based medicine originally focused on *clinical judgment*; that is, decisions about patient care. Much of the literature on evidence-based practice continues to concern evidence for clinical judgments. Clinical judgment does not generate the puzzle just described because it is propositional: the current best evidence and patient preferences justify propositions about patient care. Not all of nursing practice, however, involves clinical judgment in this sense. The *activities* of clinical practice should be evidence based too. Nurse leaders have rightly thought that practices should not be reproduced simply because "we have always done it that way." Insofar as nursing activities can be expressed in clinical guidelines or standards of care, they can be subject to evaluation by evidence. The puzzle of evidence-based practice arises when we try to link guidelines to activities. How do guidelines or standards of care make a difference to what nurses do?

It might seem as if the answer is straightforward: guidelines and standards of care give nurses reasons to act. Such an answer must conceptualize nursing action as instrumental. In this view, when a person acts, they have some goal they wish to achieve. They perform the action because they believe it is the best available way to bring about their goal. Intentional action is thus instrumental in the sense that the action is a means to an end. Evidence-based guidelines give the nurse justified beliefs about the best ways to achieve their goals. For example, consider a nurse caring for a patient with a tracheostomy tube. One of the nurse's goals will be to keep the tube clear. To do so, the nurse will perform tracheal suctioning. As a trained professional, the nurse will know the guidelines regarding catheter selection, infection control, pressure, duration, and so on. These are the means by which the nurse tries to attain the goal of keeping the tube clear. Evidence-based practice is really just evidence-based policy put to use.

Justifying practice guidelines by research is plain common sense but it does not resolve our puzzle. Instrumental action is not know-how. Suppose I want to take a walk and believe that to do so I need footwear. So, I tie up my boots and go. Describing my action instrumentally obscures the crucial moment: I tie my bootlaces. Can this be understood as instrumental action as well? Tying bootlaces is a sequence of actions. When children are being taught to tie their shoes, the sequence must be broken down, and each action treated as a means to the next. But when I put on my hiking boots, I no longer recite "over, under, around, and through; meet Mr Bunny Rabbit, pull and through." I am able to do it without thinking about the steps. The point is familiar to readers of *From Novice to Expert* (Benner, 1984). Expert know-how cannot be understood as acting on the basis of explicit rules. The problem with treating evidence-based guidelines as justifying instrumental beliefs is that it turns expert nursing into novice rule following.

The puzzle of evidence-based practice, then, is how (expert) practice could be based on or informed by evidence. Our puzzle is a particular instance of a much broader question of how propositional knowledge and practical know-how are related. We should not be misled by the word "knowledge" here. As Gweneth Doane and Coleen Varcoe have argued, the theory–practice gap with which we are concerned is an ontological problem, not an epistemological one (Doane and Varcoe, 2008). Ultimately, the issue turns on how we understand ourselves as agents.

Know-how and instrumental action

What is wrong with understanding expert practice in terms of instrumental, rule-following actions? Two famous arguments from twentieth-century philosophy support a differentiation of instrumental action from practical abilities: the regress of rules argument and the embodiment argument. These arguments open the onto-logical gap between theory and practice. To understand whether the gap can be bridged, we must look at these arguments in detail.

The regress of rules argument is usually attributed to Ludwig Wittgenstein. Section 198 of the *Philosophical Investigations* is a well-known prompt:

> "But how can a rule show me what I have to do at this point? Whatever I do is, on some interpretation, in accord with the rule." – That is not what we ought to say, but rather: any interpretation still hangs in the air along with

what it interprets, and cannot give it any support. Interpretations by themselves do not determine meaning.

(Wittgenstein, 1953: 80)

As an example of the problem worrying Wittgenstein, consider a recent analysis
of published evidence recommending that nurses use "the lowest possible suction
pressure during endotracheal suctioning, usually 80–120 mmHg" (Pedersen *et al.*,
2009: 28). How does knowledge of this rule help the nurse to know what to do
with the patient? Suppose the nurse chooses 130 mmHg pressure; was this in
accord with the rule? It was, if the nurse interpreted "lowest possible" as requiring more pressure than the normal range permitted. The problem is that the same
kind of argument could be used to support any choice of pressure: "Whatever I
do is, on some interpretation, in accord with the rule."

One might respond that the problem lies in the vagueness of the rule. It relies
on words like "lowest possible" and "usually." Unfortunately, we cannot solve the
problem by eliminating such words. The rule needs to be applicable to a variety
of contexts and suction pressure depends on contextual factors like the thickness
of the secretions. We might try to solve the problem by adding these factors to the
rule, for example "and use higher pressure when the secretions are thicker."
Wittgenstein points out that the very same problem will occur all over again. How
thick is thick enough to justify an increase (and of how much)? The problem is
not vagueness but correctness. A rule must be correctly applied, and rules cannot
state their own conditions of correct application. Nothing in the rule itself can
determine whether it has been correctly applied. Invoking a second rule to determine whether the first has been correctly applied raises the problem all over
again, since we may ask whether the second rule been correctly applied. On pain
of regress, correct application of rules cannot be a matter of rules alone; "any
interpretation still hangs in the air along with what it interprets, and cannot give
it any support."

The regress of rules argument has been taken to show that following rules
requires practical ability in addition to the cognitive recognition of the rule. Rule
following depends on something like habits (Kripke, 1982), practical attitudes
(Brandom, 1994), or embodied coping (Dreyfus, 1972, 2007). Close scrutiny of
the embodied character of human action has led to further arguments that at least
some significant forms of human action cannot be understood as the deliberate
application of rules or other propositional knowledge. Martin Heidegger was,
perhaps, the first twentieth-century philosopher to appreciate this point
(Heidegger, 2010). Hubert Dreyfus has drawn from Heidegger's work a clear
version of the embodiment argument (Dreyfus, 1972, 2007) and it is this version
of the argument that underlies Benner's (1984) *From Novice to Expert*.

Dreyfus's presentation of the embodiment argument often begins from a
phenomenological description of fluidly performed action, like the actions of
expert nurses reported in *From Novice to Expert*. Benner's exemplars are all cases
where the nurse recognized salient elements of the situation – the patient's mood,
comportment or complexion – and responded appropriately. The nurses did not

report thinking about any guidelines. Dreyfus argues that this is because the salient elements of a situation cannot be represented in rules or procedures. Procedures must break a situation into discrete factors, like suction pressures or catheter diameters. But the total situation cannot be divided into independent elements. An aspect of the context becomes a factor only as it is relevant to the task at hand. Relevant aspects of the context are perceived as "affordances"; that is, in terms of the possibilities they present for action. The nurse experiences the viscosity of the patient's secretions and the reading on the manometer in the light of the need to safely clear the patient's airway. To experience mucus as *thick enough to warrant higher pressure* is to recognize an affordance.

Affordances are motivating. As nurses recognize, the affordances of a situation solicit action as an interrelated whole. The holistic character of affordances is well illustrated by Pedersen *et al.*'s discussion of suctioning guidelines:

> The negative pressure that is actually applied to the lungs during suctioning cannot be reliably assessed on the manometer dial of the suctioning equipment; it depends on the suction catheter–ET tube ratio, the duration of the procedure, and the volume and viscosity of the secretions.
>
> (Pedersen *et al.*, 2009: 24)

An expert nurse must be directly responsive to all of these features together as soliciting bodily responses. This is what Heidegger called a "world." Representation in guidelines abstracts away from precisely those aspects of the whole context that motivate action. They draw us away from a direct responsiveness to the world (being in the world) and toward a representation of it. Any representation must be reapplied, leaving us again with the problem of what to do. Clinical expertise and other forms of know-how, therefore, cannot be the application of procedures to a context. Such is the mode of instrumental action, and any instrumental application of rules already requires practical know-how. Clinical expertise is embodied engagement with a world of solicitations.

Expertise and evidence-based practice

If expert practice is embodied engagement with the world, then how can it be informed by evidence? A number of nursing scholars have recognized this problem and tried to address it. In *From Novice to Expert*, Benner (1984) used the Dreyfus and Dreyfus (1986) five-stage model of skill acquisition to show how nursing practice can be improved by evidence. The five stages –novice, advanced beginner, competent, proficient, and expert – describe a progression by which explicit rules and procedures are first learned as propositional knowledge, and then mastered as practical knowledge. At the early stages of learning, the nurse bases their action on checklists and guidelines. As the nurse gains experience recognizing situations and applying the rules, the rules are replaced by a direct responsiveness to the affordances of the situation. In this model, basing expert practice on evidence is a matter of basing nursing education on evidence.

Evidence-based guidelines determine novice actions and these gradually become embodied.

There are two problems with the Benner/Dreyfus model. First, according to the model, nurses begin by learning the rules and acting on them. They act only on the basis of the context-free elements of the situation described in the guideline (Benner, 1984: 21). They do not respond to the aspects of the world made relevant by the current activity. This means that, at the novice stage, the nurse is not engaged in embodied coping. The novice stage is instrumental action. We have already seen why there must be a difference between instrumental action and know-how. If the instrumental model generally fails to connect guidelines to practice, then it will fail to do so in the novice stage of skill acquisition.

To see the second difficulty with the five-stage model, consider a pair of studies by Tina Day and her colleagues on tracheal and endotracheal suctioning (Day *et al.*, 2001, 2002). These studies revealed a disjuncture between nurses' propositional knowledge and their practice. Both studies triangulated non-participant observation with questionnaires and semi-structured interviews. The 28 subjects of the tracheal suctioning study (Day *et al.*, 2002) were nurses in acute and high-dependency wards in an English teaching hospital. Subjects were observed twice during regular tracheal suctioning procedures on patients. Observers scored their performance against the guidelines. The nurses' knowledge of the guidelines was then measured by a questionnaire and a semi-structured interview. The difference between the nurses' knowledge of clinical guidelines and their implementation of these guidelines in practice was striking. For example, while ten subjects correctly reported that the correct suctioning pressure should be between 80 and 150 mmHg for tracheal suctioning, only two of the subjects were observed using suction pressure within this range. And while 18 were able to state the accurate catheter size, only nine were observed using it. Not all of the discrepancies were mistakes in practice: while almost all of the subjects (27) *incorrectly* reported that saline use was acceptable, none of the subjects was observed actually using it. In other words, the nurses followed the guideline in practice, but did not have explicit knowledge of it. The Day studies show that, in this context, nurses' propositional knowledge of guidelines does not line up with their practice.

The Day studies show that even if knowledge of the guidelines could inform novice action, propositional knowledge does not always influence expert action. In some cases – but not all – the nurses of Day's study represented the rule but it did not guide their actions. Why do some procedures become embedded in practice, while others do not? The five-stage model provides no account of how the propositional knowledge of early stages is converted into the expertise of the later stages. Hence, the model cannot explain why some expert practice follows the guidelines and some does not. It can provide no advice about how to bring practice into accord with the guidelines. This problem undermines our confidence that the five-stage model's "experts" are truly expert practitioners.

A different approach to making evidence relevant to practice calls for qualitative research (for example, Rycroft-Malone *et al.*, 2004; Porter, 2010). The argument begins with the idea that there is knowledge embedded in practice.

Existing practice might be improved, then, by eliciting the tacit knowledge of expert nurses and making it explicit. Once articulated, it can be evaluated and then disseminated. While there are important questions about how such knowledge should be evaluated, there is wide agreement that the elicitation of tacit knowledge will require qualitative research.

The question of whether qualitative research provides good evidence for nursing practice is an epistemological question. Again, our problem is ontological: how are propositional and practical knowledge related? Using qualitative research to make tacit knowledge explicit does not answer this question. Once tacit knowledge is made explicit, it becomes propositional knowledge. Tacit knowledge is embedded in the nurse's ability, for example, to provide care for patients with tracheotomies. A *description* of good care is propositional knowledge. Even if qualitative evidence made tacit knowledge explicit, we remain stuck with the problem of how to re-embed it into practice.

A third answer comes from Doane and Varcoe's article, "Knowledge Translation in Everyday Nursing" (2008). Explicitly adopting a Heideggerian stance on practical action, they reconceptualize the problem as primarily a question about what kind of nurse one wants to be, and only secondarily a question of knowledge. Their way of addressing the ontological gap between theory and practice, then, involves "inquiry-based nursing:"

> *Inquiry-based nursing involves a conscious tuning into this implicit, intricate* [embodied] *knowing process as a way-of-being in nursing situations.* Within inquiry-based practice, the first function of understanding is to orient within a possible situation. ... The epistemological ground – the ground of knowing – is each person's tacit experiential presence in the world in relation with everyone and everything in the world.
>
> (Doane and Varcoe, 2008: 291)

Doane and Varcoe are not recommending a new kind of research. They are recommending a kind of stance or practical attitude, a "way-of-being in nursing situations." It involves not just acting on auto-pilot but consciously "tuning into" one's practical interactions with the world. The goal is to "attend to the possibilities [of a situation] in the light of a particular theory" (Doane and Varcoe, 2008: 291).

While Doane and Varcoe have understood the puzzle of evidence-based practice more deeply than most other authors, their positive solution fares no better than the other attempts we have surveyed in this section. Their conception of inquiry-based nursing holds onto a language of self-conscious action and experience. Unfortunately, people are not reliable reporters on the characteristics of their own action. The Day studies illustrate this vividly; the practice of the subject nurses was (sometimes) the opposite of their representation of the rule. There is no reason to believe that a conscious tuning-into one's own action will yield a reliable representation. Moreover, the idea that subjects have a transparent or incorrigible understanding of their own action is in tension with the Heideggerian conception of action that underpins Doane and Varcoe's analysis of the problem (cf. Paley, 1998).

One might reply to the forgoing argument by reading Doane and Varcoe slightly differently. They are not presupposing that agents have a reliable understanding of their own action. A world is an interlocking system of affordances revealed by the agent's purposeful activity. In this sense, agents create their own worlds. Doane and Varcoe may be read as proposing that nurses become more self-conscious about those creations. Inquiry-based nursing should lead nurses to "purposefully attend to the interconnection of ontology ('who I want to be') and epistemology ('how/what knowledge might I enlist as a knower')" (Doane and Varcoe, 2008: 292). This reading fares no better than the first. It founders on Benner's insight that expert practice is direct engagement with the world. To re-inject self-conscious deliberation about how one wants to be would bump a nurse's engagement down the ladder of expertise.

In sum, while there have been several attempts to grapple with the ontological problem of evidence-based practice, none has been successful. All three views discussed in this section share a common fault. They hang onto two ideas that are inconsistent with the conception of practical know-how as embodied coping: that agents are self-conscious and that intentional action is deliberate. The two ideas are blended in a common picture of action. An intentional action is one done for reasons, and this requires an agent to have particular properties. To have reasons, an agent must be aware of his or her values, goals, or preferences. The agent also must be consciously aware of the environment, and this awareness is constituted by a system of representations or beliefs. An agent is a being who can choose a goal and be aware of the means toward that goal; these are the agent's reasons for action. Intentional action is thus deliberate, in the sense that the action results from a choice of end and deliberation about best means. The views discussed in this section accept the idea that practical know-how is distinct from the sort of instrumental action expressed in this picture. At the same time, they preserve the idea of self-consciousness and intentionality, simply augmenting the picture with the idea of embodied know-how. If we are to make progress on the ontological problems of evidence based practice, we will have to radically revise the whole image of action and agency.

The ecological conception of agency

The radical reorientation made necessary by the idea of embodied coping is nicely expressed by Dreyfus: "When we are at home in the world, the meaningful objects embedded in their context of references among which we live are not a model of the world stored in our mind or brain; *they are the world itself*" (Dreyfus, 1972: 177–8, italics in original).

This quotation contains two important ideas. First, the world of affordances is not consciously represented in the agent's mind. The connotations of experience and perception suggested by the word "phenomenology" are actually quite misleading. To say that an object presents an affordance of a lever is not to suppose that the agent has a picture, sentence, or anything similar consciously (or "unconsciously") in his or her mind. The anti-Cartesianism of Heidegger, Wittgenstein, and many other twentieth-century philosophers, rejects the conception of the mind as a repository of representations that mirror the world. An embodied mind is directly engaged with the world itself.

Of course, "the world itself" is a world of interrelated opportunities for action: "meaningful objects embedded in their context of references." Aspects of this world are meaningfully interrelated only in the light of the agent's purposes. Purposes cannot be mere representations in the mind either. The Cartesian view must be entirely rejected. At the same time, purposes are not simply "out there" among the tables and chairs. Purposes are relationships between an animal and its environment. This means that to be an agent is not to have a special property (like rationality, subjectivity or consciousness). To be an agent is to stand in relation to the world. This ecological conception of agency is the second central idea in the quotation above.

To be an agent is to be responsive to the environment in a particular way. I have suggested elsewhere that the responsiveness can be fruitfully analyzed into three capacities:[1] the capacity to be *attuned* to action-relevant aspects of the environment, the capacity for recognizing *affordances* of the environment, and a capacity for *meta-cognition* (Risjord, 2014). Where an affordance is the recognition of the possibilities for action present in the environment, an attunement is the capacity to keep track of particular features of the environment. For a driver, the on-ramp (slip road), the lines marking the lanes, and the turns in the road are recognized as presenting certain possibilities for action. At the same time, a driver must track specific aspects of the environment, such as the sound of the engine and tires. These latter do not (or do not necessarily) present possibilities for action but they must be perceived and tracked. In action-related perception, then, we both track specific features of the environment (attunement) and recognize the possibilities for action provided by the environment (affordances).

It should be emphasized that neither attunements nor affordances are *experiences*. We do not have direct access to the cognitive systems that permit us to track specific elements of the environment or to see what action opportunities are presented. When I tie my shoes, I do not know to what aspects of the laces my eyes and hands are attuned, nor am I aware that my fingers pinch the laces with a pressure appropriate to their texture. We can, of course, reflect on our actions and thereby form judgments about what aspects of the environment we are attending to. The important point is that such consciousness is not necessary. Indeed, it often impedes expert practice, as Benner and Dreyfus have pointed out. Because we are not self-conscious of affordances and attunements, our action can have the smooth, intuitive character highlighted by the later stages of the five-stage model.

Many of our everyday actions – probably the vast majority – proceed from our capacities to track aspects of our environment and to recognize its affordances. All embodied skills rely on these two capacities. They constitute our fundamental embodied capacity to respond to the environment. At the same time, even embodied skills are not thoughtless. We have the capacity to reflect on our actions, make deliberate choices, and to recall guidelines, plans, or orders. These latter capacities are *meta-cognitive* in the sense that they are responsive to both the lower-level recognition of attunements and affordances (as well as the output of the motor control cognitive functions) and to the contents of memory. The meta-cognitive capacities are conscious in the sense that we can verbally report on them. In human action, all three capacities are normally engaged.

The ecological conception motivates a very different picture of action and agency than the one sketched at the end of the previous section. The standard picture treats deliberate, instrumental action as the paradigm of intentionality, and then tries to make room for know-how. The ecological picture treats embodied engagement as the norm and deliberate action as a particular manifestation of know-how. In a deliberate action, the agent has planned the action in advance, deciding on the best means to satisfy the agent's goals. As the action unfolds, the agent monitors their continuing performance and adjusts so that the plan is carried through. The monitoring function is conducted by the agent's meta-cognitive capacities, while ability to carry through engages the capacities for attunements and affordances. The vast majority of our daily activities are not deliberate in this sense. They require attunement and recognition of affordances, but memory of a decision, plan or rule plays no role. This does not mean that the meta-cognitive capacities are disengaged. I know what I am doing as I slow down and change lanes in response to changing road conditions, even if I am not following plans or making conscious choices. Hence, the ecological conception of agency provides a different way of understanding the self-consciousness of agents. I need not be aware of how I became aware of the opportunity to change lanes, and I may not consciously recognize that there is an opportunity until the action is underway. Nonetheless, my meta-cognitive capacities permit me to monitor my action and consciously make plans or decisions if necessary. Agents are self-conscious, and, at the same time, are not aware of all of the factors that influence their actions.

Reconceptualizing agency in ecological terms provides a slightly different take on the process of moving from novice to expert. In the Benner/Dreyfus model, the novice depends entirely on the criteria set by the rule. The rule is the novice's only reason for action. Only in the later stages does the nurse become sensitive to the network of affordances. By contrast, the ecological model holds that agents are always sensitive to the network of affordances. A novice nurse can learn tracheal care because they already have a vast repertoire of relevant practical abilities. The movement from novice to expert is constituted by the tuning and refining of these same abilities.

At the earliest stages, guidelines let the agent use their meta-cognitive capacities to guide the capacities for attunement and affordance recognition. The guidelines provide an indication of what needs attention and what needs to be done. The classroom instruction tells the nursing student to pay attention to the depth of the catheter and the reading on the manometer. The nurse doing their first tracheal suctioning will keep these things in mind (or try to!) in the sense that their meta-cognitive ability to compare the outcome of the action with the plan permits both control of the action and learning from mistakes. The process progresses as the capacities for attunement and affordance recognition become trained and can work autonomously from the meta-cognitive capacity. In some cases, like the example of shoe tying, the original instructions may be entirely lost to memory. It is also important to bear in mind that there is no stage where the meta-cognitive capacities are turned off. Even experts guide their action with consciously remembered maxims and previously devised plans, and they reflect on their successes and failures to achieve their goals. The ecological model thus explains the relationship of explicit rules to practical know-how without recourse to an instrumental stage.

Evidence for practice

The ecological conception of agency opens two routes for systematic research to improve nursing practice; what we might call an internal and an external path. On the internal path, explicit instructions and guidelines bring evidence to bear on practice, as they do on the five-stage model. We saw in the previous section that the ecological conception of agency can do so without reducing practical know-how to instrumental action. Moreover, the ecological conception of agency provides a more explicit account of the mechanisms that underlie the transition from novice to expert. This means that we can explain why guidelines do not get translated into practice, and thereby look for new solutions.

Consider, for example, one of the problems uncovered by Day's research on tracheal suctioning. Of the 28 subjects, 18 knew to use the correct size of catheter. Guidelines recommend that the "external diameter of the suction catheter should not exceed one-half of the internal diameter of the tube" (Day *et al.*, 2002: 37). Day found that only nine subjects used the correct size of tube and 18 used catheters that were too large. The ecological model of agency suggests a possible explanation for this gap between theory and practice. The guideline requires nurses to calculate the proper size of the catheter. This means that the nurse must engage their meta-cognitive capacities in each tracheal suctioning episode. The nurse must remember the recommendation, do the calculation and deliberately choose the catheter. Such processing is slow and it gets in the way of expert performance. Given the need for quick, efficient action in a suctioning procedure, the capacities for attunement and affordance recognition take over. The result is actions that are not in accord with the agent's conscious knowledge of the guideline.

The standard recommendation for addressing the discrepancy between action and guideline is more education. Reminding nurses of the guidelines would presumably increase the percentage of nurses who could correctly state them. However, Day's data and the explanation suggested above indicates that education about the guideline will not necessarily increase the percentage of nurses who both know and follow the guideline. Since performance will not be improved by further education about the rule, the internal path from propositional knowledge to practical know-how is blocked. We need another way to make evidence relevant to practice.

The ecological conception of agency emphasizes its relational character: to be an agent is to be responsive to the environment. This entails that performance can be changed by modifying the environment. We can change what people do by changing the affordances or modifying the features of the environment to which they are attuned. With regard to the catheter size problem, the ecological model suggests that the gap between theory and practice arises because of the meta-cognitive processing load imposed by the need to calculate the correct size. A change in the environment that let the nurses recognize the appropriate size directly would probably help. Since Day's studies, some manufacturers have begun color-coding tracheal tubes and the right sized catheters. By being attuned to the color, the nurse can directly recognize some catheters as appropriate and others as inappropriate. Of course, research would be required to determine whether such a change in the environment really changes practice. If it did, we would have followed an "external" path from scientific knowledge to practical know-how. Note how, on this external path, evidence is used to change practice directly, without the mediation of guidelines.

In order to use the external path from scientific knowledge to practice, we need a different kind of research than is standardly undertaken. While we must educate nurses with validated guidelines and standards of care, we have seen that the internal path is not always the best way to link evidence and practice. We there-fore need a form of research that is not a test of guidelines; we need evidence that will help modify practice directly. The research required for the external path has three parts or phases. First, we must discover some way in which nursing practice needs improvement. Day's studies provide one model for this, but standard outcome-based research might be used as well. Once we have identified a prob-lematic area of nursing practice, the researcher must look closely at what aspects of the environment nurses actually track and what affordances they actually recognize. This second phase could not take the form of a randomized controlled trial, and we have seen that the typical forms of qualitative research would not work either. The research might be observational; something like the non-partic-ipant observation used in Day's studies. It might also be experimental or quasi-experimental, manipulating the environment in different ways and deter-mining the effects on nurses' performance. The goal of this second phase would be to explain why the nurses act as they do by understanding the attunements, affordances and meta-cognitive reflection involved in their performance. These explanations (like the one proposed above) would suggest possible modifications to the nursing environment. The third phase of research would be to experiment with changes in the environment and determine their effect on the quality of nurs-ing care. In this kind of research programme, evidence would be brought to bear directly on practice by motivating changes in the nurses' world.

The solution to the puzzle of evidence-based practice requires us to think differ-ently about human agency and action. Agency is a complex bundle of interacting, but partially autonomous, embodied capacities with which we engage the envi-ronment. Some of these capacities are conscious, in the sense that we can report them to others; some of these capacities are not penetrable by self-reflection. It follows that evaluating and improving practice guidelines and standards of care is only one form of research supporting evidence-based practice. Another is research into the way in which nurses engage their environment. Evidence about the effects of modifying the nursing environment can lead to direct changes in nursing outcomes, independent of guidelines and education. Evidence-based practice may be something of an oxymoron but it need not be a paradox.

Note

1 Each of these "capacities" is properly thought of as a suite of functional relationships between various cognitive systems and the environment. To be attuned to a feature is to have groups of neurons in the parietal lobe responding to that feature in ways that enable the agent to interact with the environment.

References

Benner, P. (1984) *From Novice to Expert*, Menlo Park, CA: Addison-Wesley.

Brandom, R. (1994) *Making It Explicit*, Cambridge, MA: Harvard University Press.

Day, T., Farnell, S., Haynes, S., Wainwright, S. P. and Wilson-Barnett, J. (2002) Tracheal Suctioning: An Exploration of Nurse's Knowledge and Competence in Acute and High Dependency Ward Areas. *Journal of Advanced Nursing*, 39, 35–45.

Day, T., Wainwright, S. P. and Wilson-Barnett, J. (2001) An Evaluation of a Teaching Intervention to Improve the Practice of Endotracheal Suctioning in Intensive Care Units. *Journal of Clinical Nursing*, 10, 682–96.

Doane, G. H. and Varcoe, C. (2008) Knowledge Translation in Everyday Nursing: From Evidence-Based Nursing to Inquiry-Based Practice. *Advances in Nursing Science*, 31, 283–95.

Dreyfus, H. L. (1972) *What Computers Can't Do: The Limits of Artificial Intelligence*, New York: Harper and Row.

Dreyfus, H. L. (2007) The Return of the Myth of the Mental. *Inquiry*, 50, 352–65.

Dreyfus, H. L. and Dreyfus, S. E. (1986) *Mind over Machine*, New York: Free Press.

Heidegger, M. (2010) *Being and Time*, Albany NY: State University of New York Press.

Kripke, S. A. (1982) *Wittgenstein on Rules and Private Language*, Cambridge, MA: Harvard University Press.

Paley, J. (1998) Misinterpretive Phenomenology: Heidegger, Ontology, and Nursing Research. *Journal of Advanced Nursing*, 27, 817–24.

Pedersen, C. M., Rosendahl-Nielsen, M., Hjermind, J. and Egerod, I. (2009) Endotracheal Suctioning of the Adult Intubated Patient – What is the evidence? *Intensive and Critical Care Nursing*, 25, 21–30.

Porter, S. (2010) Fundamental Patterns of Knowing in Nursing: The Challenge of Evidence-Based Practice. *Advances in Nursing Science*, 33, 3–14.

Risjord, M. (2014) Structure, Agency, and Improvisation. In: Zahle, J. and Collin, F. (eds) *Rethinking the Individualism-Holism Debate*, Dordrecht: Springer.

Rycroft-Malone, J., Seers, K., Titchen, A., Harvey, G., Kitson, A. and McCormack, B. (2004) What Counts as Evidence in Evidence-Based Practice? *Journal of Advanced Nursing*, 47, 81–90.

Wittgenstein, L. (1953) *Philosophical Investigations*, New York: Macmillan.

7 Evidence-based nursing and the generalizability of research results

Robyn Bluhm

It seems obvious that clinical research has an important role to play in improving clinical care. Beyond this claim, however, things rapidly become more controversial. It is not at all clear what *kinds* of research should be conducted, or how to best link research and practice.

The most influential approach to answering these questions originally comes from a group of physicians (and, later, other clinicians and health researchers) at McMaster University, in Hamilton, Ontario, Canada. Their approach, known as evidence-based medicine (EBM) was first introduced in the early 1990s and then spread rapidly from internal medicine to other areas of clinical care. In 2005, members of the group published a guide to evidence-based nursing (EBN; DiCenso *et al.*, 2005), which was closely modeled on their previous guide to EBM (Guyatt and Rennie, 2002), which itself was based on a series of papers originally published in the *Journal of the American Medical Association*. This guide presents the fundamental skills required to practice EBN, particularly those that allow nurses "to discriminate high quality research from that which is flawed and to interpret the results of research studies" (DiCenso *et al.*, 2005: xxv).

There is much to be lauded in EBM and its extension to other areas of clinical practice; however, there is also much that could be improved. My aims in this chapter are to clearly lay out both the strengths and the weaknesses of this approach, as it is applied to nursing, and to suggest ways in which these weaknesses can be addressed. In doing so, I draw on philosophical criticisms of EBM's approach, showing that they are also applicable to EBN. Like Banner *et al.* (Chapter 2 of this volume), I am concerned that much research evidence may not be directly applicable to practice; I aim to show that EBM does not take this problem seriously enough.

I begin by outlining the basic approach given to EBN by DiCenso and colleagues. While theirs is not the only approach to EBN, I have chosen to focus specifically on their exposition for several reasons. First, the authors' association with the original EBM Working Group has meant that their work has both authority and influence. Second, other expositions of EBN are very similar in their main points, to the methods laid out by this group, so the guide by DiCenso *et al.* presents the main – and generally accepted – features of EBN (see, for comparison, Pope *et al.*, 2004; Melnyk and Fineout-Overholt, 2005, Cullum *et al.*, 2008).

After presenting the basics of EBN, I argue that, although the critical appraisal skills taught in the guide are extremely valuable, the approach is much weaker when it comes to teaching nurses how to use the results of their critical appraisal in clinical practice. As I show in this chapter, these limitations arise in large part because of the *kind* of research that is held to provide the best evidence, specifically randomized controlled trials (RCTs) with high internal validity. In the third part of the paper, I turn from EBN to other areas of the nursing literature, to identify ways in which nursing researchers can study the best ways to use research in clinical care.

EBM, EBN, and critical appraisal

The core idea behind both EBM and EBN is that there are clear criteria for identifying high-quality evidence. These criteria have two main parts: first, one should see where a study falls on the hierarchy of evidence. Second, the study should be appraised to determine whether it is valid. I address each of these in turn.

The hierarchy of evidence is intended to rank different kinds of study, or more broadly, sources of evidence, with the most trustworthy sources on top. The top two levels of the hierarchy consist of RCTs, with systematic reviews or meta-analyses of multiple studies ranking above a single RCT. Below this come systematic reviews of nonrandomized ("observational") studies, then a single nonrandomized trial. All of these levels refer to epidemiological research, which compares the frequency of (good or bad) outcomes in a group of patients receiving the intervention being studied with outcomes in a control group that receives a different intervention (including placebo interventions). These epidemiological methods are held to provide the best evidence that an intervention is effective (and, to a certain extent, that it is safe).[1]

By contrast, the bottom two levels of the hierarchy consist of sources of evidence that may indicate effectiveness, but about which some caution is required. The second lowest level consists of studies that examine physiology; such studies may provide a "pathophysiologic rationale" for believing that a treatment is effective, but these studies are not as good a source of evidence as ones that use the controlled, epidemiological methods of the higher levels of the hierarchy. Alternatively, these studies may be RCTs, but ones that use physiological "surrogate endpoints" (such as lowered blood pressure), testing the effects of an intervention on laboratory or physiological measures that are "used as a substitute for an endpoint that directly measures how a patient feels, functions, or survives" (DiCenso *et al.*, 2005: 237). EBN says that one should be cautious of these studies because surrogate endpoints may not adequately predict clinically important outcomes.

The lowest level of the hierarchy is that of the clinical experience of an individual nurse (or a small group of nurses) of using an intervention in practice. These "unsystematic" observations may indeed be valuable "and experienced nurses develop a healthy respect for the insights of their senior colleagues in issues of clinical observation and relations with patients and colleagues" (DiCenso *et al.*, 2005: 13); however, they do not include enough data points, or sufficiently control for other factors that may affect patient outcomes, to be considered high quality research.

Although the hierarchy "is not absolute" and there are (rare) cases in which evidence from lower levels is sufficient to guide clinical practice, "[the] hierarchy of evidence implies a clear course of action for nurses considering alternative interventions to address patients' problems: nurses should look for the highest level of available evidence from the hierarchy of study designs relevant to their clinical question" (DiCenso *et al.*, 2005: 14). All other things being equal, RCTs provide the best evidence about the effectiveness of an intervention.

Yet, of course, not all RCTs are well conducted. This brings us to the second set of criteria relevant to EBN; these criteria assess whether the results of a study are valid. The criteria look at the design and execution of a study in order to assess the extent to which the results of the study are unbiased. More specifically, they look at whether and how the study randomized patients to the treatment or control groups, whether patients, clinicians, and other outcome assessors were unaware of the group to which patients had been assigned, and whether follow-up in in both the treatment and the control groups was reasonably complete. I next briefly describe the rationale for each of these criteria, in preparation for introducing the major philosophical criticism of EBM in the next section.

Randomization serves two major purposes in a clinical study. First, it is held to be the best way to ensure that the patients in the treatment and the control group are, on average, similar with regard to characteristics that might influence the outcome(s) being measured in the study. Ideally, all of these characteristics will be "balanced" across the study groups, so that the only difference between them will be receipt (or not) of the study intervention. These characteristics include both factors that are known to influence patients' responses to treatment, and factors that do have such an influence, despite the fact that it is not known that they do. This distinction, between known and unknown confounding factors, is made to underscore the fact that, while it may be possible to ensure balance between the treatment and the control groups with regard to factors that are known, or suspected, to have an effect on outcomes, only the chance element introduced by random allocation balances (at least in most cases) unknown confounders. Although EBM recognizes that randomization may *not* balance confounding variables (and in fact cautions that readers of a study should check to see whether clinical and demographic variables are balanced across groups), it is held to be the best way of doing so.

Moreover, random allocation prevents the influence of bias (either deliberate or unconscious) in allocating patients to groups. For example, a clinician cannot assign sicker patients to an active treatment group, rather than a placebo group, so that they are sure to get treatment. Doing so would quite likely result in the treatment looking less effective, compared with placebo, than it actually is. This point is closely related to a second reason for random assignment of participants to the treatment or control groups. Not only must allocation be concealed at the beginning of a study, it must remain so throughout the course of the study. Randomization helps to ensure that participants' group allocation is concealed – from them and from anyone else who may be assessing outcomes in the study. This is important because knowing that a patient is receiving the experimental therapy or the control intervention may bias the outcome assessment. Patients may genuinely feel better knowing that they are receiving a treatment they believe to be effective, even when that treatment does not actually have any biological effect. Similarly, clinicians associated with the study may be unconsciously biased in their clinical assessments if they know the group to which a patient belongs.

In addition to random allocation and allocation concealment, which are features of study design, there are issues relevant to the execution of the study that may affect its validity. These have to do with the availability of outcome data for study participants. It is not uncommon for patients who enroll in a study to drop out of the trial. Moreover, failure to complete the study is more common in patients who are not benefitting from the intervention (whether because they do not respond to the treatment or because they experience side effects). This means that "patients who are lost to follow-up often have different prognoses than those who are retained" (DiCenso *et al.*, 2005: 57). For similar reasons, preserving the validity of the study requires including the (known) outcome data from these patients in analyses of the study, whether or not they received the intervention.[2]

In summary, the criteria by which EBN says that the validity of a study should be assessed address the quality of random allocation, allocation concealment, and follow-up of patients. These criteria are intended to ensure that the treatment and the control groups both "begin the study with a similar [average] prognosis" and "retain a similar prognosis after the study has started" (DiCenso *et al.*, 2005: 51). Two points are worth noting about the criteria, which are relevant to the criticisms of EBM discussed in the next section. First, they reinforce the hierarchy of evidence in that they focus centrally on randomization. Second, the kind of validity with which they are concerned is *internal* validity. That is, they are intended to assess the possibility that the results of the study are biased, owing to systematic differences between the treatment and the control groups. A study with high internal validity is one in which: (1) the groups are balanced with respect to potential confounders at the beginning of the study; (2) the assessment of outcomes during the study is not biased by knowledge of which intervention participants are receiving; and (3) there are no differences in the number of dropouts during the study that would tend to favor one group over the other.

EBN's approach to the critical appraisal of clinical research is designed primarily to ensure that the research that is used to influence clinical practice has high internal validity. Moreover, it does this very well. I show, however, that focusing on internal validity actually limits EBN's ability to help nurses to use the results of research to inform patient care. In making this case, I begin by surveying the existing philosophical criticisms of EBM. Given that EBN has been modeled explicitly on EBM, they apply equally to EBN. I then turn to the third question that the evidence-based approach says is important when assessing the research literature, "How can I apply these results to patient care?", and show that, unlike the first question, this one is not well answered by EBN.

Philosophical criticisms of EBM

Philosophers have been interested in EBM for a number of reasons. Some of these are epistemological; because EBM makes claims about what counts as good evidence, it is relevant to longstanding questions in the philosophy of science about the nature of evidence and the empirical support of scientific hypotheses. Others are concerned with both epistemology and ethics, and reflect a more recent interest among philosophers of science in the relationship between science and values (broadly construed). These issues emphasize that the epistemological choices made by EBM (for example, to privilege certain kinds of research over others and to focus on particular traits of studies) have ethical implications, as they affect the care delivered to patients.

There are two main epistemological criticisms of EBM that have been raised by philosophers and that are particularly relevant to my discussion of EBN in this chapter.[3] The first is that EBM oversells the importance of randomization. The second is that EBM does not pay sufficient attention to the external validity of studies; that is, to the question of whether their results are generalizable to clinical contexts that do not resemble the ones in which the study was conducted. I briefly review these arguments and show that the first problem actually exacerbates the second.

As described above, the two main functions of randomly allocating study participants to the treatment or control group are that it balances potential confounders across groups, tending to result in groups that, for example, contain roughly the same proportion of women versus men, and that have a similar average age and severity of illness. The second is that random allocation facilitates allocation concealment, which in turn prevents bias in outcome assessment from the assessor's expectations about how patients in each group will respond to treatment.

Philosophers have argued that the first virtue of randomization essentially mistakes the methods for the results. That is, what actually matters is that the groups *are* balanced, not how they got that way. Balance could also be achieved by listing the factors that are known or suspected to affect treatment outcomes and then deliberately assigning patients to groups in such a way that these characteristics are evenly balanced. Granted, this way of balancing potential confounders does not help either with the balancing of unknown confounders (factors that do affect treatment outcomes, even though we have no suspicion that they do), or with allocation concealment. To address the second of these problems first, all that would be required to ensure that outcome assessors are unaware of study participants' group status is to have someone who will not be participating in outcome assessment do the group assignments. By contrast, the possibility that at least one unknown confounder is more common in the treatment than the control group (or vice versa) cannot be solved by deliberately balancing the groups. But we cannot know whether random allocation has done so either, since (by definition) we cannot test to see whether unknown and unsuspected factors are balanced. This, then, is a solid argument in favour of random allocation. But note that, even here, random allocation does not necessarily balance *known* confounders, either. The instructions for critically appraising research therefore advise that readers of an RCT check to see whether the different groups actually were similar with regard to sex, age, and so on. Often, this is not the case. Therefore, there is also no guarantee that a study is balanced with respect to unknown confounders.

Moreover, there is empirical evidence to show that, all other aspects of study design being similar, nonrandomized and randomized studies have similar outcomes (Concato *et al.*, 2000; Benson and Hartz, 2000). Thus, while randomization is a useful strategy in trial design, it is not essential, and the important advantages of random allocation can be secured in other ways.

Having said all of this, I want to make it clear that I am not arguing *against* randomizing. In fact, I agree that it is a useful tool of clinical research. The problem, however, is that in elevating it to the top of the hierarchy of evidence, EBM has cast doubt on the usefulness of all studies that are not randomized. In the most extreme cases, advocates of EBM have claimed that, when one has both randomized and nonrandomized studies that examine the same intervention, the first thing to do is discard the nonrandomized studies (see, for example, Straus *et al.*, 2005: 118). Even when nonrandomized studies are considered, EBM claims that their results should be interpreted with caution: not only are they lower on the hierarchy, but they fail to exhibit many of the aspects of (internal) validity described above.

The problem with the message that randomized studies are significantly better than all other types of evidence from clinical trials is this: while evidence from RCTs with high internal validity and narrow confidence intervals does provide clear evidence about whether the experimental intervention is better than the control, they are the *least* generalizable source of evidence when what is required is to determine whether the intervention will be effective outside of that contest. In other words, they lack *external* validity. Recall that RCTs are designed to test whether, on average, a group of patients receiving an experimental intervention experience (statistically significantly) better outcomes than a group that receives a control intervention. In order to provide the clearest test of the hypothesis that the experimental intervention is better, RCTs are generally designed to minimize the potential influence of confounding variables on the effects of the intervention. This means that patients who participate in clinical trials tend not to have comorbid conditions, or to be taking other medications or using other therapies that might confound the estimate of the effects of the drug. This means, however, that they do not tend to resemble patients who are seen in clinical practice (Humphreys *et al.*, 2013). As a result, it is not obvious that the results of these studies are generalizable to clinical practice. In the next section, I return to the exposition of EBN provided by DiCenso *et al.* (2005), and begin to show the limits of EBN's approach when it comes to using the results in of one's critical appraisal in clinical practice.

"Using the results in clinical practice"

Critically appraising the results of studies examining health care interventions requires the would-be evidence-based nurse to ask three sets of questions: "Are the results valid?", "What are the results?", and "How can I apply the results to patient care?" I addressed the first set of questions in section 1, above; here, I focus on the third set.[4] Determining the extent to which to which the results of a clinical trial (or of a number of trials of the same intervention) is useful requires considering several further questions. These are: "Were the study patients similar to the patients in my clinical setting?", "Were all important outcomes considered?" and "Are the likely intervention benefits worth the potential harm and costs?" (DiCenso *et al.*, 2005: 48).

The first question is the one that I think EBN has the most trouble with, for reasons directly relevant to the philosophical criticisms I outlined in the previous section. The proponents of EBN acknowledge that this is a challenge, saying that "[o]ften, your patient has different attributes or characteristics from those enrolled in the trial. He or she may be older, sicker, or may have comorbid disease that would have excluded him or her from enrollment in the study" (DiCenso *et al.*, 2005: 65). They further acknowledge that, even if the patient would have qualified for the study, this does not guarantee that she or he would benefit from an intervention that had been shown by the study to be effective: "[i]nterventions are not uniformly effective in every individual patient ... RCTs estimate average intervention effects. Applying these average effects means that clinicians will likely expose some patients to the cost, inconvenience, and potential side effects of an intervention without benefit" (DiCenso *et al.*, 2005: 65). These two points indicate that it is not always the case that an RCT is evidence that an intervention is effective, is a license to infer that it will be effective for a given patient. I see this as the central problem of EBM/EBN.

I also believe that EBN does not take this problem seriously enough. DiCenso *et al.* 2005 respond to each of the points they raise in the previous paragraph. First, they claim that if a patient seen in clinical practice would have met all of the inclusion criteria and violated none of the exclusion criteria of a study, then "you could apply the results with considerable confidence" (DiCenso *et al.*, 2005: 65). This, however, ignores the point raised at the end of the previous paragraph, which shows that patients do vary in their response to an intervention. Moreover, they continue, even if the patient would *not* have qualified for the study, they suggest that most of the time this would not matter. For example (and this is indeed a reasonable example), they suggest that a patient who is two years too old to have qualified for a study will most likely be similar *enough* to the study participants (on average) to expect similar results (or at least to be as justified in expecting similar results as if the patient had been two years younger). Yet this example of dissimilarity does not justify the conclusion drawn in their next statement:

A better approach than rigidly applying a study's inclusion and exclusion criteria is to ask whether there is some compelling reason that the results should *not* be applied to the patient. A compelling reason usually will not be found, and often you can generalize the results to the patient with confidence.

(DiCenso *et al.*, 2005: 65)

In summary, then, if the patient in question would have qualified for the study in question, the results can be generalized with considerable confidence, if not, then one's confidence cannot be considerable. But this sanguine view ignores that fact that the reason that studies set inclusion and exclusion criteria in the first place is that they take into account exactly those factors (severity of illness, presence of comorbid conditions, or use of concomitant therapies) that are *likely* to affect treatment outcomes. Moreover, even if it is true in some instances that the patients a nurse sees in their own clinical setting will respond the same way to an intervention as did dissimilar patients who participated in a study, it seems contrary to the spirit of EBN not to require evidence that this is indeed the case. A truly evidence-based approach will not assume that (barring *compelling* evidence to the contrary), a well-designed, internally valid RCT is a sufficient guide to practice.

In fact, a closer look at what DiCenso *et al.* (2005) say about the role of the scientific literature in clinical practice suggests that they are more aware of the need to think critically about the role of RCT results than their remarks quoted above might suggest. A later chapter provides more information about the kinds of circumstances that may provide compelling reasons not to be confident in applying the results of a study to one's patients. According to DiCenso *et al.* (2005), the results of a study may not apply to a patient in cases where biological, sociological, or epidemiological factors are significantly different than the average in a study. Biological differences may include variations in patient physiology (such as differences in immune response, or in exposure to environmental factors affecting health), or differences in the agent that causes the disease (such as drug-resistant pathogens). The socioeconomic factors they consider are those that might affect patients' adherence to treatment, or the ability of providers to properly implement the study protocol. Epidemiological factors to consider are the prevalence of other health conditions in a population (though the example given here is of a diagnostic, rather than a treatment intervention). Yet even after introducing these complexities, DiCenso *et al.* (2005) remind readers that these kinds of compelling exceptions are relatively rare (DiCenso *et al.*, 2005: 482), again dismissing the problem of generalizability.

A second discussion of the role, and limits, of clinical research in EBN occurs in the introductory sections of the book. Here, DiCenso *et al.* (2005) stress that evidence-based practice is not simply a matter of applying the results of clinical trials in caring for patients. They describe evidence-based practice as "the integration of best research evidence with clinical expertise and patient values to facilitate clinical decision-making" and note that "a key element of evidence-based clinical decision-making is personalizing the evidence to fit a specific patient's circumstance" (DiCenso *et al.*, 2005: 4). This approach is also illustrated approach graphically in a Venn diagram with four "dimensions" that need to be taken into account in making clinical decisions: (1) research evidence; (2) clinical state, setting, and circumstances; (3) patient preferences and actions; and (4) health care resources (DiCenso *et al.*, 2005: 5).[5] Clinical expertise is represented in this diagram as the area of overlap of these dimensions.[6]

Yet, in practice, the strength of EBM/EBN has always been in the critical appraisal of research – and by far the majority of the information presented in this book addresses critical appraisal. The other three components and the clinical expertise that is supposed to bring them all together are addressed only briefly, and generally in the context of working through sample cases, rather than being taught as an explicit set of skills the way that critical appraisal is taught. Instead, this integration is supposed to be done by the individual nurse, using her clinical expertise, which is defined as "our ability to use clinical skills and past experiences to identify the health state of patients or populations, their risks, their preferences and actions, and the potential benefits of interventions; to communicate information to patients and their families; and to provide them with an environment they find comforting and supportive" (DiCenso *et al.*, 2005: 5).

My criticism of EBN is not that it leaves an important role for clinical expertise. Rather, my argument is that the evidence base provided by EBN is not providing the best kind of evidence to inform clinical decision-making. As I argued in the previous section, the goal of using research to inform patient care is not best served by internally valid RCTs. As a result, there is a gap between the available research base and clinical practice. Moreover, in attempting to use an individual nurse's "clinical skills and past experiences" to bridge this gap, EBN is jumping from the highest level of the hierarchy of evidence right to the lowest. It is not clear why a nurse's individual experience is supposed to equip her to know when the results of a study apply in specific cases that she encounters in practice, when it is, according to EBN, too limited to allow her to predict that an intervention will be effective in general.

Situation-specific theories and the (limited) generalizability of research results

There is, however, a way to bridge, or at least to narrow, the gap between clinical trials and clinical practice. In this section, I draw on the account of situation-specific theories presented by Im and Meleis (1999) in order to sketch a framework by which these theories can strengthen the evidence-base for EBN. Situation-specific theories were developed in part to bridge a different gap, that between abstract "grand theories" in nursing and clinical practice. They have a number of features that suggest that they can perform a similar function in EBM. Im and Meleis describe these theories as having six properties, all of which are relevant to the question of how to generalize the results of clinical trials to other clinical contexts. These properties are: a low level of abstraction (especially compared with grand theories); reflection of specific nursing phenomena; context (especially that provided by the clinical setting or client population of interest); connection to research and practice; incorporation of diversity; and limited generalizability (Im and Meleis, 1999: 16–20). In addition, situation-specific theories have clear implications for practice; they can provide "blueprints" for action (Im and Meleis, 1999: 13).

How might nurses develop situation-specific theories about how an intervention might work in their clinical setting or with their clients? Im and Meleis emphasize that these theories may draw from a variety of philosophical and scientific perspectives, so they do not give a single method. Yet they do note that "[s]ituation-specific theories may emerge from synthesizing and integrating research findings and clinical exemplars" (Im and Meleis, 1999: 16). These theories are also "developed to answer a set of coherent questions about situations that are limited in scope and in focus" (pp. 17–18). The approach that I am suggesting here picks up on these ideas, looking for differences between the context in which an RCT was conducted and the current clinical situation, and then relating these differences to variability in clinical outcomes. As described above, patients may differ from clinical trial participants in a number of ways. DiCenso *et al.* (2005) discuss biological and socioeconomic factors (the latter with reference to their impact on compliance), as well as patient preferences and characteristics of the setting within which care is provided. Im and Meleis (1999) focus primarily on cultural and broader social factors. Any of these may be relevant. Developing a theory of how these factors affect outcomes requires, first, simply taking very seriously the possibility that they may do so; this is a possibility downplayed by EBN, but central to situation-specific theory's focus on context and diversity. Second, observed outcome differences in clinical practice can be used, together with knowledge of context, to develop and test theories about when to implement, to modify, or to ignore, the results of clinical trials in particular clinical populations.

In order to have the maximal impact on nursing practice, these theories should themselves be published, and become part of the evidence base relevant to the intervention as originally tested. While such studies may not rank high on EBN's hierarchy of evidence, they do fit within a tradition in nursing research. It may therefore be easier to solve the "generalizability" problem in nursing than it has proven to be in the context of EBM.

Notes

1 Although RCTs do (and should) track the frequency of adverse events, EBN claims that the harmful effects of treatments are often best identified using long-term observational studies.

2 There are several ways of doing this, discussion of which is beyond the scope of the chapter.

3 Detailed discussion of the criticisms summarized in this section can be found in Worrall 2002, 2007; Cartwright, 2007; Grossman and Mackenzie, 2005; Borgerson 2009; Bluhm 2009, 2010. For a philosophical defense of EBM, see Howick 2011.

4 The second set of questions examines the actual results of the study; the more precise the results (that is, the narrower the reported confidence interval), the more confident we can be about the true effect.

5 The kinds of biological, socioeconomic, and epidemiological factors described above would fall under one of the last three dimensions.

6   Placement of "clinical expertise" in this diagram suggests that it is the element that does the integrating, while on the previous page it is described as one of the factors to be integrated. It does not matter for my argument which of these descriptions is accurate.

References

Benson, K. and Hartz, A. J. (2000) A comparison of observational studies and randomized, controlled trials. *New England Journal of Medicine* 342(25), 1878–86.

Borgerson, K. (2009) Valuing evidence: Bias and the evidence hierarchy of evidence-based medicine. *Perspectives in Biology and Medicine* 52(2), 218–33.

Bluhm, R. (2009) Some observations on "observational" research. *Perspectives in Biology and Medicine* 52(2), 252–63.

Bluhm, R. (2010) The epistemology and ethics of chronic disease research: Further lessons from ECMO. *Theoretical Medicine and Bioethics* 31(2), 107–22.

Cartwright, N. (2007) Are RCTs the gold standard? *BioSocieties* 2, 11–20.

Concato, J., Shah, N. and Horwitz, R. I. (2000) Randomized, controlled trials, observational studies, and the hierarchy of research designs. *New England Journal of Medicine* 342(25), 1887–92.

Cullum, N., Ciliska, D., Haynes, R. B. and Marks, S. (2008) *Evidence-Based Nursing: An Introduction*. Oxford: Wiley-Blackwell.

DiCenso, A., Guyatt, G. and Ciliska, D. (2005) *Evidence-Based Nursing: A Guide to Clinical Practice*. St. Louis, MO: Elsevier Mosby.

Grossman, J. and Mackenzie, F. (2005) The randomized controlled trial: Gold standard, or merely standard? *Perspectives in Biology and Medicine* 48(4): 516–34.

Guyatt, G. and Rennie, D. (eds) (2002) *Users' Guides to the Medical Literature: A Manual for Evidence-Based Practice*. Chicago: AMA Press.

Howick, J. (2011) *The Philosophy of Evidence-Based Medicine*. London: Wiley-Blackwell, BMJ Books.

Humphreys, K., Maisel, N. C., Blodgett, J. C., Fuh, I. L. and Finney, J. W. (2013) Extent and reporting of patient nonenrollment in influential randomized clinical trials, 2002 to 2010. *JAMA Internal Medicine* 173(11), 1029–31.

Im E-O and Meleis A I (1999) Situation-specific theories: philosophical roots, properties, and approach. *Advances in Nursing Science* 22(2), 11 –24.

Melnyk, B. M. and Fineout-Overholt, E. (2005) *Evidence-Based Practice in Nursing and Healthcare: A Guide to Best Practices*. Philadelphia: Wolters Kluwer Health.

Pope, R., Graham, L. and Jones, P. C. (2004) Randomised controlled Trials: Illustrative Case Studies in *Shaping the Facts: Evidence-Based Nursing and Health Care* Smith, P., James, T., Lorenzon, M., Pope, R. (eds) (pp. 89–110). Edinburgh: Elsevier Science.

Straus, S. E., Richardson, W. S., Glasziou, P. and Haynes, R. B. (2005) *Evidence-Based Medicine: How to Practice and Teach EBM*. Toronto: Elsevier.

Worrall, J. (2002) What evidence in evidence-based medicine? *Proceedings of the Philosophy of Science Association* 69(3), S316–30.

Worrall, J. (2007) Evidence in medicine and evidence-based medicine. *Philosophy Compass* 2(6), 981–1022.

8 Evidence-based practice and practice-based evidence

Gary Rolfe

Introduction

'Evidence-based practice' is a deceptively simple term for a difficult, contested and multi-faceted concept, which has been developed and expanded over a period of more than 20 years by a diverse collection of disciplines and professions. The fact that these three words are required to cover so much conceptual ground opens up the possibility that, as Wittgenstein warned, discussions and debates about seemingly substantive and important issues turn out to be little more than squabbles over the meanings attached to words. In situations such as these, Wittgenstein suggests that the job of the philosopher is not to *solve* problems but simply to *dissolve* them by revealing that many of the contestations and disputes about what evidence-based practice *is* and *is not* (to paraphrase the title of two influential papers on the topic) are based on using the term in different ways. With this thought in mind, this chapter begins with an exploration of the origins and early development of the idea of evidence-based practice, followed by an examination of the various ways in which each of the three words which make up the term are used in the seminal literature. Particular attention is paid to concept of practice, and two distinct approaches are identified, each with their own associated notion of 'best evidence'. The chapter concludes with an exposition of the richness and strangeness of nursing practice and suggests that best practice should dictate what counts as best evidence rather than vice versa.

A short history of evidence-based practice

The idea that practice should be underpinned by research findings has a long history in most health care disciplines, including nursing. However, evidence-based practice, as it was originally conceived, proposed something a little different. The concept of evidence-based practice has its origins in medicine, and the paper that first brought it to the wider attention of the profession was published in 1992 by the self-styled Evidence-Based Medicine Working Group (EBMWG), a team of 30 writers based predominantly at McMaster University in Canada and led by Gordon Guyatt (EBMWG 1992). It is important to note the full title of this seminal paper: 'Evidence-Based Medicine – A New Approach to

Teaching the Practice of Medicine' and to recognise that it was not addressed primarily to practitioners of medicine but to educators. The authors identified a common problem for junior medical residents, whereby the practice they encountered on their clinical placements was often directed and dictated by senior physicians, based largely on their own clinical experience, which junior staff were unable to challenge. The purpose of evidence-based medicine (EBM) as an educational intervention was therefore to teach medical students to search for and appraise 'evidence from clinical research' in order to confront practice based on 'intuition, unsystematic clinical experience and pathophysiological rationale'. As the authors pointed out, EBM 'puts a much lower value on authority. The underlying belief is that physicians can gain the skills to make independent assessments of evidence and thus evaluate the credibility of opinions being offered by experts' (EBMWG 1992: 2421).

The authors made it clear that the term 'evidence' refers solely to the findings from research studies, and that the critical appraisal of evidence is based almost entirely on methodological criteria, with randomised controlled trials considered to be the gold standard. Whilst they proclaimed EBM to be 'a new paradigm for medical practice', the basic principle of 'using the medical literature more effectively in guiding medical practice' was neither new nor revolutionary, even in the 1990s. If their claim that EBM represented a paradigm shift holds water, it is in the field of medical education rather than practice. What was arguably new about EBM as an educational intervention was the emphasis it placed on teaching literature searching and research appraisal skills to undergraduates, and on encouraging and empowering them to use these newly acquired abilities to challenge current practice. However, the authors were somewhat cautious about the reach and scope of EBM, since 'many aspects of clinical practice cannot, or will not, ever be adequately tested'. Furthermore, they conceded that the practice of EBM was not and might never itself be evidence-based, since 'no long-term randomised trials of traditional and evidence-based medical education are likely to be carried out'. Nevertheless, the clear message from the EBMWG was that the skills of efficient literature searching and the critical appraisal of research findings can be of greater relevance in arriving at a correct diagnosis and prescribing best treatment than clinical experience and pathophysiologic rationale.

As might have been expected, this challenge to established ways of working was met with resistance from those clinicians whose power and authority was perceived to be under threat. This led several members of the EBMWG to publish a short paper entitled 'Evidence-Based Medicine: What It Is and What It Isn't' (Sackett *et al.* 1996) in a bid to reassure senior physicians that EBM was not a 'cookbook approach' to practice and that clinical experience and expertise was not being undermined. Thus, the earlier and more radical approach to EBM as a direct challenge to expert opinion was downplayed in this later paper and EBM was recast as 'the conscientious, explicit, and judicious use of current best evidence in making decisions about the care of individual patients. The practice of evidence based medicine means integrating individual clinical expertise with the best available clinical evidence from systematic research' (Sackett *et al.* 1996: 71).

As before, the term 'evidence' continued to refer only to the findings from research. The quality of that evidence continued to be appraised according to the methods by which it was produced, with randomised controlled trials (RCTs) remaining as the gold standard. However, it was no longer considered appropriate simply to make clinical decisions based solely on the findings from RCTs. Evidence had to be used 'judiciously' and 'conscientiously' and clinicians were now expected to integrate the evidence with 'individual clinical expertise'. Sackett added that:

> external clinical evidence can inform, but can never replace, individual clinical expertise, and *it is this expertise that decides whether the external evidence applies to the individual patient at all* and, if so, how it should be integrated into a clinical decision.
>
> (Sackett *et al.* 1996: 72, my emphasis)

Sackett's statement remains probably the most cited definition not only of EBM but of evidence-based practice more generally. However, in his attempt to reassure his critics, Sackett's amended version of EBM severely limited the very challenge to clinical authority that it was originally devised to instigate. Whereas the EBMWG (1992) outlined an educational programme to equip students and junior physicians with a strategy for challenging expert opinion with research-based evidence, Sackett's revised definition of EBM allowed senior clinicians simply to dismiss any research evidence with which they disagreed. Since 'individual clinical expertise' is described merely as 'the proficiency and judgment that individual clinicians acquire through clinical experience and clinical practice' (Sackett *et al.* 1996), any challenges to that expertise are extremely difficult to articulate and sustain. Furthermore, since students presumably lack the prerequisite experience required for clinical expertise, they themselves are not equipped to practice evidence-based medicine. Thus, whereas the original EBMWG paper claimed that EBM constituted a 'new paradigm for medical practice' which de-emphasised intuition and clinical experience in favour of evidence from research, Sackett and colleagues' later paper reinstated the power and authority of senior clinicians to assert their expertise in order to dismiss any research evidence with which they disagreed.

Early developments: from evidence-based medicine to evidence-based practice

It is probably fair to say that 'evidence-based' has by now come to be used almost as a synonym for 'best quality'. As Feinstein and Horwitz (1997) noted, a mere five years after the term was first introduced, it had already 'acquired the kind of sanctity often accorded to motherhood, home, and the flag', and as such, was almost unassailable. As we have seen, however, EBM was not quite the 'new paradigm' claimed by the EBMWG, but merely added evidence from research to the list of considerations to be taken into account when arriving at a clinical decision, without explicitly stating how such decisions might be reached. Indeed, Sackett's revised definition of EBM is arguably nothing more than a restatement of an already established tradition of research-based practice, where it is left to the judgment of individual practitioners to decide whether and how to incorporate research findings into their clinical decisions. In the decade following the declaration of the new paradigm, EBM was developed, modified and broadened out into a variety of interpretations and definitions as different professional groups adapted it to their own specific needs, with nursing being one of the first to do so. Some writers attempted a more or less direct translation of the principles and tenets of EBM to the practice of nursing. For example, Ingersoll's (2000) paper 'Evidence-Based Nursing: What It Is and What It Isn't' not only mimicked the title of Sackett *et al.*'s (1996) earlier paper but it closely mirrored the wording of his definition. For Ingersoll, '[e]vidence-based nursing practice is the conscientious, explicit and judicious use of theory-derived, research-based information in making decisions about care delivery to individuals or groups of patients and in consideration of individual needs and preferences' (Ingersoll 2000: 152).

The most notable modification to the original medical definition is the addition of the term 'theory-derived ... information', presumably in recognition of the work of the American nurse theorists, although the extent to which that body of work could be described as 'evidence' is perhaps debatable. In contrast to this attempt to create an evidence-based approach to nursing in the image of EBM, Mulhall (1998) made the plea that 'tiptoeing in the wake of the movement for evidence-based medicine, however, we must ensure that evidence-based nursing attends to what is important for nursing'. Arguably, this entails attending not only to the differences between medical and nursing *practice*, but also to differences in what constitutes best *evidence* and what it means for practice to be *based* on evidence. Each of these elements of evidence-based practice will now be discussed in turn with particular reference to nursing.

Evidence and expertise

The debate concerning whether and to what extent alternatives to the 'gold standard' experimental methods should be considered as valid forms of evidence on which to base nursing practice is long-standing and continuing, and is addressed in several other chapters in this book. In response to Mulhall's point that nursing is distinct and different from medicine, discussions initially revolved around the relevance and importance of qualitative methods to the practice of nursing. However, a more fundamental question which was often overlooked concerns the disagreement and confusion over the status of expert opinion or clinical expertise as a form of evidence.[1] We have seen that Sackett made a clear distinction between evidence and expertise, where *evidence* refers solely to the findings from research, with the RCT being 'the "gold standard" for judging whether a treatment does more harm that good' and where the expertise of the practitioner determines whether and how the evidence should be applied in any specific situation. However, we have also seen that Sackett's distinction challenges the simple and perhaps simplistic formulation of evidence-based practice as the straightforward application of 'gold standard' research findings by suggesting that the evidence can be *overridden* by the clinical judgment of the practitioner. Even the most avid advocate of evidence-based practice would probably allow that, on occasion, the experienced practitioner might decide that a particular patient could benefit from an intervention that is not supported by the best evidence from research. However, if the practitioner continues to override the evidence in more and more cases, at what point would we wish to say that their practice could no longer be described as evidence-based? If the full implications of Sackett's definition are accepted, *evidence*-based practice is, in fact, *expertise*-based practice, insofar as the expert opinion of the practitioner is *always* the determining factor in coming to a clinical decision.

In response to the dilemma raised by the role of expert opinion in evidence-based practice, some writers chose to recast clinical expertise as simply *another source of evidence* rather than, in Sackett *et al.*'s (1996) words, as 'the proficiency and judgment' about if and when to *apply* evidence. For example, Evans (2003) broadened out the principles of EBM to apply them more generally to health care and offered three separate hierarchies of evidence depending on whether the clinical question relates to effectiveness, appropriateness or feasibility (Table 8.1). In all three cases, systematic reviews, multi-centre studies and RCTs are at the top of the hierarchy and expert opinion is at the bottom, alongside 'studies of poor methodological quality' (Evans 2003), a pattern that is replicated in many other

Table 8.1 Hierarchy of evidence: ranking of research evidence evaluating healthcare interventions

	Effectiveness	*Appropriateness*	*Feasibility*
Excellent	Systematic review Multi-centre studies	Systematic review Multi-centre studies	Systematic review Multi-centre studies
Good	Randomised controlled trials Observational studies	Randomised controlled trials Observational studies Interpretive studies	Randomised controlled trials Observational studies Interpretive studies
Fair	Uncontrolled trials with dramatic results Before-and-after studies Non-randomized controlled trials	Descriptive studies Focus groups	Descriptive studies Action research Before-and-after studies Focus groups
Poor	Descriptive studies Case studies Expert opinion Studies of poor methodological quality	Expert opinion Case studies Studies of poor methodological quality	Expert opinion Case studies Studies of poor methodological quality

Source: Evans 2003

hierarchies of evidence (see, for example, Long 1996, Ellis 2000, Thompson and Dowding 2002). Whereas, for Sackett, individual clinical expertise is the key to evidence-based practice and the most important factor in deciding whether or not to apply research evidence, Evans considers expert opinion to be 'at the greatest risk of error and inadequate for evaluating the effectiveness of an intervention'. Although Evans quotes Sackett approvingly, his somewhat mechanistic view of EBP could be considered as directly opposing Sackett's reassurance that it is not simply the 'cookbook' application of research findings.

Clearly, the issue of whether expertise is a lowly form of evidence or the key factor in determining if the evidence applies is more than just semantics. Whilst Evans sidestepped Sackett's challenge to integrate evidence and expertise, other writers have responded to it by representing the relationship in the form of a Venn diagram of overlapping circles. For example, rather than accepting Sackett's assertion of expertise as the key element in formulating an evidence-based decision, DiCenso *et al.* (1998) presented evidence-based nursing more simply as a combination of research evidence, resources, patients' preferences and clinical expertise (Figure 8.1). Unfortunately, they offered no clear indication as to how these factors might be integrated to arrive at a clinical decision, beyond the vague instruction that research evidence might be overridden by one or more of the other factors.

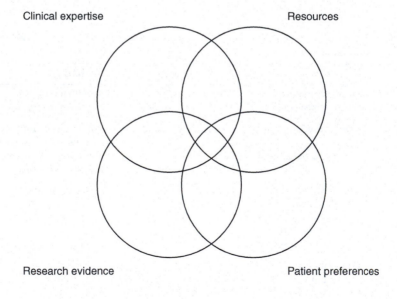

Figure 8.1 A model for evidence-based clinical decisions
Source: DiCenso *et al.* 1998

Rycroft-Malone *et al.* (2004) produced a similar diagram (Figure 8.2) but, whereas DiCenso retained Sackett's distinction between evidence and expertise, this model followed Evans by regarding experience/expertise as a source of evidence. Unlike Evans, however, they did not relegate it to the bottom of the hierarchy of evidence but suggested that all four elements represented in their Venn diagram should be 'melded together in the real-time of clinical decision-making' (Rycroft-Malone *et al.* 2004: 88). They conceded that they had no clear idea as to how this might happen, although they postulated 'a form of professional artistry including critical appreciation, synchronicity, balance and interplay'. However, they continued: 'As we are not entirely clear how this occurs, we also do not know how best it could be facilitated'.

We can see the same discrepancies and disagreements being played out in this book. For example, Thorne distinguishes between 'evidential knowledge' (knowledge derived from quantitative and some qualitative research) and 'non-evidential knowledge' (other forms of knowledge which do not meet her criteria for being regarded as evidence). In contrast, Garrett's chapter argues that not all evidence is derived from research and is concerned explicitly with a discussion of 'non-research evidence'. Many of the other chapters adopt one or other of these positions on what constitutes evidence, whilst one or two appear to mix and match or fail to make any distinctions.

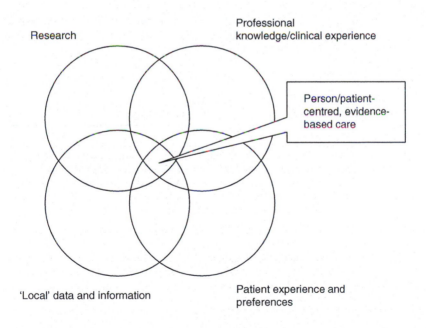

Figure 8.2 Four sources of evidence for patient-centred, evidence-based practice
Source: Rycroft-Malone *et al.* 2004

Evidence as the basis for practice

In addition to disputes and disagreements about what counts as evidence, the literature reveals a number of differences of interpretation in what it means to *base* practice on evidence. We have already seen that certain writers suggest that research evidence should always override expert clinical opinion (for example, Evans 2003, Paley 2006), whereas others argue that research and expertise should be considered together (e.g. DiCenso *et al.* 1998, Rycroft-Malone *et al.* 2004), with Sackett *et al.* (1996) going so far as to claim that clinical expertise always determines whether and how research evidence should be applied. I refer to the former view as the 'hard' approach and the latter as the 'soft' approach to the application of evidence. In some cases, expertise is recognised as a form of evidence in its own right whereas, in others, evidence and expertise are regarded as separate factors. In addition, some writers argue that only the 'best' available evidence should be used. Thus: 'if no randomised trial has been carried out for our patient's predicament, we must follow the trail to the next best external evidence and work from there' (Sackett *et al.* 1996: 72). In contrast, others suggest that evidence from across the hierarchy can be used together, providing that it is appropriately weighted (Hewitt-Taylor 2003) or 'melded together' (Rycroft-Malone *et al.* 2004). I refer to these as exclusive and inclusive[2] hierarchies respectively (Table 8.2).

These four interpretations of what it means to *base* practice on evidence could also be organised as a continuum from rationality to reasonableness, where the hard exclusive approach represents the most *rational* model of evidence-based nursing and the soft inclusive approach is the most reasonable.[3] We can see, then,

Table 8.2 Different approaches to basing practice on evidence

Approach	Exclusive	Inclusive
Hard	Only evidence from highest in the hierarchy should be used. Evidence will always override expert clinical opinion (e.g. EBMWG 1992, Evans 2003)	Evidence from anywhere in the hierarchy can be used. Will always override expert clinical opinion[1]
Soft	Only evidence from highest in the hierarchy should be used. Evidence should be considered together with expert opinion (e.g. Sackett 1996, DiCenso *et al.* 1998)	Evidence from anywhere in the hierarchy can be used. Should be considered together with expert opinion (e.g. Rycroft-Malone *et al.* 2004)

Note:
[1]   It should be noted that whilst a hard inclusive approach to evidence-based practice is possible in theory, it is difficult to find any writers who admit all forms of research evidence but omit expertise from evidence-based decisions

that when practitioners are urged to *base* their interventions on evidence, it is not altogether clear quite what they are being expected to do.

Nursing practice in the swampy lowlands

To complicate matters further, there are at least two quite distinct concepts of practice described in the literature, each of which, arguably, has a different relationship to evidence. Some writers refer exclusively to one or other of these concepts when arguing the merits and demerits of different types of evidence, others consider practice only in vague and abstract terms, while yet others make no direct reference to it whatsoever. The original paper by the EBMWG focused on practice as a planned and methodical intervention over the course of a treatment programme. For example, the authors provide a clinical scenario in which a junior medical resident responds to a question from a patient by visiting the library to conduct a literature search. This view of evidence-based practice as searching for evidence in order to plan interventions in advance can be seen in medicine in Rosenberg and Donald's (1995) four steps of formulating a clinical question, searching the literature, evaluating the evidence and implementing the findings in clinical practice. It is also apparent in evidence-based nursing practice in Hek and Moule's (2006) five stages of identifying a problem, searching the literature, appraising the evidence, taking the patient's needs and preferences into account and evaluating the effects of the intervention. This carefully measured approach might appear familiar to some doctors, for whom practice is largely a matter of formulating a diagnosis and prescribing a treatment programme. However, the practice of nursing is often of a quite different nature. Most nurses rarely have the luxury of being able to drop in and out of the practice situation in such a planned way; they are present in the clinical setting for an eight-hour shift and have to respond on the spot to whatever situations and problems present themselves. This is what Rycroft-Malone *et al.* (2004) were referring to when they spoke of the 'professional artistry' which takes place in 'the real time of clinical decision-making'. Of course, some nursing decisions, such as deciding to place a patient on a pressure-relieving mattress, deciding whether or not to give 'when necessary' medication or deciding to refer a patient to a dietician, can be carefully considered over an extended period, with reference to the research literature. However, nurses will often be called upon to make on-the-spot decisions in response to unique and unexpected situations and developments. Schön frames these two approaches to practice in the following way: 'In the varied topography of professional practice there is a high, hard ground where practitioners can make effective use of research-based theory and technique, and there is a swampy lowland where situations are confusing 'messes' incapable of technical solution' (Schön 1983: 42).

Practice in the 'swampy lowland' constantly presents us with unexpected and unanticipated challenges, which demand an instant response with no time to consult text books or research journals. Not only is there no evidence base to hand for these messy problems but, as Schön tells us, these are problems which, in any case, are simply not amenable to research-based technical solutions.

This distinction between practice as a pre-planned methodical intervention from the 'high hard ground' and as a spontaneous and messy response to whatever confronts us in the 'swampy lowland' brings us full circle to a reconsideration of the nature of evidence. On the high hard ground, evidence is amassed from research studies prior to the practice intervention and is employed in order to plan how the practitioner will act. Down in the swampy lowland, evidence is uncovered during (or sometimes after) the practice intervention in order to make sense of what has already happened and to shape the ongoing situation. This evidence is not generated by researchers but by practitioners reflecting critically on their unique and singular encounters with each of their unique and singular patients in a process which Schön (1983) refers to as 'reflection-in-action' or 'on-the-spot experimenting'.

Furthermore, Schön suggests that the collection of evidence through reflection-in-action cannot be separated from practice. Evidence is not something that is applied to practice but which emerges from practice as an integral part of practice itself. Reflection-in-action is a form of experimentation in which hypotheses are generated and tested on-the-spot in the practice situation:

> When someone reflects-in-action, he becomes a researcher in the practice context. He is not dependent on the categories of established theory and technique, but constructs a new theory of the unique case. His inquiry is not limited to a deliberation about means which depends on a prior agreement about ends. He does not keep means and ends separate, but defines them interactively as he frames a problematic situation. He does not separate thinking from doing, ratiocinating his way to a decision which he must later convert to action. Because his experimenting is a kind of action, implementation is built into his inquiry. Thus reflection-in-action can proceed, even in situations of uncertainty or uniqueness, because it is not bound by the dichotomies of Technical Rationality.
>
> (Schön 1983: 68–9)

As Schön tells us, practice in the swampy lowlands does not separate thinking from doing. Rather, practice is a form of research; evidence about the effectiveness of a practice intervention is immediately and reflexively applied back into practice.

I am suggesting, then, that the term 'practice' can be used to refer to at least two distinct and quite different nursing activities. On the one hand, nursing practice can sometimes be a rational procedure that can be planned in advance and implemented on the high hard ground more or less as expected. On the other hand, a great deal of everyday nursing practice takes place in the swampy lowlands where messy problems must be dealt with on the spot, and where evidence about what is and is not effective only emerges *after* an intervention has been made. In a great deal of the debate and discussion about evidence-based nursing, this distinction is not fully (or even partially) articulated, leading often to exaggerated and inflated claims about the benefits or otherwise of qualitative or quantitative research methods as sources of 'best evidence', with little or no consideration of the nature of the practice to which this evidence will be applied. Indeed, some of the more assertive and emphatic statements from the 'high hard ground' which promote the rigorous and at times rigid application of 'gold standard' quantitative research findings appear to be written by professional researchers and academics with little or no first-hand experience of the messy world of nursing practice.

In contrast to the criticism that some advocates of evidence-based nursing are too detached from the realities of practice, others have objected that practitioners down in the swampy lowlands are perhaps too immersed in practice and are therefore blind to the fallibility of their own professional judgment in comparison to the rigorous application of hard research evidence (for example, Paley 2006). Paley argues firstly that experiential knowledge resulting from reflection does not qualify as bona fide evidence because it does not meet certain criteria, particularly the systematic elimination of error. Secondly, he claims that even in clinical situations which the practitioner knows to be messy and singular, 'playing the percentages' by applying the evidence from quantitative research will still have a statistically greater chance of being successful than an intervention based on expertise or experience.

I suggest that practice based on reflection-in-action, as described above, addresses both of these objections. Firstly, the process of systematically adjusting practice as it is taking place through the accumulation of evidence from the practice setting itself is an effective way of minimizing error by testing the practice intervention against reality. Secondly, Paley's dismissal of experience or expertise as less effective than simply applying the research-based solution in each and every case does not take into account Schön's notion of expertise as a process of systematically learning from the situation as part of the act of responding to it. Paley's 'evidence' for the superiority of 'playing the odds' is based on a static view of expertise as simply the accumulation of knowledge from previous experience rather than the dynamic process of generating and testing evidence in the here-and-now. As he admits: 'There are, of course, numerous variations on the theme [of expertise], especially following the incorporation of reflective practice … However, *my preference here is to use a broad brush, dispensing with the subtleties*' (Paley 2006: 88, my emphasis).

Paley's broad brush effectively paints out the differences between the subtle and not-so-subtle theories of expertise and presents them all as merely variations on a single theme. However, the model of expert practice based on reflection-in-action addresses Paley's 'error criterion' by immediately testing the evidence against the real world of practice and adjusting practice and evidence accordingly, although there are no comparative studies to determine whether it is more effective than 'playing the odds'.

Conclusion

I have argued in this chapter that a great deal of the disagreement surrounding the theory and practice of evidence-based nursing stems from misunderstandings about definitions and the use of words. Much of the dispute focuses on the question of what counts as 'best evidence', particularly in relation to qualitative and quantitative research methods, clinical experience and other forms of nursing knowledge. Attempts to answer this question have generated far more heat than light but, in any case, I have suggested that this is neither the most interesting question about evidence-based nursing nor the most important. Furthermore, any answers to this question depend on the answers we give to two prior questions: *What do we understand by practice?* and *What do we mean when we claim that practice is based on evidence?* Indeed, I would go so far as to say that it is meaningless to discuss the nature of evidence without relating it directly and explicitly to the nature of practice.

The term 'nursing practice' covers a wide range of activities which often have only a family resemblance to one another and these varied activities can stand in a number of different relationships to the evidence; indeed, the idea of evidence will take on different meanings depending on the nature of the practice with which it is associated. I therefore consider it to be misleading and misguided to advocate a single best approach to evidence-based nursing, if for no other reason than there is no single idea or concept that covers the entirety of nursing practice. Even the most junior nurse with the most limited experience knows that the term 'practice' covers a wide variety of activities, including medical and quasi-medical nursing interventions, such as intubating a patient or giving an injection, psychological interventions such as reassuring a frightened patient or comforting a bereaved relative, public health interventions such as educating patients about diet and exercise or persuading mothers to have their children vaccinated, and intensely personal interventions such as bathing a patient of the opposite sex or comforting someone who is dying. Nursing usually involves complex combinations of these different types of intervention in one and the same act, it is (among other things) part motor skill, part problem solving and part relationship building, and it is therefore partially invisible to the naked eye; nursing is concerned with *being* and with *relating* as much as with *doing*. There are also moral, ethical, professional and human considerations to the practice of nursing which suggest that, under the circumstances, the most rational intervention might not be the most reasonable one (and vice versa).

These are all aspects of the daily job of the nurse and all are subsumed under the general term 'nursing practice'. In the case of technical interventions, the 'best evidence' for practice will usually be based on the findings from quantitative, experimental research. If there has been a randomised controlled trial which has determined the most effective method of intubating a patient, then that is the method I would want for myself and my family. Having said that, I know of many experienced nurses who have modified so-called best practice through careful experimentation in response to feedback from their patients and have demonstrated measurably better outcomes as a result. In other cases, particularly in the psychosocial domain of nursing practice, the most important and relevant nursing questions can usually best be answered through naturalistic research methods such as participant observation and in-depth interviews. Even when quantitative research findings are available, it is often qualitative research which provides the necessary knowledge and information to understand and empathise with the distressed, frightened, embarrassed, confused, aggressive, unpleasant or uncooperative human being confronting the nurse. Indeed, it is important to remember that the purpose of research is not only to instruct nurses on what to do; it also helps them to understand and comprehend the practice situation so that they might decide for themselves how best to act. In addition, there will be instances when the intervention that best meets the technical demands of the situation does not best meet the human needs, when 'best practice' is not necessarily that which is dictated by research but rather by our empathic human response and accumulated professional wisdom. This, I suspect, is what Sackett was suggesting when he claimed that external clinical evidence can never replace individual clinical expertise, and 'it is this expertise that decides whether the external evidence applies to the individual patient at all' (Sackett *et al.* 1996).

In some cases, however, there simply *are* no research findings because there are times in the swampy lowlands when technical rationality fails altogether, when research simply cannot provide the answers that the nurse requires. Sometimes this will be because the questions which practice poses cannot be answered by researchers and sometimes it will be because it is not even clear to the nurse what the questions are. Sometimes nurses must simply do what feels right and modify their responses according to the evidence that their interventions generate from the midst of the unfolding practice situation. Whether or not we regard this as bona fide evidence and whether or not we refer to it as evidence-based practice might appear to be a question of semantics but, in reality, it matters greatly. At a time when the pressures on nurses to base their practice on 'the evidence' is intense, it is important that they are able to justify the full range of interventions open to them in terms of evidence-based practice.

The practice of nursing, whatever else it might be, is a series of human encounters which can never be rationalised into an algorithm for 'best practice'. In the words of the song, people are strange; that is, they are often unpredictable and sometimes completely unknowable. To imagine that the simple and straightforward application of research-based evidence into 'best practice' is the norm, or in some cases is even possible, is to have forgotten the richness and strangeness of practice. If we in the academic community wish to have a sensible, meaningful and, above all, useful conversation about evidence-based practice, we must firstly learn to speak a common language and then enter into a dialogue with our practice colleagues and listen to what they are telling us about the rich and strange world of nursing.

Notes

1   When I refer to expert opinion or expertise in this chapter I am using the term in Sackett's non-technical sense of the proficiency and judgment acquired through experience and practice. In this sense, the terms expertise and experience are largely interchangeable.

2   My use of the term 'inclusive' should not be confused or conflated with Paley's term
    'inclusionist' used in this book and elsewhere (Paley 2006). In particular, I do not
    wish to imply that the 'inclusive' approach that I am outlining here is a political or
    ideological move but, rather, it is a sincere attempt by its advocates to promote best
    nursing practice.

3   For a detailed discussion of reason and rationality in medical practice, see Toulmin
    (2001), particularly Chapter 7 'Practical Reason and the Clinical Arts', which distin-
    guishes 'between a practitioner's reasonable judgments and a theoreticians rational
    computations'. Gadamer (1996) also explores the limitations of rationality in the prac-
    tice of medicine, arguing that health is fundamentally 'enigmatic' and its restoration
    and maintenance is as much an art as a science. We could also apply Heidegger's
    (1966) distinction between calculative and meditative thinking.

References

DiCenso, A., Cullum, N. and Ciliska, D. (1998) Implementing evidence–based nursing:
some misconceptions. *Evidence-Based Nursing*, 1(2), 38–40.

Ellis, J. (2000) Sharing the evidence: clinical practice benchmarking to improve continu-
ously the quality of care. *Journal of Advanced Nursing*, 32(1), 215–25.

Evans, D. (2003) Hierarchy of evidence: a framework for ranking evidence evaluating
healthcare interventions. *Journal of Clinical Nursing*, 12, 77–84.

EBMWG (1992) Evidence-based medicine – a new approach to teaching the practice of
medicine. Evidence-Based Medicine Working Group. *JAMA*, 268(17), 2420–5.

Feinstein, A. R. and Horwitz, R. I. (1997) Problems in the 'evidence' of 'evidence-based
medicine'. *American Journal of Medicine*, 103, 529–35.

Gadamer, H.-G. (1996) *The Enigma of Health*. Cambridge: Polity.

Heidegger, M. (1966) *Discourse on Thinking*. New York: Harper Row.

Hek, G. and Moule, P. (2006) *Making Sense of Research*. London: Sage.

Hewitt-Taylor, J. (2003) Reviewing evidence. *Intensive and Critical Care Nursing*, 19, 43–9.

Ingersoll, G. L. (2000) Evidence-based nursing: what it is and what it isn't. *Nursing
Outlook*, 48, 151–2.

Long, A. (1996) Health services research: a radical approach to cross the research and
development divide? In M. Baker and S. Kirk (eds) *Research and Development for the
NHS: Evidence, Evaluation and Effectiveness* (pp. 51–63). Oxford: Radcliffe.

Mulhall, A. (1998) Nursing, research, and the evidence. *Evidence-Based Nursing*, 1(1),
4–6.

Paley, J. (2006) Evidence and expertise. *Nursing Inquiry*, 13(2), 82–93.

Rosenberg, W. and Donald, A. (1995) Evidence-based medicine: an approach to clinical
problem-solving. *British Medical Journal*, 310, 1122–6.

Rycroft-Malone, J., Seers, K., Titchen, A., Harvey, G., Kitson, A. and McCormack, B.
(2004) What counts as evidence in evidence-based practice? *Journal of Advanced
Nursing*, 47(1), 81–90.

Sackett, D. L., Rosenberg, W. M. C., Gray, J. A. M., Haynes, R. B. and Richardson, W. S.
(1996) Evidence-based medicine: what it is and what it isn't. *British Journal of
Medicine*, 312, 71–2.

Schön, D. (1983) *The Reflective Practitioner*. London: Temple Smith.

Toulmin, S. (2001) *Return to Reason*. Cambridge, MA: Harvard University Press.

Thompson, C. and Dowding, D. (2002) *Clinical Decision Making and Judgement in
Nursing*. Edinburgh: Churchill Livingstone.

9 Non-research evidence

What we overlook (but shouldn't)

Bernie Garrett

In this chapter, I explore some aspects of evidence-based practice (EBP) that often get overlooked in the narrative. As explored in the previous chapters, there have been some rather inflammatory and even polemic attacks on the nature of EBP within nursing over the past decade (for example, Holmes *et al.*, 2006, 2012). Outside the ontological and epistemological arguments over the fundamental nature of knowledge and evidence, much of the critique is based on an interpretation of EBP that focuses upon the formulation of research questions, the relative merits of different research methodologies and the use of research findings. Indeed, some textbooks and chapters on EBP designed for undergraduate students almost entirely focus on the research methods and the hierarchy of evidence, presenting EBP in a manner that largely ignores non-research forms of evidence (for example, Levin and Feldman, 2013). Nevertheless, the original conception of EBP proposed by Archie Cochrane (1972), and later David Sackett *et al.* (1996, 2000), identified a far wider context for evidence. It is important to explore the implications of this focus on research evidence, particularly in nursing education, for its impact on the understanding of EBP that nurses develop through their education and the care they subsequently offer. In this chapter I compare all the forms of evidence inherent in the EBP process and review how the limitations in curriculum time devoted to EBP and how an over-emphasis on research (or discovery based) evidence in EBP impacts the level of scientific literacy that can be realistically expected of students in contemporary nursing programs.

Context

Before we explore the nature of non-research forms of evidence, it is worthwhile to briefly reflect on the nature of EBP, and why its grounding in empirical scientific research is viewed as being central to the approach. EBP represents a highly significant positive innovation in healthcare provision, and arguably is one of the best examples of the benefits of the application of science in modern society over the twentieth century. However, the term "evidence-based" probably also represents one of the most poorly understood adjectives in professional nursing (Garrett, 2013; Melnyk and Fineout-Overholt, 2011; Smyth and Craig, 2002).

Modern EBP is recognized to have developed over the last thirty years from the evidence-based medicine (EBM) movement (although many of its ideas are much older), and particularly from the original work of the Scottish physician Archie Cochrane (1972). Cochrane originally sought to overthrow the dominance of medical authority and expertise in the provision of medical care. He outlined a systematic approach to healthcare decision making that involved the practitioner asking: "what is the best solution to this particular health issue?" His ideas suggest that we consider the following aspects as evidence to support our clinical decisions: the scientific evidence of a demonstrated positive (or negative) effect of a specific intervention/approach, the specific clinical situation, and the economic viability. Particularly, he went on to develop the principles behind modern systematic reviews and meta-analyses that are argued to provide the best quality of research evidence. Following Archie Cochrane's innovative ideas, the work of David Sacket and his colleagues helped develop the EBM movement at the turn of the century (Sacket *et al.*, 2000). In their model for EBM, they identified finding and evaluating research evidence in stages 2 and 3 of the process outlined in Table 9.1, but building on Cochrane's earlier ideas, they also outlined the importance of clinical expertise and patient values here also, in stage 4. This recognized the uniqueness of the specific clinical situation, and patient autonomy in the process. However, often these aspects are less prominent or even absent in other models, as they are considered in the implementation or integration phases of the process.

Table 9.1 Models of evidence-based practice implementation

Stage	Evidence-based medicine[1]	Iowa model[2]	Diffusion of innovation[3]	ACE Star model[4]	PICO model[5]
1	Ask a question	Ask a question	Acquire knowledge	Discovery	Ask a PICO question
2	Find the best evidence	Literature search	Persuasion	Summary	Collect evidence
3	Evaluate the evidence	Appraise evidence	Decision	Translation	Appraise evidence
4	Application in combination with clinical expertise and patient values	Implementation	Implementation	Implementation	Integration
5	Evaluate	Evaluate	Confirmation	Evaluate	Evaluate

Notes:
[1]   Sacket *et al.*, 2000
[2]   Titler *et al.*, 2001
[3]   Rogers, 2003
[4]   ACE Star Model of Knowledge Transformation®; Stevens, 2004
[5]   Problem/population, intervention, comparison, and outcome model; Melnyk and Fineout-Overholt, 2011

The semantics of EBP

The interpretation of the term evidence is key in some of the concerns raised about EBP. Practically, evidence may be thought of as the proof supporting a particular claim or belief and, in the case of public health interventions, evidence typically refers to the effectiveness of an intervention in achieving a particular outcome that will create health benefits for an individual or population. A simple and generally well-accepted example being that brushing our teeth regularly is believed to decrease the risk of dental disease, although one study revealed a wide diversity between recommendations on tooth brushing techniques, how often people should brush their teeth and for how long (Wainright and Sheiham, 2014). On the other hand, on related research into the value of fluoridated water to prevent dental decay, systematic reviews of the value of fluoridation have suggested it does result in a reduction of dental caries, but that its value in over-all dental health is much less clear (McDonagh *et al.*, 2000; Yeung, 2008). These studies also found that there was no significant evidence that it represents the major health risk some anti-fluoridation proponents have claimed (Fluoride Action Network, 2014). As these examples demonstrate, in EBP, the use of the term 'evidence' is firmly grounded in empirical science. For example, we can cite reviews, trials, case studies and experiments that demonstrate that those who regularly brush their teeth suffer fewer dental problems than those who do not as a basis for dental policy and patient advice. It is also important to acknowledge that this process also affords that the acquisition of new evidence may change our previously established knowledge.

EBP also presents a particular hierarchical structure for the quality of this evidence (see the discussion in other chapters, and Figure 9.1). Such evidence is usually published in scientific literature, such as in professional journals, books, or government reports. EBP is based on a particular set of epistemological values and beliefs (scientific rationalism). If your belief framework does not accept the established notion of illness, disease and health to begin with (Holmes *et al.* 2012), you are unlikely to find EBP a satisfactory paradigm upon which to base professional healthcare.

Other chapters in this volume engage with some of the semantic issues surrounding the use of the term "evidence-based," and in consideration of such arguments some academics have argued for the term "evidence-informed prac-tice" to be used to bring the focus back onto research informing nursing practice, with the nurse as the critical professional decision maker using a wider context of evidence, rather than the focus being the scientific evidence, research and quan-titative measures (McSherry *et al.*, 2002). Others have suggested an alternative term, which some may find more appealing as "research enhanced health care" (Haynes *et al.*, 2002). However, the rationale for this seems to be based on a particular view of EBP that emphasizes the research evidence component of EBP over other aspects, and also seems, a move by nursing academics to further distance the profession from the scientific paradigm adopted by medicine. This view clearly attempts to take the emphasis away from the centrality of scientific

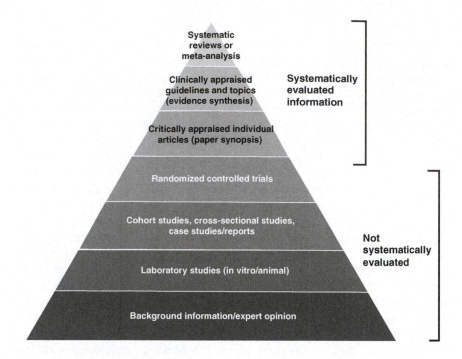

Systematic
reviews or
meta-analysis

Clinically appraised
guidelines and topics
(evidence synthesis)

Systematically
evaluated
information

Critically appraised individual
articles (paper synopsis)

Randomized controlled trials

Cohort studies, cross-sectional studies,
case studies/reports

Not
systematically
evaluated

Laboratory studies (in vitro/animal)

Background information/expert opinion

Figure 9.1 The pyramid of evidence

evidence in the process, and to focus on the way the nurse uses it, but practically seems to offer no perceptible advantage other than to apply the ideas in a slightly different context. Indeed, it is more likely to promote more room for confusion as to the underlying nature of EBP, and its scientific rationale (which as we have noted, already includes clinical judgment and patient preference). The whole rationale for EBP is the critical examination of evidence by the practitioner using experience, judgment and expertise with the best available evidence from systematic investigation. Indeed, as Sacket *et al.* identified in 1996: "without clinical expertise, practice risks becoming tyrannized by evidence" and "EBP is not restricted to randomized trials and meta-analyses." As the focus on research, practice and decision making is already clearly defined in EBP, there seems little benefit from engaging in such semantic debates, and promoting better understanding of the non-research evidence aspects of EBP would seem a more rewarding activity. EBP is about healthcare professionals using quantitative and qualitative information, together with other forms of knowledge, wisely in a clinical context. EBP incorporates other forms of knowledge, including patient preferences, and clinical expertise, so let us explore all the different forms of evidence inherent within EBP, and particularly those non-research evidence components in more detail.

The centrality of clinical research

One of the central features of EBP is the attempt to identify what represents the best research evidence to support clinical decisions. Therefore, the theoretical development of EBP has mainly been based in three key areas; firstly, developing information systems and tools to process and support the acquisition and dissemination of research evidence; secondly, on clinical research question development to support EBP; and thirdly on devising a consensual hierarchy of best evidence.

Probably the largest area of work in the EBP field has been in the development of centralized research dissemination systems. For example, following Cochrane's original work the UK National Health Service led to the establishment of the Cochrane Centre in Oxford (ukcc.cochrane.org) at the end of 1992, with the aim of making up-to-date and accurate information about the effects of healthcare interventions available worldwide. Interest in EBP has increased exponentially and other Cochrane centres and similar EBP organizations have developed throughout the world.

EBP questions most usually come directly from clients, or from practitioners as they provide and evaluate care in terms of the treatment options, effectiveness, appropriateness, or efficiency of specific interventions and practices. They may also arise from reviewing traditional practices, or from the professional literature. One approach to understand the nature of clinical questions has been to collect and classify actual clinical queries (Ely *et al.*, 2000; Jerome *et al.*, 2001). Such analyses have yielded a wide variety of clinical questions. Sackett *et al.* (2000) suggest that, for medicine, these may be classified as either background questions, related to physiology, pathophysiology, epidemiology and disease/condition progression or foreground questions relating to which treatment is most effective for condition X in patient Y. These foreground questions have been the focus for most published work in this area, and led to suggested formats for asking EBP questions such as the well-known: problem/population, intervention, comparison, and outcome (PICO) format; for example, for chest pain immediately following a myocardial infarction, is it better to give an intravenous bolus of morphine or the thrombolytic drugs first, to best support long-term cardiac function? There are varying different forms of this format and the exact origins of its development remain rather unclear, but it is firmly rooted in medicine, and likely developed form the ideas of Scott Richardson and colleagues (1995), Mark Ebell (1999) and Eamon Armstrong (1999).

This approach has been widely promoted by some nursing researchers such as Melnyck and Finout-Overholt (2011). Nevertheless, designing EBP questions is fundamentally the same as for any other research activity, and an evaluation study of PICO as an appropriate form of knowledge representation for clinical questions undertaken by Huang *et al.* (2006) concluded that whilst a useful format for some types of question, there were significant problems in employing PICO-framed questions as a useful tool for other clinical issues. For example, inductive research questions such as "What are rheumatoid arthritis patients most common symptomatic complaints?" do not fit the format, or even questions such as "What protective effects do vitamins E, C, and beta carotene have on the cardiovascular system?" as there is no space in the PICO framework for capturing systems. Capturing clinical questions is a highly complex undertaking, and there is a realistic concern that this format is not a good fit for EBP in terms of nursing, and there is a danger that by focusing on teaching this particular aspect of EBP we engender an over-simplification of the nature of EBP, and more importantly of its value to real-world nursing practice. Nevertheless, once a nurse has identified the specific parameters of their own practice question, they may search, acquire and appraise the evidence, and then integrate the selected intervention(s) into their practice using non research-based evidence, as we explore further below.

Another key area of focus for EBP theory has been the development of a hierarchical taxonomy of best research. A contemporary version is illustrated in Figure 9.1 (after Sackett *et al.*, 2000).

Where research has provided evidence of the quantifiable (statistically significant) effectiveness of specific therapeutic interventions for specific problems, it is clear to see the value of this. However, this is not always the case or even possible. Sufficient high-level quantitative research studies may not have been undertaken, and so other forms of available evidence may need to be considered. Nevertheless, EBP inevitably involves a taxonomic hierarchy of evidence, as the scientific philosophy inherent in its design is based upon examining competing hypotheses, and determining the best explanation through empirical means. A number of different versions of these taxonomic hierarchies have evolved over time, and which one represents the best classification is a matter of academic debate. Most present a similar overall hierarchy, and generally we can categorize published research evidence into two broad categories: evidence from multiple sources that has been systematically and rigorously evaluated, and evidence that has not. We can think of this as information that has been filtered to produce the best possible results, and information that remains unfiltered, but may still be valuable.

Much of the critique on the value of EBP for nursing care has also arisen over the assumptions inherent in this pyramid of evidence that it does not reflect other ways of knowing (Nairn, 2011). Many modern nursing curricula (particularly in graduate education) seem to focus on this aspect of EBP. However, these often seem to ignore the practical successes of EBP in improving health outcomes, and more importantly the other non-research aspects evidence included in the EBP framework.

Different forms of evidence

These debates of the relative merits of various forms of research evidence, and research questions or even ontological and epistemological arguments on the merits of science seem to have led to some academics here in Canada and elsewhere viewing EBP in terms of a "tyranny of evidence" (Bonnisteel, 2009) or, even worse, "fascist" (Holmes *et al.*, 2006). Putting such hyperbole aside, it is more useful to explore Cochrane's original practical conceptualization, in that EBP is about supporting our clinical decision making in a systematic way, which reflects the best evidence available to provide the best care solution. It emphasizes the value of scientific research in this process, but also considers other evidence. We can summarize the key elements that should be considered in EBP as:

- scientific evidence of a demonstrated positive (or negative) effect of a specific intervention or approach to care;
- economic viability of the intervention/approach to care;
- clinical expertise (expert appraisal of the specific clinical situation); and
- patient preferences.

Let us explore a few examples of the non-research factors further, as these are as much a part of EBP as discovery-based scientific knowledge.

Economic viability

Economic viability is probably one of he most significant factors affecting the deployment of any clinical intervention. Medications are frequently too expensive for practical clinical use, despite excellent evidence of good efficacy. In 2014, the National Institute for Health and Care Excellence (NICE), which provides national guidance and advice to improve health and social care in the UK, rejected a treatment that has been demonstrated to extend the lives of some women with an advanced breast cancer because it was too expensive. The drug, Kadcyla® (trastuzumab emtansine), costs about £90,000 per patient, and even though its makers, Roche, offered a discount, NICE Chief Executive Andrew Dillon said in a statement: "Although Roche proposed a discount to the full list price of Kadcyla, it made little difference to its value for money, leaving it well above the top of our specially extended range of cost effectiveness for cancer drugs" (NICE, 2014). Even the simple consideration of where a patient is cared for provides another example. The use of mixed-sex wards still occurs in some hospitals, although patient surveys have provided good evidence that although not the most significant patient issue, patients have a preference for single sex wards (Spiessl *et al.*, 2001; Hadden *et al.*, 1993). Most UK hospital wards are now single-sex but those mixed-sex units that remain would not be cost-effective to convert (such as coronary or critical care units), although the NHS has committed to completely phasing out mixed-sex general wards (NHS Choices, 2012). In the UK, NICE has the overall responsibility of exploring the costs associated with EBP, and for making decisions on the economic viability of different therapies for the NHS. Economic analysis and research can also be found in the Cochrane repositories, although most research in these databases is clinically focused. In considering economic evidence, it is useful to differentiate between cost-benefit, cost-effectiveness and cost-efficiency.

- Cost-benefit: a measure in economic terms of the worth of the intervention to the individual and society, in terms of the rate of return to the individual and to society as a whole. A cost-benefit analysis is useful when both cost and effects can be measured in monetary terms.
- Cost-effectiveness: a measurement of the extent to which an intervention produces outputs that are relevant to the needs and demands of its clients. Cost-effectiveness is useful when costs are expressed in monetary terms and effects are measured in non-monetary terms.
- Cost-efficiency: a relative measure of comparison to another system; where the output costs less than the other system per unit of input. An intervention increases its cost-efficiency when it maintains output with a less than proportional increase in input (Boardman, 2006).

Overall, these studies are extremely complex to perform, and certainly infrequent in the literature of nursing practice. Historically, sociopolitical influences seem to have a greater impact on the adoption or rejection of treatments rather than economic evidence. A recent example was the NHS's continued support for homeopathy, despite numerous studies that have demonstrated no significant efficacy when compared with placebo, and an influential health committee condemning it as medically unproven, and a waste of resources (House of Commons Science and Technology Committee, 2010). The total costs of homeopathy to the NHS are thought to be in the region of 3–4 million a year (NHS Choices, 2010). On the global scale, there are good reasons why we should try to estimate the economic and other costs associated with healthcare decisions as well as research evidence. A key historical example is represented by the use of the anti-malarial pesticide dichlorodiphenyltrichloroethane (DDT), which was effectively banned from use in 1972 by the US Environmental Protection Agency over growing public fears of its environmental safety. At the time, the global incidence of malaria was about 60,000 deaths a year (Carter and Mendis, 2002). Currently, Malaria incidence is at about 600,000 deaths a year (World Health Organization, 2014), but has been much higher (nearly one million deaths a year in 2000) and DDT has been demonstrated as much less toxic than originally argued (Wildavsky, 1997; Agency for Toxic Substances and Diseases Registry, 1994). That represents a global increase of around 30 million deaths since the ban), alongside multi-million dollar economic costs associated with trying to prevent and treat the disease (Carter and Mendis, 2002). Although this occurred well before the rise of EBP, it illustrates the complexity of predicting the longer-term costs and benefits of any particular health intervention.

On a smaller scale, in terms of providing evidence-based nursing care, nurses have little choice but to operate within the financial constraints present in their clinical environment, and this will affect their day-to day decision making regarding care provision. For example, a mixed-sex unit might be all that is available for admitting a patient, or the best evidence-based drug, wound dressing, or piece of equipment might be unavailable. Managers and clinicians have to base care decisions upon economic evidence, and that requires consideration of both the economic constraints, and clinical expertise, the next factor in the provision of EBP.

Clinical expertise

The value of clinical expertise, as a source of evidence in EBP is another area often neglected in the discourse over EBP in nursing. The use of clinical expertise as evidence is central to day-to-day clinical decisions. For example, a nurse may know why a particular alginate dressing is optimal for use on a particular patient's moist wound, based on the research evidence, and economic evidence that it is a prudent choice. However, if they also have knowledge that the patient is also suffering from dementia and pulls off the dressing several times a day, they may elect to use another material that is less costly, as the positive effects of the alginate will not be realized in short-term exposure.

In any given situation, clinical expertise regarding the patient's clinical condition and circumstances will affect the treatment options available to the nurse, who will have to decide upon the best course of action. For instance, a nurse encountering a person who has experienced a fractured clavicle while out in a rural community setting may have to settle for acetaminophen (paracetamol) and immobilization as the only effective treatments immediately available, whereas once back in an urban centre, they will likely have access to far better resources. An evidence-based decision about the appropriate use of anticoagulant therapy for a patient with a stroke is not only determined by research evidence on the efficacy of anticoagulation and its potential adverse effects, but will vary from one patient to another according to individual clinical situation (for example, the patient's age and history of bleeding) and their personal preferences (see below).

The way in which nurses use their expertise to make such decisions has been studied extensively but, to date, a consensus on how it occurs has yet to emerge. The research broadly reveals two major discourses with regard to clinical decision-making, firstly the intuitive humanistic espoused by Patricia Benner, based on Dreyfus's model of skills acquisition (Thompson, 1999; Benner and Tanner, 1987; Dreyfus and Dreyfus 1980), and, secondly, a systematic positivistic approach as exemplified in information processing theory (Garrett, 2005; Ellis, 2002; Bench-Capon, 1990; Putzier *et al.*, 1985; Elstein *et al.*, 1981). The systematic positivistic approach is concerned with established cognitive reasoning theory (such as deductive, inductive and abductive reasoning processes), while the humanistic school embraces the value of expert intuition in the reasoning process. The problem is these two discourses also seem to present us with diametrically opposed paradigms for clinical decision making. Thompson (1999) suggested a theoretical stance involving a cognitive continuum that probably better represents the nature of real-world clinical decision making. Here, the systematic positivistic and intuitive humanistic schools of thought are seen to occupy polar positions at either end of a continuum (as opposed to being on separate theoretical planes). As clinical expertise and decision making is central to EBP these differing perspectives are worthy of some further exploration.

Ellis (2002) observed that the systematic positivistic approach to clinical decision making in nursing makes use of two cognitive processes: goal-directed processes and rule-out processes. The rule-out processes determine the problem, the cause, and the action to be taken (forward chaining reasoning using inductive and deductive steps) while goal-directed processes involve taking actions to reach a specific goal (working backwards from the desired goal). These can be seen as analogous to the forward and backward chaining decision making pathways used by information scientists in constructing expert systems to mimic human behaviours (Bench-Capon, 1990; Jackson, 1999).

In their widely publicized work, Benner and Tanner (1987) explored the use of intuition in decision making by expert nurses defining it as "understanding without a rationale," and associated it with pattern recognition and what was termed "common sense understanding." However, the nature of intuitive reasoning processes, as used in the intuitive humanistic approach, remains unclear as the exact processes involved remain to be established (Garrett, 2005; Myers, 2002; Effken, 2001; Tewes, 2001; Buckingham and Adams, 2000; Rew, 2000).

This is an area of concern in that, as the cognitive processes involved with such expert intuitive reasoning remain unclear, they cannot be guaranteed to be truth-preserving processes. Therefore, without a clear understanding of the mechanisms, it remains logically difficult to validate intuition as a rationale for clinical decision making, even when the empirical evidence suggests positive results. Experienced nurses are known to use more intuitive reasoning processes (King and Clark, 2002), or a combination of techniques in their decision making (Redden and Wotton, 2001). Reddon and Wooton's small interpretive study explored experienced critical care and gastrointestinal surgical nurses' decision making. They proposed that the qualifications and the culture of the critical care unit promoted a more systematic positivistic approach, whilst the surgical nurses used more intuitive humanistic methods. It has also been noted that intuition plays a significant part in clinical decision making amongst experienced psychiatric nurses (Rew, 2000).

Therefore, we know experts use this type of decision making as evidence for interventions in their practice, but cognitively it has the characteristics of a black-box approach. That is to say, we can observe the inputs, outputs, and results but cannot explain what happens in-between. Modern neuroscience is beginning to shed some light on this (Gupta *et al.*, 2011; Jarcho *et al.* 2011; Naqvi *et al.*, 2006;) but we are still a long way from understanding how expert intuition works. This presents us with rather a dilemma in our EBP framework, as the use of evidence is central to the process, and yet, if we support the intuitive humanistic approach for clinical decisions, we once again find ourselves resorting to expert intuitive knowledge that cannot be easily quantified as a source of evidence. We should also consider that junior or student nurses may lack the necessary experience to use pattern recognition and associative reasoning techniques effectively, the use of intuitive humanistic approaches may be particularly problematic (Garrett, 2005).

Overall, as our example above demonstrates, evidence from clinical expertise must be considered as a central part of the clinical decision-making process.

Evidence does not make decisions, people do, and EBP was never designed to imply that research evidence overrides all else. Both Cochrane and Sacket recognized this in their original work. As a professional practitioner, the nurse will always use their clinical experience as a source of evidence in the clinical-decision making process, based upon what they know will work from prior experience and expert clinical rationale. This also involves consideration of our final source of evidence: the patient's preference.

Patient's preference

Another piece of the evidence puzzle that needs consideration (and as proponents of patient-centered care, this should prevail over all of the above for adult patients who are mentally competent to able to make their wishes known) is consideration of the patient's own desires with respect to their care. One criticism directed at EBP is that it binds the hands of practitioners and robs patients of their personal choices in reaching a decision about optimal care (DaCruz, 2002). Nevertheless, there may be many barriers to implementing health research in practice, but patient preferences were incorporated into the very first model of evidence-based medicine devised (EBMWG, 1992), and the importance of this aspect has been underscored in depictions of the process, such as the one illustrated in Figure 9.2.

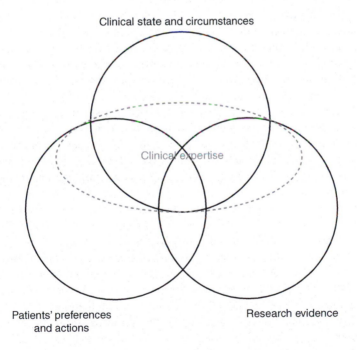

Figure 9.2 Model of the process of evidence-based medicine

Clinical decisions must include consideration of the patient's clinical condition, supported by research evidence concerning the efficacy, effectiveness, and efficiency of the intervention options available. Also, given the likely consequences associated with each option, the clinician must also consider the patient's preferences and likely actions (in terms of what interventions they are ready and able to accept). Finally, clinical expertise is used to bind these considerations together and recommend the treatment that the patient is agreeable to accepting (Haynes *et al.*, 2002).

Patient preference often overrides evidence of best practice. A commonly used example is an adult experiencing a life-threatening haemorrhage who holds a religious belief that dictates against receiving a blood transfusion. After informing the patient of their treatment options and likely consequences, the patient's choice is the overriding factor that determines whether the transfusion may be given, or whether other acceptable, but less effective intravenous substances are used. Despite all of the evidence and clinical expertise that suggests blood transfusion is the best option, EBP supports the patient's decision not to have it.

Sometimes patient preferences are not easily known, and this is an area in which we could use EBP techniques to establish a better understanding of patient perceptions with regards to treatment. One 2001 study demonstrated that patients varied widely on the risk of haemorrhage they were prepared to accept in return for anticoagulant therapy for a reduction of stroke risk (Devereaux *et al.* 2001). Additionally, patients in this study were reported as being much less averse to bleeding as an adverse consequence of anticoagulant prophylaxis than the doctors treating them. In another example, outcome measurement in arthritis have undergone a major shift during the last twenty years, moving from process measures (such as plasma viscosity) to patient-centered outcome measures (like pain and function). A recent paper reviewed evidence on the correspondence of patients with arthritis and doctors' views of their health outcomes, and reported considerable variation between them (Hewlett, 2014). This review demonstrated significant differences between the patients' and doctors' assessments of their priorities in terms of functionality and pain in many cases, and physicians' willingness to take risks for improving health, with doctors rating their patients' health status as better than patients, and being less willing than patients to take risks to achieve good outcomes.

EBP was developed to encourage practitioners and patients to consider current best evidence in making clinical decisions, and that includes evidence from the patient. However, providing evidence to patients in a way that allows them to make an informed choice is probably one of the most challenging aspects of modern health care, and represents an excellent focus for modern nursing research. By exploring the alternative therapeutic interventions available using the best evidence of effectiveness (Does it work?), pragmatic evidence (Will it work in this case? Is it readily available, legally approved, affordable and usable in this context?), and the patient's preference (Will the patient accept it?): EBP is a process that supports the nurse to help make the best care decision.

Curricular challenges

If nursing students are to fully grasp the complexities and nature of EBP, and to produce nurses who are EBP literate, there is a need to provide education that provides an understanding of its original basis in post-positivist science, of the broader remit of EBP, of its pragmatic value to contemporary health care, along-side the often-cited critique of its epistemological standing. The original aims and objectives of EBP are important to consider alongside postmodern nursing perspectives and ontological considerations on the nature of evidence that pervade modern nursing education (particularly here in North America). Otherwise, nursing students are likely to receive a very one-dimensional view of EBP in their education, one that equates it with the promotion of quantitative techniques and randomized controlled trials, and where it becomes seen as simply another way of knowing that they may take or leave.

As nursing education has aligned itself more with the social rather than phys-ical sciences, this has led to something of an identity crisis in modern nursing education. Nurses are being taught EBP from a fundamentally research-based evidence approach on the one hand, and encouraged to adopt postmodern rela-tivist epistemologies rejecting the domination of an empirical approach, on the other. Much of the nursing research conducted over the last twenty-five years has been characterized by this move towards more interpretive, postmodern, and crit-ical practices, many of which, do not represent scientific forms of inquiry, or worse are typically anti-science (Frazier, 2009; Guba and Lincoln, 2005; Gutting, 2000; Kermode, 1996). Such approaches are sometimes rather represented as post-positivist thinking, in that they reject the positivists' ideas that systematic inquiry should be the same across both natural and social sciences and research findings can only be proved by empirical and testable means. However, this label is rather simplistic and misleading given that classical positivist thinking really died off in the 1930s and that modern post-positivist science (such as espoused by Thomas Kuhn) supports an empirical basis for its archetype.

There is then, a strong trend in North American nursing curricula over recent years to represent EBP as a straw man confection of positivist thinking, the evidence-based tyranny of medicine, and advocating for consideration of other ways of knowing (Garrett and Cutting, 2014; Holmes *et al.*, 2012). This anti-science trend is well established in modern nursing here in Canada and beyond. Australian nursing educator Stephen Kermode warned of the implications of this back in 1996, when he noted that "Science is under threat from a number of sources. In nurse education a range of discourses have been attempting to margin-alize science and to replace it with epistemologies which are deemed to be more appropriate."

He observed that arguments supporting postmodern approaches to nursing produce an epistemological anarchy that keeps ideas in play so that explanatory and predictive theory does not emerge. Walker (1994: 164) provided a good example of this type of thinking, when he noted that nurses thinking was limited by accepting "congealed dualistic categories such as subjective/objective;

quantitative/qualitative; hard data/soft data and theory/practice that have constrained the ways we think and do research."

In this world view, explanatory frameworks such as EBP are seen as hegemonic and oppressive. The result of nursing adopting this line of postmodern thought has been the growth of nurses supporting some very non evidence-based practices, including therapeutic touch (Jaimet, 2012; Glazer, 2002), homeopathy (Mantle, 2008) and other mystical interpretations of healthcare (Parse, 1992).

Unfortunately, educating students in this way is unlikely to prove beneficial in preparing them for the realities of working within public healthcare systems that remain primarily directed by medical science, nor to equip them with the skills to challenge their professional status in this system, or even to produce graduates able to deal with the complexities of clinical decision making using EBP. It seems that nurse educators now stand at rather a crossroads for our future disciplinary development, and need to consider how we best prepare future nurses to take the profession forward. To this end, a more expansive evaluation of EBP, exploring all the forms of evidence it entails would seem highly appropriate in all undergraduate nursing curricula. Education that presents the complexity, benefits and flaws inherent in EBP is needed, rather than epistemological approaches that do not align well with the science-based nature of modern medical care, or reflect the clinical challenges that students will experience in real-world practice once they graduate.

Fundamentally, we can choose to espouse a view of health care that rejects the consideration of competing hypotheses and methods of establishing best evidence to make decisions, in favor of a postmodern nominalist approach that moves we embrace multiple truths. EBP then becomes an irrelevancy, and medical science becomes the domain of an oppressive profession. The trouble is, that does not explain the overwhelming success of medical science over the last century, mesh with the current public support and demand for medical services, or actually prepare nurses adequately to work in contemporary public healthcare systems.

Conclusion

The primary value of EBP is that it is a client/patient-centered approach focused on using the best evidence to support practice, not simply the imposition of research evidence on practice as it is frequently mischaracterized; sometimes even by its proponents. The development of a systematic framework for the evaluation of evidence using an empirical scientific approach represents a significant landmark in the progress of health care. Nevertheless, the persistence of the myth by some academics in nursing education that the focus of EBP is solely upon research, and that studies with certain research designs (primarily quantitative) represent the only significant high-quality evidence is damaging the potential for nurses to fully realize the potential of EBP.

In reality, the application of rigorous critical appraisal criteria across studies inherent in EBP identifies the strengths and weaknesses in all kinds of research methods, and provides a systematic basis for resolving disagreements about the most favourable approaches to client care. This approach makes it important for individual practitioners to think independently about the validity, importance, and precision of results from empirical studies when applying them to clinical care. The clinician's task is to interpret the best current evidence from systematic research in relationship to the individual client/patient, including consideration of that individual's preferences, culture, the environment of care, and their personal values regarding health and wellbeing.

There remain significant barriers to EBP such as practitioners having insufficient time to research the best interventions, or nurses having to make decisions where there is little high-quality evidence available. Internet access to high-quality sources and sites is now significantly decreasing the time needed to locate current best evidence, in both qualitative and quantitative work, and we can promote the acquisition of new knowledge through research to help improve the evidence-base we can use for care. Furthermore, if we do not support an EBP approach to health care, then the question arises, how do we best justify our practice decisions? Those who have been critical of EBP, have yet to demonstrate a more effective alternative for professional practice and public healthcare policy.

To return to the original motives behind EBP, Cochrane moved that clinical disciplines should be able to summarize the scientific evidence concerning healthcare practices, and that patients should only accept health care that is based on scientific evidence. The key advantage of EBP is that it attempts to establish substantive reliable evidence as the basis for practice, rather than relying on practice informed by established tradition, intuition, expert opinion or authority or what we might term eminence-based practice. The goal of EBP is to provide optimal clinical service to that client/patient on an individual basis, not the broad imposition of empirical research findings.

These are important issues and nurses are challenged to think about the assumptions embedded in the concept and practice of EBP, and nurse educators their role in preparing nurses adequately to meet the demands of contemporary practice. EBP is a continuing dynamic process integrating the current state of health knowledge with clinical expertise and into everyday practice, and it is important to remember there are four distinct forms of evidence inherent in the EBP framework, not one. Overall, EBP is far from perfect, but it represents the best framework currently devised for the implementation of effective and efficient health care. It is neither the panacea for all of our healthcare needs, nor the tyrant that some academics have proposed. Rather, it offers us a set of tools by which we can systematically improve our clinical practice, and as such I would argue we should embrace and further develop the principles embodied within it.

References

Agency for Toxic Substances and Diseases Registry (1994) Toxicological Profile for 4,4'-DDT, 4,4'-DDE, 4, 4'-DDD (Update). Atlanta, GA: US Public Health Service.

Armstrong, E. C. (1999) The Well-built Clinical Question: The key to finding the best evidence efficiently. *Wisconsin Medical Journal*, 98(2): 25–8.

Benner, P. and Tanner, C. A. (1987) How Expert Nurses Use Intuition. *American Journal of Nursing*, 87, 23–31.

Bench-Capon, T. (1990) *Knowledge Representation*. London: Harcourt Brace Jovanich.

Boardman, N. E. (2006) *Cost-benefit Analysis: Concepts and Practice* (3rd ed.). Upper Saddle River, NJ: Prentice Hall.

Bonisteel, P. (2009) The tyranny of evidence-based medicine. *Canadian Family Physician Médecin de Famille Canadien*, 55(10), 979.

Buckingham C. D. and Adams, A. (2000) Classifying Clinical Decision Making: Interpreting nursing intuition, heuristics and medical diagnosis. *Journal of Advanced Nursing*, 324, 990–8.

Carter, R. and Mendis, K. N. (2002) Evolutionary and Historical Aspects of the Burden of Malaria. *Clinical Microbiology Reviews*, 15(4), 564–94.

Cochrane, A. L. (1972) *Effectiveness and Efficiency: Random Reflections on Health Services*. London: Royal Society of Medicine Press.

DaCruz, D. (2002) You have a Choice, Dear Patient. *BMJ*, 323(4432), 324, 67.

Devereaux, P. J., Anderson, D. R., Gardner, M. J., Putnam, W., Flowerdew, G. J., Brownell, B. F., Nagpul, S. and Cox, J. L. (2001) Differences between perspectives of physicians and patients on anticoagulation in patients with atrial fibrillation: observational study. *BMJ (Clinical Research Education)*, 323(7323), 1218–22.

Dreyfus, S. E. and Dreyfus, H. L. (1980) *A Five-Stage Model of the Mental Activities Involved in Directed Skill Acquisition*. Washington, DC: Storming Media.

Ebell, M. (1999) Information at the Point of Care: Answering clinical questions. *Journal of Family Practice*, 12(3), 225–35.

EBMWG (1992) Evidence-based medicine – a new approach to teaching the practice of medicine. Evidence-Based Medicine Working Group. *JAMA*, 268(17), 2420–5.

Effken, J. A. (2001) Informational Basis for Expert Intuition. *Journal of Advanced Nursing*, 342, 246–55.

Ellis, P. A. (2002) Clinical Decision-making: A process. Doctoral Dissertation. Southern Illinois University, Carbondale.

Elstein, A. S., Shulman, L. S. and Sprafka, S. A. (1981) Medical Problem Solving. *Journal of Medical Education*, 561, 75–6.

Ely, J. W., Osheroff, J. A., Gorman, P. N., Ebell, M. H., Chambliss, M. L., Pifer, E. A. and Stavri, P. Z. (2000) A Taxonomy of Generic Clinical Questions: Classification study. *BMJ*, 321(7258), 429–32.

Fluoride Action Network (2014) Broadening Public Awareness on Fluoride. Available online at http://fluoridealert.org (accessed 11 March 2015).

Frazier, K. (2009) *Science Under Siege, Defending Science, Exposing Pseudoscience*. New York: Prometheus.

Garrett, B. (2005) Student Nurses' Perceptions of Clinical Decision-Making in the Final Year of Adult Nursing Studies. *Nurse Education in Practice*, 5(1), 30–9.

Garrett, B. (2013) *Science and Modern Thought in Nursing: Pragmatism and praxis for evidence-based practice*. Victoria, BC: Northern Lights Media.

Garrett, B. and Cutting, R. (2014) Ways of knowing: realism, non-realism, nominalism and a typology revisited with a counter perspective for nursing science. *Nursing Inquiry*. doi: 10.1111/nin.12070.

Glazer, S. (2001) Therapeutic Touch and Postmodernism in Nursing. *Nursing Philosophy*, 2, 196–212.

Guba, E. G. and Lincoln, Y. S. (2005) Paradigmatic Controversies, Contradictions, and Emerging Influences. In N. K. Denzin and Y. S. Lincoln (eds), *The Sage Handbook of*

Qualitative Research, 3, 191–215. Thousand Oaks, CA: Sage.

Gutting, G. (2000) A House Built on Sand: Exposing postmodernist myths about science. *British Journal of Philosophical Science,* 51(51), 191–5.

Gupta, R., Koscik, T. R., Bechara, A. and Tranel, D. (2011) The Amygdala and Decision-making. *Neuropsychologia,* 49(4), 760–6.

Hadden, D. S., Dearden, C. H. and Ross, G. (1993) Mixed-sex Wards: A survey of patient's opinions. *Archives of Emergency Medicine,* 10(4), 354–6.

Haynes, R. B., Devereaux, P. J. and Guyatt, G. H. (2002) Physicians' and Patients' Choices in Evidence Based Practice. *BMJ (Clinical Research Education),* 324(7350), 1350.

Hewlett, S. A. (2003) Patients and Clinicians have Different Perspectives on Outcomes in Arthritis. *Journal of Rheumatology,* 30, 877–9.

Holmes, D., Murray, S. J., Perron, A. and Rail, G. (2006) Deconstructing the Evidence-based Discourse in Health Sciences: Truth, power and fascism. *International Journal of Evidence-Based Health Care,* 4(3), 180–6.

Holmes, D., Roy, B. and Perron, A. (2012) The Use of Postcolonialism in the Nursing Domain: Colonial patronage, conversion, and resistance. In P. G. Reed and N. B. Crawford Shearer (eds), *Perspectives on Nursing Theory* (6th ed.), pp. 257–64. Philadelphia, PA: Wolters Kluwer/Lippincott, Williams and Wilkins.

House of Commons Science and Technology Committee (2010) *House of Commons Science and Technology Committee – Fourth Report. Evidence Check 2: Homeopathy.* London: TSO. Available online at www.publications.parliament.uk/pa/cm200910/cmselect/cmsctech/45/4502.htm (accessed 11 March 2015).

Jackson, P. (1999) *An Introduction to Expert Systems,* (3rd ed.). Harlow: Addison-Wesley.

Jaimet, K. (2012) Energy at Work. *Canadian Nurse,* 108(7) 33–6.

Jarcho, J. M., Berkman, E. T. and Lieberman, M. D. (2011) The Neural Basis of Rationalization: Cognitive dissonance reduction during decision-making. *Social Cognitive and Affective Neuroscience,* 6(4), 460–7.

Jerome, R. N., Giuse, N. B., Gish, K. W., Sathe, N. A. and Dietrich, M. S. (2001) Information Needs of Clinical Teams: analysis of questions received by the Clinical Informatics Consult Service. *Bull Medical Library Association,* 89(2):177–84.

Kermode, S. (1996) Science and Not Science in Nurse Education. Keynote Speech: Proceedings of Supporting Sciences: Facts or Frameworks for Nursing Practice, Conference on Science in Nursing Education (COSINE '96), Queensland University of Technology and Science in Nursing Education, Brisbane, Queensland, Gold Coast, Australia.

King, L. and Clark, W. (2002) Intuition and the Development of Expertise in Surgical Ward and Intensive Care Nurses. *Journal of Advanced Nursing,* 374, 322–9.

Levin, R. and Feldman, H. R. (2013) *Teaching Evidence-Based Practice in Nursing* (2nd ed.). New York: Springer.

Mantle, F. (2008) Homeopathy. *Nursing Times,* 21 July. Available online at www.nursingtimes.net/homeopathy/1736863.article (accessed 11 March 2015).

Melnyk, B. M. and Fineout-Overholt, E. (2011) *Evidence-based Practice in Nursing and Healthcare: A guide to best practice.* New York: Wolters Kluwer.

Myers, D. G. (2002) The Powers and Perils of Intuition. *Psychology Today,* November/December, 42–52.

McDonagh, M., Whiting, P., Bradley, M., Cooper, J., Sutton, A. and Chestnutt, I. (2000) A Systematic Review of Public Water Fluoridation. *BMJ,* 321(7265), 855–9.

McSherry, R., Simmons, M. and Abbott, P. (2002) *Evidence-informed Nursing: A guide for clinical nurses.* Abingdon: Routledge.

Nairn, S. (2012) A critical realist approach to knowledge: implications for evidence-based practice in and beyond nursing. *Nursing Inquiry*, 19(1) 6–17.

Naqvi, N., Shiv, B. and Bechara, A. (2006) The Role of Emotion in Decision Making: A cognitive neuroscience perspective. *Current Directions in Psychological Science*, 15(5), 260–4.

NHS Choices (2010) NHS Homeopathy. Available online at www.nhs.uk/news/2010/July07/Pages/nhs-homeopathy.aspx (accessed 11 March 2015).

NHS Choices (2012) Will I be offered a same-sex hospital ward? Health Questions. Available online at www.nhs.uk/chq/Pages/903.aspx?CategoryID=69andSubCategory ID=695 (accessed 11 March 2015).

NICE (2014) Kadcyla: NICE disappointed by manufacturer's decision. National Institute for Clinical Excellence [press release]. Available online at www.nice.org.uk/news/press-and-media/kadcyla-nice-disappointed-by-manufacturers-decision (accessed 11 March 2015).

Nurse, P. (2011) Opinion: Stamp out Anti-science in US politics. *New Scientist*, (2830), 4–5.

Parse, R. R. (1992) Human Becoming: Parse's theory of nursing. *Nursing Science Quarterly*, 5(35), 35–42.

Putzier, D. J., Padrick, K. P., Westfall, U. E. and Tanner, C.A. (1985) Diagnostic Reasoning in Critical Care Nursing. *Heart and Lung*, 14 (5), 430–5.

Redden, M. and Wotton, K. (2001) Clinical Decision Making by Nurses when Faced with Third-space Fluid Shift: How well do they fare? *Gastroenterology Nursing*, 244, 182–91.

Richardson, W. S., Wilson, M. C., Nishikawa, J. and Hayward, R. S. (1995) The Well-built Clinical Question: A key to evidence-based decisions. *American Clinical Practice Journal Club*, 123(3), A12–13.

Rew, L. (2000) Acknowledging Intuition in Clinical Decision Making. *Journal of Holistic Nursing*, 182, 94–113.

Sackett, D. L., Rosenberg, W. M. C., Muir Gray, J. A., Haynes, R. B. and Richardson, W. S. (1996) Evidence-based Medicine: What it is and what it isn't. *British Medical Journal*, 312, 71–2.

Sackett, D. L., Straus, S. E., Richardson, W. S., Rosenberg, W. and Hayes, R. B. (2000) *Evidence-based Medicine: How to practice and teach EBM* (2nd ed.). Edinburgh: Churchill Livingstone.

Smyth, R. L. and Craig, J. V. (2002) *The Evidence-based Practice Manual for Nurses.* Edinburgh: Churchill Livingstone.

Spiessl, H., Frick, U., von Kovatsits, U., Klein, H. E. and Vukovich, A. (2001) [Single Sex or Mixed sex Treatment in the Psychiatric Clinic from the Viewpoint of Patients]. *Der Nervenarzt*, 72(7), 515–20.

Stevens, K. R. (2012) ACE Star Model of Knowledge Transformation. Academic Center for Evidence-Based Practice (ACE), University of Texas Health Science Center at San Antonio. Available online at www.acestar.uthscsa.edu/acestar-model.asp (accessed 18 March 2015).

Tewes, R. (2001) Magic in Nursing: Some ideas about unexplainable situations. *Creative Nursing*, 74, 10–11.

Thompson, C. (1999) A Conceptual Treadmill: The need for 'middle ground' in clinical decision making theory in nursing. *Journal of Advanced Nursing*, 305, 1222–9.

Wainwright, J. and Sheiham, A. (2014) An Analysis of Methods of Toothbrushing Recommended by Dental Associations, Toothpaste and Toothbrush Companies and in Dental Texts. *British Dental Journal*, 217(3), E5.

Walker, K. (1994) Research with/in nursing: 'troubling' the field. *Contemporary Nurse*, 3(4):162–8.

World Health Organization (2010) *World Malaria Report 2010*. Geneva: WHO.

World Health Organization (2014) *Malaria*. Factsheet No. 94. Geneva: WHO. Available online at www.who.int/mediacentre/factsheets/fs094/en (accessed 11 March 2015).

Wildavsky, A. (1997) *But is it True? A Citizen's Guide to Environmental Health and Safety Issues*. Cambridge, MA: Harvard University Press.

Yeung, C. A. (2008) A systematic Review of the Efficacy and Safety of Fluoridation. *Evidence-Based Dentistry*, 9(2), 39–43.

10 Evidence and the qualitative research analogous structure

John Paley

Introduction

Hierarchies of evidence, it is often said, 'privilege' quantitative research in general and the randomized controlled trial in particular. This is usually attributed, as the word 'privilege' implies, to ideology and dogma; for example, the dominant political culture (Colyer and Kamath 1999), logical positivism in the NHS (Welsh and Lyons 2001), the dominant medical perspective (Fawcett *et al.* 2001), research agendas driven by the post-positivist paradigm (Holmes *et al.* 2006), indoctrination in nurse education (Mitchell 2013), a biomedical narrative which has dominated health care but whose concepts can be 'troubled' by queer theory (Zeeman *et al.* 2014), the values traditionally associated with masculinity (Lines 2001) and overcompensation/penis envy (Freshwater and Rolfe 2004). Very few of these writers, given their postmodern, post-structuralist, constructivist and phenomenological perspectives, concern themselves with the logical reasons why quantitative and experimental evidence might legitimately be preferred to other kinds, preferring to see evidence-based practice as an arbitrary imposition by political, economic, managerial, philosophical, biomedical, male, straight or Freudian forces.

One of the more popular reactions to this iniquitous situation is to argue that the evidence derived from qualitative research should have higher status, given that 'conventional hierarchies of evidence exclude many knowledge forms that are meaningful to nurses' (Thorne 2009: 569). This argument, which is a direct descendant of Carper's (1978) 'patterns of knowing in nursing', points towards a more inclusive concept of evidence, one which incorporates 'meaning as well as measurement' (Upshur *et al.* 2001). This is the position that I have previously termed 'inclusionist' (Paley 2006). Many authors adopt a broadly similar view, including Kitson (2002), Rycroft-Malone *et al.* (2004), Jack (2006), Booth *et al.* (2007), Mantzoukas (2008), Freshwater *et al.* (2010), Leeman and Sandelowski (2012), all of whom would agree that it is necessary 'to legitimize evidence derived from qualitative studies' and put it on 'an equal footing with other forms of research' (Upshur *et al.* 2001: 95).

The terms of the inclusionist campaign ensure that qualitative research gets a free pass. Because the hierarchy of evidence is taken to be ideologically driven, the objective is to secure equal opportunities for a favoured but 'marginalized' method, without reference to the merits of different research designs. The possibility that qualitative research, or certain forms of it, might deserve a comparatively low place in the hierarchy is simply not countenanced. In particular, the critical question has not been answered (Paley 2005). Given that, in quantitative research, statistical procedures and experimental protocols are designed to minimize the risk of inferential error (Mayo 1996), what are the corresponding procedures and protocols in qualitative studies? Without a convincing answer to this question, there is no way of discriminating between legitimate inference in qualitative research and various forms of cognitive bias: observer expectancy effects, belief bias, illusory correlation, availability cascade, selective perception, congruence bias, motivated reasoning or outright wishful thinking.

Always ready to tell an indignant story about the 'hegemony' of quantitative research, the advocates of qualitative health research have been somewhat less critical of methodological developments in their own field, and have exhibited little curiosity about the origins of its routines and rhetoric. Here, I can provide only a rough sketch of several interesting aspects of that history.

I begin (a) with a short account of the evolutionary pressure exerted by academic environments on qualitative methodology, and (b) define the qualitative research analogous structure (QRAS), which is the template for a significant number of qualitative studies. This will lead (c) to a review of popular but unpersuasive arguments, followed by some sceptical comments (d) on the idea that people's meanings are crucial to understanding their behaviour. Finally, I return to the claim that qualitative evidence should be 'on an equal footing', with evidence derived from quantitative and experimental designs, and (e) suggest that, for QRAS studies at least, it is unwarranted.

Evolutionary pressures on qualitative methods

For the past thirty years, methodological discussion in qualitative health research, as in several other disciplines, has been subordinated to the requirements of postgraduate study. The need to maximize publication output has resulted in even master's level research – supposedly a display of entry-level competence rather than a contribution to knowledge – appearing routinely in the journals. This has necessitated the legitimation of methods suited to the time-limited, resource-constrained, 'bums-on-seats' MSc enterprise. The process is akin to Darwinian evolution. The academic environment has selected for whatever can be achieved in a year full-time or two years part-time, and methodologists have borrowed various philosophical ideas to provide a corresponding theoretical justification.

What conditions does the scene of postgraduate study impose on methodology? Here are some of the most obvious. It must be possible to carry out the research in a limited and predictable period of time, defined by the deadline for dissertation submission. It must be possible for one person to conduct the study, and for that person to be able to do so with virtually zero resources. Given that most students obtained their first degree in nursing or some other health-related field, it must be possible to design the study, and to analyse the findings, in the absence of any grounding in relevantly adjacent disciplines such as psychology or sociology. In view of vastly increased postgraduate numbers and severe restrictions on time, the intellectual demands must not be too challenging. However, if the study is to be publishable, it must be possible to claim clinical relevance for the research, and to imply (if only obliquely) that the findings are generalizable.

These conditions are likely to select for designs and methods with the following characteristics:

- *Interview-based*. Other methods, such as participant observation, require a great deal of organization and are difficult to accommodate to fixed timetables and deadlines. Interviews and focus groups are an efficient alternative, being more manageable and more predictable.
- *Small samples*. The time available to an MSc student permits only a limited number of interviews to be conducted. In qualitative studies published in nursing journals the average sample size is about eleven. Single-figure samples are commonplace.
- *Tabula rasa*. Some methodological texts recommend that the field of study be approached without any 'preconceived theory' (for example, Glaser and Strauss 1967, and, for different reasons, phenomenology). This conveniently limits the amount of reading required, reducing the overall burden on the student.
- *Study of experience*. By the same token, a focus on experience absolves the student from having to dig into a lot of theoretical background. The respondent's experience, described retrospectively in his or her own words, is independent of academic theory, so can be approached without an in-depth study of potentially relevant material.
- *Meaning*. An idea associated with the concept of experience, and espoused for similar reasons. The meanings which respondents attach to phenomena or to their own experiences can also be identified independently of prior academic theory, and eliciting them does not require any theoretical preparation.
- *Description*. According to Sandelowski (2000), descriptive studies are the 'least theoretical' examples of qualitative research. Consequently, they make fewer demands on the student, who is relieved of the responsibility of tracking relevant theory in adjacent, non-health disciplines.
- *Emergent themes*. The student burden is further alleviated by an approach to analysis which permits concepts to be generated (internally) from the data, rather than (externally) from statistics, theoretical sources or a systematic review of the relevant literature.
- *Induction*. Since it is impossible to justify generalizing from tiny samples on statistical grounds, it is necessary to invent alternatives such as transferability, the phenomenological nod and the formulation of essences, to permit generalization by another name. These alternatives are used, implicitly or explicitly, to justify the publication of small-sample MSc research.

- *Recipes*. Methods which can be reduced to recipes are likely to be preferred to those which require the exercise of independent thought. Recipes can be applied to all phases of the research process, including the design stage, interviewing, and data analysis.

One particularly important recipe determines the formulation of a research aim. It amounts to a kind of pro forma template for a popular type of qualitative study (Figure 10.1) This is a relatively undemanding exercise, which takes the pain out of thinking about research and is therefore admirably suited to postgraduate study. Instead of a meticulous analysis of the literature to identify a clinical question to which we do not already know the answer – and to justify the claim that an answer to it would be of value – the student merely has to identify a group of people who have not yet been asked to: 'Tell me about your experience of …'. In other words, the template revises (and dumbs down) the concept of a 'gap in the literature'.

I am not, of course, claiming that anybody devised this pro forma or that students and supervisors ever consciously decide to adopt it. I am claiming that, in the current academic environment, studies which take this form – and which incorporate several of the characteristics outlined above – will be strongly selected for. They will be the default option. Moreover, they will be the default option, not just for MSc research but for qualitative health research generally. Once the template has evolved – and once it has spawned hundreds of publications, and acquired countless off-the-peg, cheap-and-cheerful, quick-and-dirty philosophical justifications – it becomes available to everybody undertaking qualitative studies.

The qualitative research analogous structure

Extend the natural selection analogy. Convergence occurs when, thanks to the selective pressures of the same environment, unrelated species acquire similar biological traits, called 'analogous structures'. The wing, for example, evolved

To	explore / illuminate / identify / elucidate[1]	*<description>*
the	experience / phenomenon / meaning[1]	*<experience>*
of	*insert situation, treatment or condition[1]*	*<state of affairs>*
from the perspective of	patients / nurses / health professionals[1]	*<perspective>*
in	insert location	*<location>*

[1] Select one

Figure 10.1 Recipe for determining the formulation of a research aim

separately in birds, bats and insects. In the case of qualitative methods, a number of different species – phenomenology, grounded theory, ethnography, narrative enquiry, and so on – have all acquired identical traits as a result of adaptation to the postgraduate environment. Although they retain their respective philosophical frameworks and their respective technical vocabularies, these approaches have converged on the following analogous structure of research practice:

> The *retrospective description* of *experience* and *meaning* through *small-sample interviewing*, both data collection and analysis being carried out *in the absence of theoretical preconceptions*, with the implicit aim of *inductively* generalizing to a population while explicitly disowning the concept of generalization.

From here on, I refer to this as the qualitative research analogous structure (QRAS). I should emphasize that the rest of the chapter is exclusively concerned with QRAS. It is not about qualitative research *tout court*.

A brief example of convergent evolution. Glaser and Strauss (1967) show *no* interest in 'experience' and their examples are fieldwork studies based on extensive observation of behaviour rather than a series of interviews. They do not restrict themselves to description but propose theoretical explanations linking variables (for example, the quality of nursing care is a function of the nurse's assessment of the social loss represented by the patient). Their objective is to generate theory, which can subsequently be tested, rather than to perform inductive inferences extrapolating from sample to population. Yet fifty years later, it is quite routine to classify inductive, descriptive, interview-based studies of experience as 'grounded theory' (recent examples include Gibson and Watkins 2012, Giske and Cone 2012, Van Dover and Pfeiffer 2012, Helgesen *et al.* 2013, Reisenhofer and Seibold 2013, Dlugaschi and Ugarriza 2014, Førsund *et al.* 2014, Lee *et al.* 2014); and a paper published in *Social Science and Medicine* (Greenfield *et al.* 2012) describes grounded theory as an appropriate method for the study of attitudes, motives, feelings and 'narrative-phenomenological data'.

Discourse replicator arguments

This is not to deny that there are dozens of pocket arguments used to justify the view that qualitative research should involve inductive, small-sample, interview-based description of experience and the meanings people attach to it. Just as the postgraduate environment has selected for studies with these characteristics, so it has selected for philosophical ideas which can be claimed to vindicate them. These ideas become memes – discourse replicators – endlessly copied and recycled, but evolving in a such a way as to perform the function required of them.

For example, the expression 'multiple realities' was originally used to refer to different social 'worlds': the world of work, the world of dreams, the world of the theatre, the world of science, the world of play, the world of religion, and so on (Schutz 1945). Each of these is a specific form of sociality, an intersubjective realm with its own 'rules' and its own 'cognitive style'. However, Schutz's sociological term is no longer used in that way. It has evolved into a rhetorical marker for philosophical relativism – constructivist code for the idea that, corresponding to every different experience, belief, interpretation or *Weltanschauung*, there is an ontologically independent reality. This evolution of 'multiple realities' buttresses the QRAS – and specifically research on experience – by suggesting that studying 'reality' and studying the 'experience of reality' are the same thing. It permits a flattening of the world into a single ontological category, the only thing that can ever be studied: 'experience'.

The discourse-replicator philosophical arguments are usually weak, since their function is primarily creedal. Concepts such as 'multiple realities', 'inductive-descriptive', 'essence' and 'transferability' provide no more than comic-book rationalizations of the QRAS. They are not designed to withstand critical analysis. They are based on disprovable myths or mis-readings of philosophy and some of them are vulnerable to empirical disconfirmation. In this section, I run through a few of the more popular ones, while acknowledging that the selection is far from comprehensive and that the entire discussion deserves much more depth and detail.

Experience

Consider first the attention given by qualitative methodologists to *experience*. There are several sources for this but one of the most important is the phenomenological tradition. It is assumed, and constantly repeated, that phenomenology has from its inception been the study of 'lived experience', whether as a descriptive Husserlian enterprise, or as an interpretive Heideggerian one (Smith *et al.* 2009, Teddlie and Tashakkori 2009); and this often segues into the claim that qualitative research is, by definition, a form of enquiry that focuses on people's experiences (Holloway and Wheeler 2010).

The belief that Husserl and Heidegger were both, in different ways, concerned with 'lived experience' appears to be ineradicable. Yet it is (I would argue) mistaken. Husserl wanted to break out of ordinary experience, into the realm of pure, transcendental consciousness, by means of the phenomenological reduction. The reduction is not simply a matter of 'identifying one's preconceptions' and toggling them to 'off' as a precursor to interviewing; it is rather the wholesale cancellation of every form of inference and judgment employed in the natural attitude, including those concerning the very existence of other people (Husserl 1982). Heidegger explicitly disavows the concept of 'lived experience' (*Erlebnis*), along with 'consciousness' and 'subjectivity', because it belongs to the dualism between 'experiencing subject' and 'experienced object' that he is attempting to dismantle (Heidegger 1962). Heidegger does not offer a new, improved concept of 'subjectivity'. On the contrary, he wants to undermine objectivity and subjectivity as part of a package deal. Being-in-the-world has nothing to do with 'lived experience' (Keller 1999, Carman 2003); neither does 'pure transcendental consciousness' (Philipse 1995, Smith 2007). I have said more about all this in Paley (2014).

Description

Phenomenology is also a source for the assumption that qualitative research is essentially *descriptive*. According to Husserl, it is suggested, phenomenology is an 'inductive, descriptive method', a phrase associated with Omery (1983) but standardly repeated in articles and textbooks (Burns and Grove 2015, Beck 2006). However, description is a restriction imposed by the phenomenological reduction – and this is not, as I have just noted, a matter of the researcher 'bracketing her own experience'. It is something much more radical. The phenomenological reduction is a strategy for refraining from all the forms of cognition to which we have recourse routinely in the natural attitude: judging, theorizing, speculating, testing, explaining, taking for granted, assuming, evaluating, interrogating, hypothesizing, and so on. Transcendental consciousness, which is the outcome of the reduction, is a theory-free, judgment-free, inference-free, assumption-free zone; and the only thing left that can be done in this zone is to describe. In Husserl's phenomenology, description is literally the only game in town, because every other type of inference is deliberately and strategically excluded, to escape from ordinary 'experience' in the natural attitude. That is what the phenomenological reduction *is*.

But if qualitative research takes place in the natural attitude, not in transcendental consciousness – as it manifestly does, and as even Husserlians like Giorgi (2009) admit – then there is no longer any reason to impose this restriction. Why is description still mandated when the constraint that enforced it in the first place, the phenomenological reduction, has been abandoned? Why should a qualitative researcher, positioned in the natural attitude, be confined to 'descriptive analysis' when the reason for the self-denying ordinance no longer applies? Why continue to impose a methodological restriction which the epistemological circumstances no longer make necessary? Giorgi never answers this question; nor do phenomenological researchers in nursing.

Outside phenomenology, the preference for description is motivated by the idea that whatever is being studied should not have 'alien' categories imposed upon it, although there are several variations on this theme. According to an influential paper by Sandelowski (2000), qualitative descriptive studies should aim at accounts 'unencumbered' by theory, involving no 'pre-selection of variables' and 'no a priori commitment to any one theoretical view'. They should stick to the unadorned 'facts' and 'allow the phenomenon to present itself as it would if it were not under study'.

Studying something to determine 'how it presents itself' when it is not being studied sounds a bit self-defeating, like opening the fridge door to see if the interior light is on when the door is closed. Nevertheless, this argument points to a familiar unease. There is suspicion of 'pre-selected categories' and 'theory' because they might represent a challenge to the respondent's account. It is assumed that there is a doctrinaire quality, a sort of academic paternalism, in the adoption of a theoretical perspective different from, and possibly inconsistent with, the participant's version of events. By what right, and according to what warrant, can the participant's understanding of her own experience be questioned?

Below, I argue that there *is* such a warrant and that, as a consequence, theoretical challenges to the participant's account of her experience are inevitable. For now, consider the implications of the descriptive strategy in studies of, say, patient experience. If, as a matter of principle, researchers refrain from imposing their own concepts and categories on the respondent; if they avoid specific questions for fear of imposing their own agenda; if they merely invite the participant to talk about his experience 'in his own words', without any clue as to the question they are trying to answer, then the respondent is likely to discuss whatever comes to mind, whatever is salient to him. As a result, he will almost certainly cover the same ground as other respondents in comparable studies: for example, the shock of the diagnosis, the difficulty of coming to terms with a life-limiting disease, the stress of living with the condition, the embarrassment or discomfort of certain symptoms, the psychological consequences, the attempt to maintain a semblance of normality and independence, the disruption of ordinary life, the support of family, friends or health care professionals, and so on. I certainly do not want to underplay the horror, the anxiety, the misery and, in some cases, the tragedy conveyed by these stories. But, in research terms, they are excessively familiar, excessively routine, excessively banal. The 'descriptive' template of QRAS is, in effect, a device for reproducing the same basic findings, the same basic narrative, over and over again, across hundreds of studies.

For recent studies illustrating this claim, see Waller and Pattison (2013), Subasic (2013), Monaro *et al.* (2014), Baillie and Lankshear (2014), Follan and McNamara (2014), Liljeroos *et al.* (2014), Bolejko *et al.* (2014), Cheng *et al.* (2013), Kao and Tsai (2014), Feuchtinger *et al.* (2014), and Tao *et al.* (2014). Of course, not all studies will turn out this way; but the few that do not will either have been exceptionally lucky or will have departed in some significant manner from the QRAS template.

Induction

The claim that qualitative research is inductive conceals an ambiguity. In philosophy, 'induction' refers to the process of generalizing from examined cases to unexamined cases: all observed crows are black, so all unobserved crows must be black as well. The problem of induction is to find a way of justifying this kind of inference – from the sample to the population – and the solution usually involves reference to probability theory. Presumably, this cannot be what qualitative methodologists have in mind, because most of them reject the idea of generalization based on statistics. As Lincoln and Guba (1985) say: 'The only generalization is: there is no generalization'. So 'induction' in the context of qualitative methods is not used in the philosophical sense. Instead, it is a vague reference to the idea of a bottom-up process of enquiry, starting with data, in contrast to a top-down process, starting with theories and hypotheses.

And yet, as I noted earlier, the need to publish modest postgraduate studies requires that generalization from tiny samples should appear possible, even if probability theory does not warrant it. Consequently, several arguments have appeared, designed to suggest that small-sample generalization is feasible after all. It is hard to take some of them seriously. Stake (1978), for example, invented something he called 'naturalistic generalization', based on the idea that a small sample of cases 'may be epistemologically in harmony with the reader's experience'. In other words, generalization (with the 'naturalistic' tag) is possible if the researcher's findings comply with the reader's prejudices and preconceptions. This is akin to the 'phenomenological nod', promoted by van Manen (1990). Both imply that 'generalizable' is a way of referring to findings with which the reader already agrees, or which she readily accepts when they are presented to her. This is generalizability defined as: 'what the reader already thinks'. 'That accords with my experience, so it must be right'.

'Essence' is another concept that slots into the category of convenient inventions, and can be added to the list of phenomenological myths. The view that, according to Heidegger and Husserl, 'essences' can be identified by collecting empirical data is simply wrong. For both of them, identifying essences is a philosophical enterprise. It is a form of a priori analysis and empirical data are irrelevant. If you claim to have identified the 'essence of a phenomenon' by interviewing a handful of people, you are not doing anything that Husserl or Heidegger would have recognized as legitimate. What you are doing is generalizing from a tiny sample but concealing that fact by giving it a spurious alternative name.

The best known example of generalization by another name is transferability. According to Lincoln and Guba (1985), the extent to which findings from one context (the sample cases) can be 'transferred' to another context (new cases) is a 'function of the similarity between the two contexts'. If the researcher describes the research sample in sufficient detail – a 'thick description' – then I, the reader, will be able to assess whether the new cases are similar enough to warrant a 'transfer' of findings.

Everything hangs on the idea of 'similarity', but it is an extremely vague concept. Some similarities are relevant, others presumably are not. How do I know which is which? Suppose that, in a certain research study (see box below), the sample cases have all been found to have characteristic X and I want to know whether some of my own cases, as yet unexamined, will have the same characteristic. The thick description suggests that the research sample cases also have characteristics F and G. My new cases all have F but not G.

Research sample cases	X	[F, G]
My new cases	?	[F, ~ G]

Can I infer that my cases will have X as well? Does the fact that the sample cases and my new cases both have F make them similar enough? Is F a relevant similarity? Can I 'transfer' X on the basis of F, even though G is not present?

There is only one way I can answer this question and that is by having independent statistical evidence that there is an association between X and F but not between X and G. If there is such evidence, then X is 'transferable': I can 'transfer' X to my own cases (that is, I can infer that my own cases also have X). Otherwise not. So the idea of transferability presupposes a statistical generalization to make it work. But this is precisely the claim that Lincoln and Guba reject. Like 'naturalistic generalization', the 'phenomenological nod' or 'essence', 'transferability' is merely linguistic camouflage. It conceals the fact that, despite the author's denials, a generalization is being made.

Meaning

The idea that *meaning* is crucial to the social sciences has a long history, going back to Weber at least, but its recent contribution to the ideology of qualitative methods has been pivotal. Ever since the 1960s, when the influence of Schutz (1967) began to exert itself, it has been claimed that human beings 'act on the basis of the meanings they attribute' to reality (Poggi 2006); that action can be explained 'in terms of the subjective categories of the actor – the actor's beliefs, goals and intentions' (Martin 2000). This, if true, is staggeringly important. It implies that the ultimate source of action is something going on in people's heads: their conscious meanings, interpretings, understandings and definings. Context and circumstance may be significant but only to the extent that they are themselves interpreted. If this is correct, then understanding people's interpretation of experience – the 'meanings' they attach to it – is fundamental. It is the account that counts, and small-sample, in-depth interviewing is the only way to get access to it.

The link between meaning and behaviour is so foundational for the QRAS that it deserves a section to itself. Below, I examine the claim that people act on the basis of their 'meanings' and find it wanting.

Meaning and behaviour

The claim that human beings act on the basis of the meanings they attach to their experience is often presented as if it were a philosophical thesis. However, it is clearly an empirical generalization. It says that, making all due allowance for unusual circumstances, we can explain what people do by reference to their 'meanings'. The relation between 'meaning' and behaviour is unequivocally one of cause and effect. Generally speaking, an individual's meanings and interpretations account for her behaviour and her behaviour can, very broadly, be predicted on the basis of what we understand her meanings to be. (Here and elsewhere, I use 'behaviour' as a convenient shorthand for 'behaviour, judgments, decisions, and expressions of preference'.)

Being an empirical generalization, the 'meaning' claim is open to empirical testing and conceivably to empirical disconfirmation. In this section, I argue that it *has* been empirically disconfirmed. Forty years of social psychology have shown that people's 'meanings' do not explain their behaviour, at least not reliably, and that other factors do. There is often a discrepancy between how someone explains and interprets her own actions and what actually causes them. Such discrepancies are not exceptional; they are not occasional quirks or psychological oddities. Rather, they are standard, ubiquitous, pervasive. The literature is correspondingly vast, and I make no attempt to summarize it. Instead, I offer a few brief examples.

German judges read a detailed description of a case, then rolled a pair of dice which (unknown to them) were loaded so that every roll resulted in a 3 or a 9. They were then asked how long a prison sentence they would give the offender concerned. On average, those who rolled a 9 gave her eight months; those who rolled a 3 gave her five months (Englich *et al.* 2006). The judges attached no 'meaning' to the dice roll but it clearly influenced their decisions. This illustrates the anchoring effect (Kahneman 2011), in which irrelevant environmental cues influence the outcome of a judgment or action.

Shoppers were asked to decide which type of pantyhose they thought were the highest quality. Pairs of tights were in four piles labelled A, B, C, D (from left to right) and the preferences were, respectively, 12 per cent, 17 per cent, 31 per cent and 40 per cent. When participants were asked whether the position of their preferred type had influenced their choice, all but one said, 'of course not' and explained that their preferences were based on sheerness, elasticity, and so on. But all the pairs were identical (Wilson 2002).

In a study carried out by Hall *et al.* (2010), shoppers were asked to take part in what was ostensibly a consumer survey. Participants were invited to sample two different flavours of jam and decide which they preferred. Once they had expressed their preference, they were asked to sample the selected jam again and, this time, give their reasons for choosing that particular jam. However, a covert switch was carried out before the second sampling, so that (for example) a participant who had originally preferred the grapefruit flavour was now sampling the cinnamon-apple flavour. Only 14 per cent of shoppers detected the switch. The rest proceeded to give cinnamon-apple reasons for their preference, although they had originally chosen grapefruit (or vice versa), and expressed great surprise, amounting to disbelief, when the switch was explained. In this, as in the previous example, the 'meaning' which a subject attached to their selection (jam or pantyhose) did not, and could not, account for the preference they expressed.

Bargh *et al.* (1996) gave participants a scrambled sentence test which included words related to either rudeness, politeness or neither (this is known as priming). The participants were asked to inform the experimenter when they had finished. However, when they tried to do so, they found the experimenter engaged in a staged conversation with a confederate. Of those primed for rudeness, 67 per cent interrupted; of those primed for politeness, 16 per cent interrupted. In the debriefing, none of the participants showed any awareness of a link between the sentence test and their subsequent (non)interrupting-behaviour. They did not attach any 'meaning', in this respect, to the sentence test.

Subjects primed by being asked to search for first person plural pronouns ('we', 'our', 'us') in a writing sample were more likely to report that values such as interdependence, belongingness, friendship and family acted as 'guiding principles in their lives' than subjects primed to search for first person singular pronouns ('I', 'my'), who were more likely to endorse values such as freedom and autonomy (Gardner *et al.* 1999). In similar studies, participants exhibited enhanced performance on a subsequent task when primed with 'success' words and were more cooperative during a resource dilemma task when primed with cooperation-related words (Bargh *et al.* 2001). In none of these studies did participants recognize any link between the priming experience and their subsequent behaviour.

Participants consumed more of a novel drink and rated it as more appealing, after being subliminally presented with happy faces, than participants who were subliminally presented with angry or sad faces (Winjkielman *et al.* 2005). Experimental subjects who briefly held a cup of hot coffee judged another person to be warmer, more caring and more generous than those who briefly held a cup of iced coffee (Williams and Bargh 2008). None of the participants showed any awareness of the possible link between the temperature of the coffee and their judgment about the target person's personality traits.

University staff dropped money into an honesty box whenever they helped themselves to milk from the communal kitchen. For several weeks, a poster was placed above the box, changed on a weekly basis – pictures of flowers alternating with pictures of eyes that seemed to look directly at the observer. During the 'eyes' weeks, the average contribution was £0.70 per litre. During the 'flowers' weeks, it was £0.15 per litre. The staff did not know that the experiment was taking place and were unaware of the significance of the posters (Bateson *et al.* 2006).

People invited to complete a questionnaire on life satisfaction were first asked to photocopy a sheet of paper for the experimenter. Half the respondents found a dime on the copying machine, the other half did not. When their questionnaire results were analysed, the life satisfaction scores of the first group were significantly higher than those of the second (Schwartz and Strack 2003). However, members of the first group were not aware of any connection between finding the dime and their sense of satisfaction as expressed in the questionnaire.

This study is reminiscent of an experiment in which one group of people using a telephone box found a dime that had apparently been left in it by a previous user, while another group did not. On emerging from the telephone box, the first group were much more likely to help a passer-by who had dropped a folder of papers, now scattered on the pavement, than the second group (Isen and Levin 1972). This is a further illustration of the way in which imperceptible environmental cues influence people's behaviour.

One version of a famous ethical problem involves inviting participants to decide whether it is morally acceptable to push a large man off a footbridge to stop a trolley that would otherwise kill five people further down the line (the large man will inevitably die instead). Most people say no. However, people who have watched a funny film immediately beforehand are significantly more likely to claim that pushing the man off the bridge is, in the circumstances, morally accept-able (Valdesolo and DeSteno 2006). The 'meaning' they attach to their decision reflects, so they claim, the moral requirements of the situation; it has nothing to do with the film.

Physicians asked to recommend surgery or radiation for lung cancer were given statistics pertaining to the surgery option. Half were provided with the survival rates (one month survival rate of 90 per cent) and the other half were given the same information in terms of mortality rates (10 per cent mortality rate in the first month). Eighty-four per cent of physicians opted for surgery when given the survival rate version; only 50 per cent did so when provided with the mortality-rate version (McNeil *et al.* 1982). They all based their choice on the 'meaning' they 'attached' to the statistical information they were given. None of them realized that their decision was influenced by the way the information was presented, not by the information itself. This illustrates the role of framing in preference elicitation (Lichtenstein and Slovic 2006: 1–40).

People asked to nod their heads while listening to a recorded talk through headphones (ostensibly to test the 'not slipping off your head' properties of the headphones) subsequently report a greater degree of agreement with the position being defended in the recording than people asked to shake their heads while carrying out the same task (Wells and Petty 1980). This illustrates the process of unconsciously inferring one's own beliefs by observing one's own behaviour. I am nodding my head, so I must agree with what is being said.

People were invited to eat grasshoppers by an experimenter who was either cold and distant (for half the subjects) or warm and affable (for the other half). About 50 per cent of all participants actually ate one or more grasshoppers. Those who did so at the invitation of the unfriendly experimenter subsequently reported a much more favourable attitude towards grasshoppers as food than those who did so at the invitation of the friendly experimenter (Zimbardo *et al.* 1965). The members of the first group cannot explain their eating-grasshopper behaviour by telling themselves that they were induced by a charming and persuasive experi-menter, so they infer that grasshoppers are not so bad after all. Members of the second group can explain their behaviour that way, so have no incentive to believe that grasshoppers make decent food. The mechanism here is cognitive dissonance, which involves people unconsciously inferring their attitudes by observing their own behaviour (Cooper 2007). This is, of course, the inverse of explaining an action on the basis of the 'meaning' that people attach to it.

The examples that I have described do not scratch the surface of the literature on how cognitive mechanisms influence a person's thoughts, perceptions or behaviour in ways of which they are not conscious (Kunda 1999, Eagly and Chaiken 1993, Gilovich *et al.* 2002, Wilson 2002, Hassin *et al.* 2005, Lichtenstein and Slovic 2006, Dalbert 2009, Pronin 2009, Chabris and Simons 2011, Carruthers 2011, Kahneman 2011, Vazire and Wilson 2012). If the effects of these mechanisms were exceptional, it might not matter a great deal. However, as I said earlier, the evidence demonstrates that they are ubiquitous. In fact, they are routine.

The existence of such mechanisms casts considerable doubt on the claim that people act (or formulate judgments, or make decisions, or express preferences) on the basis of the 'meanings' they attribute to experience, and suggests that the understanding of action (or judgments, or decisions, or preferences) frequently requires reference to cognitive dynamics of which the person concerned is unaware and to which they attach no 'meaning' at all. It is this 'cognitive unconscious' (Kihlstrom 1987) that provides the warrant (anticipated earlier) for challenges to the participant's account. If we are interested in the reasons why people behave as they do, or why they express particular beliefs and preferences, a study of 'meanings' will contribute little or nothing to this project.

I am not claiming that people *never* act on the basis of their attached meanings. I am claiming that, in a particular case, it is impossible to determine whether they have or have not just by interviewing them. It is 'misleading for social scientists to ask their subjects about the influence on their evaluations, choices, or behaviour' (Nisbett and Wilson 1977: 247). Similarly, 'demonstrations of respondents' lack of introspective access to the causes of their own judgments and behaviour ... forever shattered the illusion that self-reports would be a sufficient means for illuminating the workings of the mind' (Gawronski and Bodenhausen 2007: 265). The consequences of this for QRAS are potentially devastating, because it implies that interviewing people to determine their motives, reasons, desires, intentions, beliefs and preferences is likely to be fruitless.

It has been suggested to me, more than once, that this line of thought leads to behaviourism. I do not see how. Those who write about the 'adaptive unconscious' (Wilson 2002), the 'new unconscious' (Hassin *et al.* 2005) or the 'cognitive unconscious' (Kihlstrom 1987) do not omit mental states in the way that the behaviourists did. Instead, they claim that our behaviour is frequently determined – more often than we might imagine – by mental states which are below the consciousness threshold. People who dislike this idea might object to it for all sorts of reasons. But you cannot sensibly argue against a position that talks about unconscious mental states by complaining that it leaves out mental states.

Summary and conclusion

The postgraduate environment has selected for tiny-sample, interview-based studies of experience, and the meanings people attach to it, as a result of which there has been an evolutionary convergence of different research species. The environment has also selected for philosophical discourse replicators designed to justify the QRAS; but these memes – I have looked at arguments in favour of description, experience, meaning and induction – do not stand up to scrutiny. Moreover, the evidence from social psychology heavily qualifies, if it does not completely undermine, the usual assumption that people act on the basis of their 'meanings'.

I would argue that qualitative research, in any field, cannot be done adequately if the researcher does not have some familiarity with cognitive and social psychology or an understanding of the cognitive mechanisms to which I have been alluding. Some qualitative research, fortunately, meets this condition but, here, I have been concerned, not with qualitative research *tout court*, but with the qualitative research analogous structure. At this point, then, a reminder of what I take the QRAS to be might be opportune:

> The *retrospective description* of *experience* and *meaning* through *small-sample interviewing*, both data collection and analysis being carried out *in the absence of theoretical preconceptions*, with the implicit aim of *inductively* generalizing to a population while explicitly disowning the concept of generalization.

The conclusion is as follows: the claim that qualitative research evidence should be placed on an equal footing with experimental and statistical evidence is (in the case of evidence derived from QRAS) quite without warrant. In fact, I would go further and describe it as preposterous.

References

Baillie, J. and Lankshear, A. (2014) Patient and family perspectives on peritoneal dialysis at home: findings from an ethnographic study. *Journal of Clinical Nursing*, doi: 10.1111/jocn.12663.

Bargh, J. A., Chen, M. and Burrows, L. (1996) Automaticity of social behavior: direct effects of trait construct and stereotype activation on action. *Journal of Personality and Social Psychology*, 71, 230–44.

Bargh, J. A., Gollwitzer, P. M., Lee-Chai, A., Barndollar, K. and Trötschel, R. (2001) The automated will: nonconscious activation and pursuit of behavioral goals. *Journal of Personality and Social Psychology*, 81, 1014–27.

Bateson, M., Nettle, D. and Roberts, G. (2006) Cues of being watched enhanced cooperation in a real-world setting. *Biology Letters*, 2, 412–14.

Beck, C. T. (2006) Phenomenology. In *Encyclopedia of Nursing Research*, Fitzpatrick, J. J. and Wallace, M. (eds) (pp. 431–3). New York: Springer.

Bolejko, A., Zackrisson, S., Hagell, P. and Wann-Hansson, C. (2014) A roller coaster of emotions and sense: coping with the perceived psychosocial consequences of a false-positive screening mammography. *Journal of Clinical Nursing*, 23(13–14), 2053–62.

Booth, J., Tolson, D., Hotchkiss, R. and Schofield, I. (2007) Using action research to construct national evidence-based nursing care guidance for gerontological nursing. *Journal of Clinical Nursing*, 16(5), 845–953.

Burns, N. and Grove, S. K. (2015) *Understanding Nursing Research*, 6th edn. Philadelphia, PA: Elsevier Saunders.

Carman, T. (2003) *Heidegger's Analytic: Interpretation, Discourse, and Authenticity in Being and Time*, Cambridge: Cambridge University Press.

Carper, B. (1978) Fundamental patterns of knowing in nursing. *Advances in Nursing Science*, 1(1), 13–24.

Carruthers, P. (2011) *The Opacity of Mind: An Integrative Theory of Self-Knowledge*, Oxford: Oxford University Press.

Chabris, C. and Simons, D. (2011) *The Invisible Gorilla and Other Ways In Which Our Intuition Deceives Us*, London: Harper.

Cheng, C.-H., Wang, T.-J., Lin, Y.-P., Lin, H.-R., Hu, W.-Y., Wung, S.-H. and Liang, S.-Y. (2013) The illness experience of middle-aged men with oral cancer. *Journal of Child Psychology and Psychiatry*, 22, 3549–56.

Colyer, H. and Kamath, P. (1999) Evidence-based practice: a philosophical and political analysis: some matters for consideration by professional practitioners. *Journal of Advanced Nursing*, 29, 188–93.

Cooper, J. (2007) *Cognitive Dissonance: Fifty Years of a Classic Theory*, London: Sage.

Dalbert, C. (2009) Belief in a just world. In *Handbook of Individual Differences in Social Behavior*, Leary, M. R. and Hoyle, R. H. (eds) (pp. 288–97), New York: Guilford.

Dlugaschi, L. B. and Ugarriza, D. (2014) Self-monitoring of blood glucose experiences of adults with type 2 diabetes. *Journal of the American Association of Nurse Practitioners*, 26(6), 323–29.

Eagly, A. H. and Chaiken, S. (1993) *The Psychology of Attitudes*, Belmont, CA: Wadsworth.

Englich, B., Mussweiler, T. and Strack, F. (2006) Playing dice with criminal sentences: the influence of irrelevant anchors on experts' judicial decision making. *Personality and Social Psychology Bulletin*, 32, 188–200.

Fawcett, J., Watson, J., Neuman, B., Walker, P. H. and Fitzpatrick, J. J. (2001) On nursing theories and evidence. *Journal of Nursing Scholarship*, 33, 115–19.

Feuchtinger, J., Burbaum, C., Heilmann, C., Imvery, C., Siepe, M., Stotz, U., Fritzsche, K. and Beyersdorf, F. (2014) Anxiety and fear in patients with short waiting times before coronary artery bypass surgery: a qualitative study. *Journal of Clinical Nursing*, 23(13–14), 1900–7.

Follan, M. and McNamara, M. (2014) A fragile bond: adoptive parents' experiences of caring for children with a diagnosis of reactive attachment disorder. *Journal of Clinical Nursing*, 23(7), 1076–85.

Førsund, L. H., Skovdahl, K., Kiik, R. and Ytrehus, S. (2014) The loss of a shared lifetime: a qualitative study exploring spouses' experiences of losing couplehood with their partner with dementia living in institutional care. *Journal of Clinical Nursing*, doi: 10.1111/jocn.12648.

Freshwater, D. and Rolfe, G. (2004) *Deconstructing Evidence-Based Practice*. Abingdon: Routledge.

Freshwater, D., Cahill, J., Walsh, E. and Muncey, T. (2010) Qualitative research as evidence: criteria for rigour and relevance. *Journal of Research in Nursing*, 15(6), 497–508.

Gardner, W. L., Gabriel, S. and Lee, A. Y. (1999) 'I' value freedom but 'we' value relationships: self-construal priming mirrors cultural differences in judgment. *Psychological Science*, 10, 321–6.

Gawronski, B. and Bodenhausen, G. V. (2007) What do we know about implicit attitude measures and what do we have to learn? In *Implicit Measures of Attitudes*, Wittenbrink, B. and Schwartz, N. (eds) (pp. 265–86) New York: Guilford.

Gibson, J. and Watkins, C. (2012) People's experiences of the impact of transient ischaemic attack and its consequences: qualitative study. *Journal of Advanced Nursing*, 68(8), 1707–15.

Gilovich, T., Griffin, D. and Kahneman, D. (eds) (2002) *Heuristics and Biases: The Psychology of Intuitive Judgment*, Cambridge: Cambridge University Press.

Giorgi, A. (2009) *The Descriptive Phenomenological Method in Psychology: A Modified Husserlian Approach*, Pittsburgh: Duquesne University Press.

Giske, T. and Cone, P. H. (2012) Opening up to learning spiritual care of patients: a grounded theory study of nursing students. *Journal of Clinical Nursing*, 21, 2006–15.

Glaser, B. G. and Strauss, A. L. (1967) *The Discovery of Grounded Theory: Strategies for Qualitative research*, New Brunswick, NJ: Aldine Transaction.

Greenfield, G., Pliskin, J. S., Feder-Bubis, P., Wientroub, S. and Davidovitch, N. (2012) Patient-physician relationships in second opinion encounters: the physicians' perspective. *Social Science and Medicine*, 75(7), 1202–12.

Hall, L., Johansson, P., Tärning, B., Sikstrom, S. and Deutgen, T. (2010) Magic at the marketplace: choice, blindness for taste of jam and the smell of tea. *Cognition*, 117, 54–61.

Hassin, R. R., Uleman, J. S. and Bargh, J. A. (eds) (2005) *The New Unconscious*, New York: Oxford University Press.

Heidegger, M. (1962) *Being and Time*, Oxford: Basil Blackwell.

Helgesen, A. K., Larsson, M. and Athlin, E. (2013) How do relatives of persons with dementia experience their role in the patient participation process in special care units? *Journal of Clinical Nursing*, 22(11–12), 1672–81.

Holloway, I. and Wheeler, S. (2010) *Qualitative Research in Nursing and Healthcare*. 3rd ed., Oxford: Wiley-Blackwell.

Holmes, D., Perron, A. and O'Byrne, P. (2006) Evidence, virulence, and the disappearance of nursing knowledge: a critique of the evidence-based dogma. *Worldviews on Evidence-Based Nursing*, 3(3), 95–102.

Husserl, E. (1982) *Ideas I: Ideas Pertaining to a Pure Phenomenology and a Phenomenological Philosophy: General Introduction to a Pure Phenomenology*, Dordrecht: Kluwer.

Isen, A. M. and Levin, P. F. (1972) The effect of feeling food on a helping task that is incompatible with good mood. *Social Psychology*, 41, 346–9.

Jack, S. (2006) Utility of qualitative research findings in evidence-based public health practice. *Public Health Nursing*, 23(3), 277–83.

Kahneman, D. (2011) *Thinking, Fast and Slow*, London: Allen Lane.

Kao, M.-H. and Tsai, Y.-F. (2014) Illness experiences in middle-aged adults with early-stage knee osteoarthritis: findings from a qualitative study. *Journal of Advanced Nursing*, 70(7), 1564–72.

Keller, P. (1999) *Husserl and Heidegger on Human Experience*, Cambridge: Cambridge University Press.

Kihlstrom, J. F. (1987) The cognitive unconscious. *Science*, 237, 1445–52.

Kitson, A. (2002) Recognising relationships: reflections on evidence-based practice. *Nursing Inquiry*, 9(3), 179–86.

Kunda, Z. (1999) *Social Cognition: Making Sense of People*, Cambridge, MA: MIT Press.

Lee, P.-S., Lee, C.-L., Hu, S.-T. and Tsao, L.-I. (2014) Relieving my discomforts safely: the experiences of discontinuing HRT among menopausal women. *Journal of Clinical Nursing*, 23(17–18), 2481–90.

Leeman, J. and Sandelowski, M. (2012) Practice-based evidence and qualitative inquiry. *Journal of Nursing Scholarship*, 44(2), 171–9.

Lichtenstein, S. and Slovic, P. (eds) (2006) *The Construction of Preference*, Cambridge: Cambridge University Press.

Liljeroos, M., Agren, S., Jaarsma, T. and Strömberg, A. (2014) Perceived caring needs in patient-partner dyads affected by heart failure: a qualitative study. *Journal of Clinical Nursing*, 23(19–20), 2928–38.

Lincoln, Y. S. and Guba, E. G. (1985) *Naturalistic Inquiry*, Beverly Hills, CA: Sage.

Lines, K. (2001) A philosophical analysis of evidence-based practice in mental health nursing. *Australian and New Zealand Journal of Mental Health Nursing*, 10, 167–75.

Mantzoukas, S. (2008) A review of evidence-based practice, nursing research and reflection: levelling the hierarchy. *Journal of Clinical Nursing*, 17(2), 214–23.

Martin, M. (2000) *Verstehen: The Uses of Understanding in Social Science*, New Brunswick, NJ: Transaction.

Mayo, D. G. (1996) *Error and the Growth of Experimental Knowledge*, Chicago: University of Chicago Press.

McNeil, B., Pauker, S. G., Sox, H. C. and Tversky, A. (1982) On the elicitation of preferences for alternative therapies. *New England Journal of Medicine*, 306, 1259–62.

Mitchell, G. J. (2013) Implications of holding ideas of evidence-based practice in nursing. *Nursing Science Quarterly*, 26(2), 143–51.

Monaro, S., Stewart, G. and Gullick, J. (2014) A 'lost life': coming to terms with haemodialysis. *Journal of Clinical Nursing*, 23(2), 3262–73.

Nisbett, R. E. and Wilson, T. D. (1977) Telling more than we can know: verbal reports on mental processes. *Psychological Review*, 84(3), 231–59.

Omery, A. (1983) Phenomenology: a method for nursing research. *Advances in Nursing Science*, 5, 49–63.

Paley, J. (2005) Error and objectivity: cognitive illusions and qualitative research. *Nursing Philosophy*, 6, 196–209.

Paley, J. (2006) Evidence and expertise. *Nursing Inquiry*, 13(2), 82–93.

Paley, J. (2014) Heidegger, lived experience and method. *Journal of Advanced Nursing*, 70(7), 1520–31.

Philipse, H. (1995) Transcendental idealism. In *The Cambridge Companion to Husserl*, Smith, B. and Smith, D. W. (eds) (pp. 239–322). Cambridge: Cambridge University Press.

Poggi, G. (2006) *Weber: A Short Introduction*, Cambridge: Polity.

Pronin, E. (2009) The introspection illusion. *Advances in Experimental Social Psychology*, 41, 1–67.

Reisenhofer, S. and Seibold, C. (2013) Emergency healthcare experiences of women living with intimate partner violence. *Journal of Clinical Nursing*, 22(15–16), 2253–63.

Rycroft-Malone, J., Seers, K., Titchen, A., Harvey, G., Kitson, A. and McCormack, B. (2004) What counts as evidence in evidence-based practice? *Journal of Advanced Nursing*, 47(1), 81–90.

Sandelowski, M. (2000) Whatever happened to qualitative description. *Research in Nursing and Health*, 23, 334–40.

Schutz, A. (1945) On multiple realities. *Philosophy and Phenomenological Research*, 5(4), 533–76.

Schutz, A. (1967) *The Phenomenology of the Social World*, Evanston, IL: Northwestern University Press.

Schwartz, N. and Strack, F. (2003) Reports of subject well-being: judgmental processes and their methodological implications. In *Well-Being: Foundations of Hedonic Psychology*, Kahneman, D., Diener, E. and Schwartz, N. (eds) (pp. 61–84). New York: Russell Sage Foundation.

Smith, D. W. (2007) *Husserl*, London: Routledge.

Smith, J. A., Flowers, P. and Larkin, M. (2009) *Interpretive Phenomenological Analysis*, London: Sage.

Stake, R. E. (1978) The case-study method in social inquiry. *Educational Researcher*, 7, 5–8.

Subasic, K. (2013) Living with hypertrophic cardiomyopathy. *Journal of Nursing Scholarship*, 45(4), 371–9.

Tao, H., Songwathana, P., Isaramalai, S. and Wang, Q. (2014) Taking good care of myself: a qualitative study on self-care behavior among Chinese persons with a permanent colostomy. *Nursing and Health Sciences*, doi: 10.1111/nhs.12166.

Teddlie, C. and Tashakkori, A. (2009) *Foundations of Mixed Methods Research: Integrating Quantitative and Qualitative Approaches in the Social and Behavioural Sciences*, Los Angeles, CA: Sage.

Thorne, S. (2009) The role of qualitative research within an evidence-based context: can metasynthesis be the answer? *International Journal of Nursing Studies*, 46, 569–75.

Upshur, R. E. G., VanDenKerkhof, E. and Goel, V. (2001) Meaning and measurement: an inclusive model of evidence in health care. *Journal of Evaluation in Clinical Practice*, 7, 91–6.

Valdesolo, P. and DeSteno, D. (2006) Manipulations of emotional context shape moral judgment. *Psychological Science*, 17, 476–7.

Van Dover, L. and Pfeiffer, J. (2012) Patients of parish nurses experience renewed spiritual identity: a grounded theory study. *Journal of Advanced Nursing*, 68(8), 1824–44.

van Manen, M. (1990) *Researching Lived Experience: Human Science for an Action Sensitive Pedagogy*, Albany, NY: State University of New York Press.

Vazire, S. and Wilson, T. D. (eds) (2012) *Handbook of Self-Knowledge*, New York: Guilford.

Waller, J. and Pattison, N. (2013) Men's experiences of regaining urinary continence following robotic-assisted laparoscopic prostatectomy (RALP) for localised prostate cancer: a qualitative phenomenological study. *Journal of Clinical Nursing*, 22, 363–78.

Wells, G. and Petty, R. (1980) The effects of overt head movements on persuasion. *Basic and Applied Social Psychology*, 1, 219–30.

Welsh, I. and Lyons, C. M. (2001) Evidence-based care and the case for intuition and tacit knowledge in clinical assessment and decision making in mental health nursing practice: an empirical contribution to the debate. *Journal of Psychiatric and Mental Health Nursing*, 8, 299–305.

Williams, L. E. and Bargh, J. A. (2008) Experiencing physical warmth promotes interpersonal warmth. *Science*, 322(5901), 606–7.

Wilson, T. D. (2002) *Strangers to Ourselves: Discovering the Adaptive Unconscious*, Cambridge, MA: Belknap.

Winjkielman, P., Berridge, K. C. and Wilbarger, J. L. (2005) Unconscious affective reactions to masked happy versus angry faces influence consumption behavior and judgments of value. *Personality and Social Psychology Bulletin*, 31(1), 121–35.

Zeeman, L., Aranda, K. and Grant, A. (2014) Queer challenges to evidence-based practice. *Nursing Inquiry*, 21(2), 101–11.

Zimbardo, P. G., Weisenberg, M., Forestone, I. and Levy, B. (1965) Communicative effectiveness in producing public conformity and private attitude change. *Journal of Personality*, 33, 233–55.

11 The status and use value of qualitative research findings

New ways to make sense of qualitative work

Sally Thorne

In an era of in which "evidence-based" practices have become uncritically preferred over those that are not in many quarters, it is not surprising that we encounter considerable controversy over the matter of what constitutes evidence. In the wider healthcare delivery system discourse, for example, an evidence-based claim about one's services becomes conflated with impressions of excellence, integrity and credibility, thus taking on an ideological, rather than just a scientific or technical dimension. Within the public domain, where members of society are increasingly looking to evidence as a basis for their health-related decisions, formal scientific evidence is increasingly accessible and is often in competition with various forms of marketing and persuasion. These broader contextual phenomena have created an enthusiasm within many scholarly and professional quarters to find new and creative ways to expand the conventional boundaries of the evidence definition, such that systematically developed knowledge finds a rightful place within the evidence conversation. In particular, scholars using qualitative methods in the health field have contributed to this confusion by advancing the products of all such efforts "as evidence." From my perspective, there seems to have been insufficient critical reflection on the implications of expansion of this evidence idea to ensure that the qualitative research community is not inadvertently contributing to the confusion and ideological posturing that faces planners, practitioners, and patients, not to mention the general public with a legitimate interest in this matter.

Although practice and policy decision makers tend to prefer absolute certainties, such as confident claims that one treatment works better than another under comparable circumstances, researchers understand that conclusions about science are rarely that conclusive. Because of this, evidence debates swirl around matters of what does and does not get included in an evidentiary claim and, as a result, there is increasing interest in deconstructing the nature of the various knowledge forms as well as interpreting their relationship to the idea we have in mind when we use the term "evidence." In this chapter, I attempt to untangle the somewhat circular argument that underscores much of the evidence dialogue within qualitative research circles, and to propose an alternative approach to understanding the appropriate role of qualitative research processes and products in addressing the problems that the evidence based practice movement was meant to solve.

What is evidence for or against?

It may be useful to begin with a reflection on where the evidence based movement began. As it is understood today, the movement is traceable to Archie
Cochrane's (1972) treatise on *Effectiveness and Efficiency: Random Reflections
on Health Services*, published as an attempt to bridge a divide between scientific
medicine and clinical judgment that he had come to associate with social injus-
tices experienced as a medical office during a four-year period as a German
prisoner of war (Shah and Chung, 2009). Although he was not the first to question the effectiveness of medical therapies, Cochrane's book was particularly
persuasive in using an amalgamation of studies to demonstrate that the problem
of evidence was pervasive across medical contexts (Cochrane, 1989). While
Cochrane would not have challenged the sentiment of Sir William Osler's often
quoted claim that the practice of medicine had the attributes of an art of probability, based on science of uncertainty (Silverman *et al.*, 2008), he also recognized
that there was a fundamental difference between 'obvious' logic and scientifically
demonstrable likelihood. Specifically, he was motivated by clear evidence that
seemingly obvious logic is not uncommonly flawed, leading to unnecessary and
inappropriate patient morbidities (Sackett and Rosenberg, 1995).

The goal of the evidence based practice movement as it evolved from
Cochrane's initial challenge was to solidify the scientific foundation of health
care and reduce uncertainties in clinical decision making (Sackett and Rosenberg,
1995). It sought to encourage the sensible use of the best available external
evidence from systematic research assimilated with knowledge derived from clinical expertise to determine the best course of care for a patient (Sackett *et al.*,
1996). In this manner, it was designed not to diminish the importance of the "art"
of medicine, but rather to ensure that commitment to that art did not trump flawed
logic. Thus, it was a movement aimed not only at discovering better practices, but
also – and perhaps more importantly – at stopping bad practice.

Nurses are quick to recognize the value of evidence in curtailing unproven
practice when it represents a medical intervention they consider excessive (such
as the overuse of radical mastectomy for breast cancer, or heroic lifesaving measures for individuals who have expressed a desire to die with dignity), or for
care-system expectations that offend their sensibilities around what patient-
oriented care ought to look like (such as barring fathers from the delivery room
or allowing parents to comfort their post-surgical children in the recovery room).
However, they can be much less enthusiastic about applying the evidence standard to many of their own practices, typically granting considerable license to the
merits of multiple ways of knowing to inform nursing practice, including the
value of such attributes as pattern recognition clinical wisdom (Clarke, 1999;
French, 2002; Thompson, 2003). This kind of logical slippage tends to be associated with a misguided assumption that evidence based practice excludes other
forms of knowledge from being relevant to a clinical decision-making process,
rather than being a commitment to understand and be informed by the nature and
quality of evidence that exists in relation to the kind of decision one is making.

What kind of science does health care evidence require?

When we claim that practice is based on evidence, we are setting forth a claim that we have access to credible and replicable scientific confirmation that one particular approach to a designated situation works better than another. Global claims about evidence, such as "the evidence shows ..." or "there is clear evidence ..." convey to an intended audience a persuasive claim that a particular course of action has been established. In the world of marketing toothpaste, a claim that evidence exists to confirm that one brand is better than another may simply be taken by the receiving public as an exaggerated expression of confidence in one's product. In the world of professional health care practice, however, a claim about evidence is – and fundamentally must be – something quite different from an obvious logic or opinion writ large.

The idea that a particular kind of science is needed to warrant claims about evidence in relation to the nature of a problem or decision to be taken was well established in the early days of the evidence based practice movement. Sacket *et al.* (1996: 72) illustrated this using various examples. For a question about prognosis, they explained that you would require proper follow-up studies of cases assembled at a uniform point early in the clinical disease course. To determine the accuracy of a diagnostic text, you would need proper cross-sectional studies of persons clinically suspected of harbouring a particular disorder. For questions about whether certain interventions did or did not work, or whether they did more good than harm, the randomized controlled trial (RCT) had become the gold standard. However, they strongly emphasized the point that not all interventions or therapies were amenable to an RCT approach, and instead required that one look for "next best" evidence according to the nature of the question being posed. However, they specifically cautioned against using non-experimental approaches since, in their opinion, these routinely lead to false positive conclusions about efficacy.

What is qualitative research in relation to evidentiary knowledge?

Qualitative research as we know it today originated as a systematic approach to scholarly inquiry in disciplines typically characterized as social sciences and humanities, such as sociology and anthropology (Bowers, 2013). First mentioned in the French literature of the early nineteenth century, the idea inherent in the term "social sciences" was an outgrowth of philosophy (Wokler, 1995). Concerned with efforts to standardize and regularize theorizing about such matters as the opposition between animality and morality that intrigued these early scholars, they began to develop rules about scholarship and methodology that became more fully formalized toward the mid-twentieth century as a science of social theorizing (Baker, 1964). Although the term "social science" now tends to be used as an general or umbrella reference to all disciplines using rigorous scholarly approaches to analyze society and culture, its roots in the philosophical questions of social organization and the nature of humanity are important to informing an understanding of the strong alignment between its methodologies and the larger project of social theorizing (Reason, 1996).

Qualitative methods first entered the nursing research lexicon in the last three decades of the twentieth century in response to an increasing level of disciplinary awareness of the inherent limitations of conventional health science methods for addressing some of the more experiential, dynamic and complex human health phenomena of concern to nursing practice (Bowers, 2013; Dzurek, 1989). These methods allowed for an extension of formal inquiry beyond that which can be regularized, decontextualized, and quantified, opening up many of the more profoundly interesting dimensions of what concerns nurses to systematic study. The alignment with methods associated with social science, by then a well-recognized form of scholarship, served the early years of the movement quite well in that it helped build legitimacy for a version of "science" that departed from what had become normalized in the rest of the biomedical scientific world (Thorne, 2008). However, in seeking a measure of credibility through aligning its qualitative methodologies more closely to the social than the biomedical sciences, a significant number of nursing's qualitative scholars drifted away from an ethos of using the method to solve the discipline's clinical problems (Chenail, 1992; Miller and Crabtree, 1994), evolving toward more explicitly situating their scholarship as social science, or theorizing for its own sake (Thorne, 2011). Thus, through rigorous attention to the social science methodological tradition in order to sidestep the critique of fuzzy scholarship, various species of qualitative nursing research products began to appear that bore little relationship to the clinical complexities that had motivated the movement in the first place. The applied qualitative research movement in nursing and other health disciplines is now emerging to try to wrestle that emphasis back (Thorne, 2014). This becomes relevant to the conversation with respect to the role of qualitative research in evidence based practice, in that we have essentially appropriated methods designed for one purpose in an attempt to put them to use elsewhere. And that disjuncture has not yet attracted the level of rigorous and deep consideration I believe it deserves.

The qualitative health research community has long felt itself to be the "poor cousin" of more quantitative forms of health science in the evidence based practice genealogy (Denzin, 2009; Morse, 2012). In considerations of what does and does not constitute evidence for practice, not only is it eliminated from the upper rungs, but it is may not even qualify for the zones that Sackett *et al.* (1996) would have referenced as "next best," in that it is often quite difficult to distinguish it from the anecdotal knowledge that is at the core of the illogic that evidence based practice is designed to extinguish (Limb, 2011). In an effort to elevate the stature of the genre, and underscore the importance of the kinds of insights that have derived from qualitative approaches, a number of qualitatively inclined investigators have used various language manipulations, such as referencing "qualitative evidence," or have sought out integrative or meta-synthesis options for expanding upon the more tenuous claims that can be warranted on the basis of single pieces of qualitative inquiry. Having set the stage for why the evidence based practice movement exists, and the reasons that anecdotal information are quite properly considered suspect within it, I turn more directly to the complex question of why this misalignment is important at this juncture in the evolution of our disciplinary knowledge development processes.

What are the dangers of positioning qualitative findings "as evidence?"

In the civil legal sense, we are familiar with the idea that everything, whether weak or strong, that is admissible into a particular consideration may be considered as part of the "evidence," and it becomes the "preponderance" of this evidence that persuades the decision. Certainly individual pieces of evidence are considered in terms of their convincingness and their probable truth or accuracy, but it becomes the "weight" that can legitimately sway the verdict. In the context of criminal law, we see a more severe test of evidence referenced as "beyond a reasonable doubt," implying that there is no viable alternative choice (Oran, 2000).

In the medical and healthcare sense, neither of these conceptualizations of evidence is quite applicable (Upshur, 2001). Because the post-positivist scientific world orients itself toward assumptions of a theoretical truth, regardless of whether one can actually aspire to arrive at it, the evidence-building project is directed toward substantiating the body of evidence upon which one becomes ever more certain of the rightness of a particular course of action in a common set of cases. When the law considers evidence, it considers the specificities and peculiarities of the case before it; when medicine considers a case, the evidence it brings to bear is that which has been derived from other cases thought to be similar to the one at hand. Thus, the nature of evidence in the medical and healthcare sense is constructed under a much more narrow set of principles than the more generous framework of legal evidence. It is well recognized that all medical decisions are fraught with some level of uncertainty, and it is the role of evidence to reduce that uncertainty. However, even when the body of evidence is strong, the Cochrane and Sackett orientation of evidence-based practice always calls for an integration of its directionality with the expanded particularized insights that derive from clinical expertise (Traynor, 2002). Therefore the kind of knowledge that a skilled clinician brings to bear in determining the recommended course of action for any patient is not only the available evidence, but also the human and contextual understandings obtained through other knowledge forms (Sackett, 2000). It is essential, then, that the evidence aspect is quite clearly distinguished from the other aspect, to understand where they align and where they might conflict. The process of high-quality evidence-based medical practice therefore demands a clear understanding of various knowledge that may be highly important and relevant, but are not by their very nature evidence.

If we misguidedly allow for a blurring of definitional properties of evidence as a means by which to ensure that it includes all forms of knowledge from which a nurse might legitimately build a good decision, we lose track of what differentiates the various knowledge forms, creating a circularity of logic within which everything is evidence and nothing remains as a corrective for false logic. Thus, the level of confusion for what constitutes evidence for practice across the nursing literature is highly worrisome (Rolfe *et al.*, 2008; Tarlier, 2005). A review of the literature yields numerous arguments in favor of extending the evidence boundary well beyond what can be scientifically derived (Morse, 2012; Rycroft-Malone *et al.*, 2004). We see, for example, depictions of such entities as "theoretic evidence, practical evidence, expert evidence, judicial evidence and ethics-based evidence" (Buetow and Kenealy, 2000: 85). Studies of how nurses take up evidence report that they include in that definition such possibilities as professional literature tailored to their particular specialty practice and their personal experience (Profetto-McGrath *et al.*, 2010), guidance provided by other more senior clinicians (Bonner and Lloyd, 2011), internet sources and textbooks (Verhoeven *et al.*, 2009), and conveniently pre-packaged resources (O'Leary and Mhaolrunaigh, 2011). In addition to the considerable interpretive license being taken with respect to what evidence might mean among those who believe it to be valuable and appropriate, there is also a thoughtful and potentially more problematic debate in the nursing literature with regard to the very motives underlying the movement. At its worst, evidence-based practice is depicted as the essence of a dehumanizing medical reductionism and an attempt to discredit alternative forms of knowledge that ought properly to be considered in clinical decision making (Freshwater and Rolfe, 2004; Madjar and Walton, 2001; Walker, 2003). Traynor describes this tension as "a struggle between those who have promoted a discourse of nursing as a morally located activity and those who have emphasized technical expertise and autonomy of practice" as exemplifying the ideal characteristics of the profession (Traynor, 1999: 187). Reflecting the complex constellation of contextual issues affecting nursing in the modern era, in an increasingly regulated and managerial healthcare environment, including new and competing demands on professional autonomy, these discourses tend to discount the point of what the evidence-based practice movement was meant to accomplish, leaving little room for the possibility of detecting and eradicating indefensible practices (Paley, 2005; Parker, 2002). Thus, by framing the evidence-based practice movement as a seditious plot, and seeking to protect what Parker has called the 'many commonplaces of nursing practice' (Parker, 2002: 139) from the scrutiny of evidence, this line of reasoning indulges these fuzzy definitional gymnastics about the nature of evidence, accentuating its risk for being incapable of systematic self-correction.

If we return to the idea that the function of evidence is the ability to identify and reduce or eliminate error, then the measure of whether a knowledge source ought to count as evidence would be its capacity to pass the test that Paley refers to as the "error criterion" (Paley, 2005). Using this criterion, that which is evidence should include not simply that which is derived from scholarly research of one form or another, but that which has scholarly properties and the capacity to refute an untrue or erroneous conceptualization (Scott-Findlay and Pollock, 2004; Upshur, 2001). However, the conflation that so often occurs in the qualitative health research world is the idea that all scholarly products constitute evidence, rather than recognizing that that which derives from various forms of research naturally takes quite different forms (Jeffs *et al.*, 2013).

How might we more appropriately position qualitative contributions?

That which we consider to be *evidential knowledge* takes the form of *justified true beliefs* in the form of propositions that can be articulated and confirmed using systematic processes capable of substantiating the warrants for that truth value (Thorne and Sawazky, 2014). Although I am convinced that it is theoretically possible for some qualitatively derived research products to meet that standard, it seems apparent that most nursing qualitative studies have not been designed in a manner that bears any relationship whatsoever to that it. Clearly, a robust conversation is required so that we can meaningfully deliberate on the question of *when* qualitatively derived findings are or are not usefully considered to be evidence. Paradoxically, when we mistakenly broaden our definition of evidence beyond that which is reasonably generalizable in serving the error criterion, we also lose the capacity to think rigorously about the appropriate application and use of *non-evidential* forms of knowledge (Thorne and Sawazky, 2014). And it is in considering this broader knowledge world of nursing that I believe we find the best insight about how qualitative research can be most constructively put to use.

Reflecting on the qualitative contribution to evolving knowledge in the health field, Sandelowski highlighted the distinctly non-evidential nature of most qualitatively derived products. "Complicating the borderlands between methods (and the policing of these borderlands that too often passes for methodological rigor and expertise) is that in qualitative research, methodological procedures function more to trigger analytic insights than to determine or constitute them" (Sandelowski, 2010: 81). If qualitative research products are not meaningfully construed as *evidence*, then it behoves us to effectively articulate what they do represent, and how we ought to be using them in a world that seems so dominated by the evidence discourse (Morse, 2012). Recognizing the dangers inherent in failing to articulate these distinctions, a number of scholars have suggested that the responsibility to make explicit the appropriate role and contribution of their scholarship to evidence-based practice ought to lie with those disciplines most dependent upon qualitative research (Jack, 2006; Kearney, 2001; Tarlier, 2005). Clearly, this opens a space for nursing scholarly leadership.

Multiple ways of knowing

First, I believe we need a clear recognition that qualitative research produces a body of scholarly material that is far from homogeneous (Rolfe, 2006). For example, the literature reveals considerable diversity with respect to the form and texture of published qualitative research reports, their size and scope, the level of theoretical conceptualization they aspire to and achieve (Sandelowski and Barroso, 2003). While there are popular conventions on quality criteria and credibility, it is commonly understood by those who conduct metasyntheses of the qualitative literature that applying them with any consistency and accuracy is highly problematic because of this diversity (Barnett-Page and Thomas, 2009; Dixon-Woods *et al.*, 2007; Walsh and Downe, 2006). Nevertheless, those engaged within the genre are clearly convinced that meaningful distinctions with relation to quality are achievable (Mays and Pope, 2006; Tracy, 2010).

Within nursing, I believe that we have been seriously limited in our capacity to think this through, by virtue of our assumption that these are general, rather than disciplinary, problems. However, once we shift our thinking into a more applied perspective of qualitative methods serving disciplinary objects, then the alignment between our "ways of knowing" and the products of our scholarship become more apparent. And from this, we can begin to tease out issues such as how we would evaluate the quality of a qualitative study and how we would put it to use (Johnson, 2013). I propose that the general conventions of qualitative rigor and credibility are not serving us at all well, and we would do far better to take up criteria more directly aligned with disciplinary priorities for the multiple species of knowledge we bring to bear on a clinical question. These could include such evaluative dimensions as epistemological integrity, representative credibility, analytic clarity, interpretive authority as well as the more professional elements of moral defensibility, disciplinary relevance, pragmatic obligation, contextual awareness (Thorne, 2008), as well as that slippery element that nurse philosopher June Kikuchi and her colleagues would have referred to as "probable truth" (Kikuchi and Simmons, 1996). After all, nursing needs to be able to act on its knowledge, even as it appreciates that knowledge is ever changing. Thus, more effective alignment of the design and focus of our qualitative products with the full range of disciplinary knowledge options could go a long way toward undoing the unfortunate conflation between all qualitatively derived products and "evidence."

Multiple strategic motivations

Arguably, a disproportionate emphasis in qualitative nursing research attention has been on describing subjectively experienced human health phenomena (Johnson, 2013). Not that there are not good reasons for doing good description from time to time, but we tend to allow ourselves the conceit of assuming that, because any clinical phenomenon has not yet been described in exactly the manner we intend, this kind of study is always justifiable (Thorne, 2008). I believe that, to advance disciplinary knowledge, we ought to be far more scrupulous in our expectations for a truly solid argument for why we are studying a thing. While mere intellectual curiosity or abstract theorizing may have been understood as a sufficient basis for inquiry within a social science tradition, the ontological and epistemological nature of our decidedly applied health professional discipline ought to play a much more overt role in how we enact methodology.

From that perspective, it becomes possible to tease out a number of highly relevant motivational possibilities that might warrant our engaging in qualitative research. Because nursing knowledge explicitly capitalizes on a dialectic between the general and the particular (Reed, 1995; Rolfe, 2011), we need bodies of general knowledge positioned not as prescriptive or superordinate truths but, more strategically, as guides to the complex challenge of informing the considerations that will be applied in the particularities of individual nurses, patient and contexts (Thorne and Sawazky, 2014). And while pure description might be justifiable in a discipline whose intellectual project is primarily theoretical, the theorizing component of nursing scholarship is not an end in itself (Pesut and Johnson, 2013), but rather a mechanism through which to uncover the implications of how a discipline thinks about particular phenomena (Kagan *et al.*, 2009). We therefore need studies designed to actively engage and translate the link between the ideas that we hold and the actions and implications that derive from them (Johnson, 2013). This means, perhaps, that qualitative nurse scholars ought to be held to a standard that requires them to anticipate the implications of their findings in the hands of a practice audience, including guarding against the potentially untoward effects that uncritical application of general claims could have in certain instances (Cheek, 2000). Estabrooks (2001) has argued that, when one considers the question of research utilization, qualitative methods may have taken a privileged hold on clinical audiences such as ours because our study results can be understood regardless of a sophisticated knowledge of methodology or statistics. This also means that our findings are potentially exposed to more misuse and misinterpretation because of that privilege. Thus, while we have been battling to try to insert the products of our qualitative work into the evidence conversation, we seem to have overlooked the very real and different manner in which our qualitative findings may be shaping the practice world.

Multiple designs

By virtue of its efforts to appease the methodological gods of both biomedical and social science, the qualitative nursing research community has traditionally been more hesitant than has been the case in some other disciplines to bend and shape its study designs to more effectively fit its disciplinary objectives (Sandelowski, 1993; Thorne, 2014). Further, we have complicated the question by assuming, when we speak of the theoretical frameworks with which we enter our studies, that we are necessarily referring to external substantive theories rather than disciplinary knowledge. This, in part, relates to a generation of nursing theory skirmishes in which various model builders competed with others for primacy. Now that we understand that model building project as fundamentally philosophical, rather than scientific, it seems time to return to the idea that the core epistemological structure of our discipline can and should scaffold our qualitative scholarly inquiries.

The question we ought to be asking ourselves when we consider our approaches to inquiry is not whether we have conformed to the tenets of the methodology as it was constructed for some other purpose, but rather whether we have chosen and shaped study design options toward meeting the needs of the knowledge project within which we are operating. From this perspective, we open up possibilities across the full range of qualitative scholarship (not to mention quantitative scholarship and mixed methods), and orient our critical lens toward an effective argument as to the relationship between the study approach and the nature of our question. This re-inserts philosophy, or the capacity handle the ideas of the discipline in a rational and reasoned manner, as a core attribute of our disciplinary scholarship (Pesut and Johnson, 2008). Just as we are comfortable with a clinical practice that necessarily serves multiple masters simultaneously and with careful attention to integrity, I see no reason why our science should not be held to a similar standard. We are not just doing studies, we are building disciplinary knowledge.

Multiple ends in view

I have asserted here that qualitative research is unlikely to offer much by way of competition to its quantitative counterparts by way of such measures as prediction, control, population generalizability, correlation, and causality. Having invested their energies in the more human and dynamic particularities of health phenomena, qualitative scholars are well positioned to recognize the inherent limits in methods drawn from conventional science. It is this capacity to understand and deconstruct scientific method that may offer the most important contribution qualitative research can make to the evidence discourse. Beyond the traditional role of qualitative investigations in surfacing variables that can be incorporated in quantitative design, building theory that can later be tested, and gaining insight into the relationship between dependent and independent variables (Bowers, 2013), qualitative methods offer tremendous potential for building ways to understand such issues as context and condition (Morse, 2001). While quantitative methods might reliably tell us "what works" or "what works best," the truly clinically interesting collateral questions we might pose, such as "when does it work," "why does it work in this circumstance and not in another," "and what else is hindered or facilitated by its working" are the purview of qualitative scholarship (Forbes and Griffiths, 2002; Walker, 2003). And rather than grounding our inquiries in different and unrelated questions – questions whose shape and form derives directly from the scholarly traditions of our borrowed methods rather than our disciplinary knowledge agenda – I believe there is a tremendous need for nurses to directly point their research questions at the centre of what evidence based knowledge looks like in the evolving practice world. By understanding how current evidence is constructed, and inserting our qualitative inquiries directly into the fray, we don't compete with the numbers, but we increase our changes of informing what is done with them.

Conclusion

As Morse points out,

> Qualitative researchers are at the fringes of health research, but remember that it is at the fringes where the greatest advances are often made. We are addressing the confusing and uncontrollable problems that are too difficult to tackle quantitatively. But they are important problems that merit attention.
>
> (Morse, 2012: 114)

In the hands of creative disciplinary thinkers, qualitative methods can fill the gaps between what is capturable using instruments and biomarkers. It can illuminate those aspects of human health phenomena that are otherwise rendered invisible by virtue of attention to that which can be measured. They can problematize, or expose the dynamics of harm, inequity or unintended consequences of clinical realities such as interventions or approaches. They can challenge the ideologies and assumptions that become codified in our systems and structures of practice. They can humanize our gaze on that which is otherwise rendered technical and mechanical. And, perhaps most importantly, they can help us confront the inevitable standardization of quantitative evidence building with solid and rigorous depiction of the marvelous variance and diversity that is the foundation of a nursing angle of vision.

References

Baker, K. M. (1964) The early history of the term "social science". *Annals of Science*, 20(3), 211–26.

Barnett-Page, E. and Thomas, J. (2009) Methods for the synthesis of qualitative research: A critical review. *BMC Medical Research Methodology*, 9, 59. doi:10.1186/1471-2288-9-59. Available online at www.biomedcentral.com/1471-2288/9/59 (accessed 12 March 2015).

Bonner, A. and Lloyd, A. (2011) What information counts at the moment of practice? Information practices of renal nurses. *Journal of Advanced Nursing*, 67(6), 1213–21.

Bowers, B. (2013) Evidence-based practice: Contributions and possibilities for qualitative research. In C. T. Beck (ed.), *Routledge International Handbook of Qualitative Nursing Research* (pp. 405–16). London: Routledge.

Buetow, S. and Kenealy, T. (2000) Evidence-based medicine: The need for a new definition. *Journal of Evaluation in Clinical Practice*, 6(2), 85–92.

Cheek, J. (2000) *Postmodern and Poststructural Approaches to Nursing Research*. Thousand Oaks, CA: Sage.

Chenail, R. J. (1992) A case for clinical qualitative research. *Qualitative Report*, 1(4). Available online at www.nova.edu/ssss/QR/QR1-4/clinqual.html (accessed 12 March 2015).

Clarke, J. B. (1999) Evidence-based practice: A retrograde step? The importance of pluralism in evidence generation for the practice of health care. *Journal of Clinical Nursing*, 8(1), 89–94.

Cochrane, A. (1989) *One Man's Medicine*. London: BMJ Publishing.

Cochrane, A. L. (1972) *Effectiveness and Efficiency: Random reflections on health services*. London: Nuffield Provincial Hospitals Trust.

Denzin, N. (2009) The elephant in the living room: Or extending the conversation about the politics of evidence. *Qualitative Research*, 9(2), 139–60.

Dixon-Woods, M., Booth, A. and Sutton, A. J. (2007) Synthesizing qualitative research: A review of published reports. *Qualitative Research*, 7(3), 375–422.

Dzurek, L. C. (1989) The necessity for and evolution of multiple paradigms for nursing research: A poststructuralist perspective. *Advances in Nursing Science*, 11(4), 69–77.

Estabrooks, C. (2001) Research utilization and qualitative research. In J. M. Morse, J. M. Swanson and A. J. Kuzel (eds), *The Nature of Qualitative Evidence* (pp. 275–98). Thousand Oaks, CA: Sage.

Forbes, A. and Griffiths, P. (2002) Methodological strategies for the identification and synthesis of 'evidence' to support decision–making in relation to complex health systems and practices. *Nursing Inquiry*, 9(3), 141–55.

French, P. (2002) What is the evidence on evidence-based nursing?: An epistemological concern. *Journal of Advanced Nursing*, 37(3), 250–7.

Freshwater, D. and Rolfe, G. (2004) *Deconstructing Evidence-based Practice*. Abingdon: Routledge.

Jack, S. M. (2006) Utility of qualitative research findings in evidence-based public health practice. *Public Health Nursing*, 23(3), 277–83.

Jeffs, L., Beswick, S., Lo, J., Campbell, H., Ferris, E. and Sidani, S. (2013) Defining what evidence is, linking it to patient outcomes, and making it relevant to practice: Insights from clinical nurses. *Applied Nursing Research*, 26(3), 105–9.

Johnson, J. L. (2013) Politics and qualitative nursing research. In C. T. Beck (ed.), *Routledge International Handbook of Qualitative Nursing Research* (pp. 371–9). Abingdon: Routledge.

Kagan, P. N., Smith, M. C., Cowling, W. R. and Chinn, P. L. (2009) A nursing manifesto: An emancipatory call for knowledge development, conscience, and praxis. *Nursing Philosophy*, 11(1), 67–84.

Kearney, M. H. (2001) Levels and applications of qualitative research evidence. *Research in Nursing and Health*, 24, 145–53.

Kikuchi, J. F. and Simmons, H. (1996) *Truth in Nursing Inquiry*. Thousand Oaks, CA: Sage.

Limb, C. J. (2011) The need for evidence in an anecdotal world. *Trends in Amplification*, 15(1–2), 3–4.

Madjar, I. and Walton, J. A. (2001) What is problematic about evidence? In J. M. Morse, J. M. Swanson and A. J. Kuzel (eds), *The Nature of Qualitative Evidence* (pp. 228–45). Thousand Oaks, CA: Sage.

Mays, N. and Pope, C. (2006) Quality criteria in qualitative health research. In C. Pope and N. Mays (eds), *Qualitative Research in Health Care*, 3rd edn. (pp. 82–101). Oxford: Blackwell.

Miller, W. L. and Crabtree, B. F. (1994) Clinical research. In N. Denzin and Y. Lincoln (eds), *Handbook of Qualitative Research* (pp. 340–52). Thousand Oaks, CA: Sage.

Morse, J. M. (2001) Qualitative verification: Building evidence by extending basic findings. In J. M. Morse, J. M. Swanson and A. J. Kuzel (eds), *The Nature of Qualitative Evidence* (pp. 203–20). Thousand Oaks, CA: Sage.

Morse, J. M. (2012) *Qualitative Health Research: Creating a New Discipline*. Walnut Creek, CA: Left Coast.

O'Leary, D. and Mhaolrunaigh, S. (2011) Information-seeking behavior of nurses: Where is information sought and what processes are followed? *Journal of Advanced Nursing*, 68(2), 379–90.

Oran, D. (2000) Oran's Dictionary of the Law. Albany, NY: Thompson Learning.

Paley, J. (2005) Evidence and expertise. *Nursing Inquiry*, 13(2), 82–93.

Parker, J. M. (2002) Evidence-based nursing: A defence. *Nursing Inquiry*, 9, 139–40.

Pesut, B. and Johnson, J. (2008) Reinstating the "queen:" Understanding philosophical inquiry in nursing. *Journal of Advanced Nursing*, 61(1), 115–21.

Pesut, B. and Johnson, J. (2013) Philosophical contributions to nursing ethics. In J. L. Storch, P. Rodney and R. Starzomski (eds), *Toward a Moral Horizon: Nursing ethics for leadership and practice*, 2nd edn. (pp. 41–58). Toronto: Pearson.

Profetto-McGrath, J., Negrin, K., Hugo, K. and Smith, K. (2010) Clinical nurse specialists' approaches in selecting and using evidence to improve practice. *Worldviews on Evidence-Based Nursing*, 7(1), 36–50.

Reason, P. (1996) Reflections on the purposes of human inquiry. *Qualitative Inquiry*, 2, 15–28.

Reed, P. G. (1995) A treatise on nursing knowledge development for the 21st century: Beyond postmodernism. *Advances in Nursing Science*, 17(3), 70–84.

Rolfe, G. (2006) Validity, trustworthiness and rigour: quality and the idea of qualitative research. *Journal of Advanced Nursing*, 53(3), 304–10.

Rolfe, G. (2011) Practitioner-centred research: Nursing praxis and the science of the unique. In P. G. Reed and N. B. Crawford Shearer (eds), *Nursing Knowledge and Theory Innovation: Advancing the science of practice* (pp. 59–74). New York: Springer.

Rolfe, G., Segrott, J. and Jordan, S. (2008) Tensions and contradictions in nurses' perspectives of evidence-based practice. *Journal of Nursing Management*, 16(4), 440–51.

Rycroft-Malone, J., Seers, K., Titchen, A., Harvey, G., Kitson, A. and McCormack, B. (2004) What counts as evidence in evidence-based practice? *Journal of Advanced Nursing*, 47, 81–90.

Sackett, D. L. (2000) *Evidence-based Medicine: How to practice and teach EBM*. Edinburgh: Churchill Livingstone.

Sackett, D. L. and Rosenberg, W. M. (1995) The need for evidence-based medicine. *Journal of the Royal Society of Medicine*, 88(11), 620–4.

Sackett, D. L., Rosenberg, W. M., Gray, J. A., Haynes, R. B. and Richardson, W. S. (1996) Evidence based medicine: what it is and what it isn't. *BMJ*, 312(7023), 71–2.

Sandelowski, M. (1993) Rigor and rigor mortis: The problem of rigor in qualitative research revisited. *Advances in Nursing Science*, 16(2), 1–8.

Sandelowski, M. (2010) What's in a name? Qualitative description revisited. *Research in Nursing and Health*, 33, 77–84.

Sandelowski, M. and Barroso, J. (2003) Classifying the findings in qualitative research. *Qualitative Health Research*, 13(7), 905–23.

Scott-Findlay, S. and Pollock, S. (2004) Evidence, research, knowledge: A call for conceptual clarity. *Worldviews on Evidence-Based Nursing*, 1, 92–7.

Shah, H. M. and Chung, K. C. (2009) Archie Cochrane and his vision for evidence-based medicine. *Plastic and Reconstructive Surgery*, 124(3), 982–8.

Silverman, M. E., Murray, T. J. and Bryan, C. S. (eds) (2008) *The Quotable Osler*. Philadelphia, PA: American College of Physicians.

Tarlier, D. (2005) Mediating the meaning of evidence through epistemological diversity. *Nursing Inquiry*, 12(2), 126–34.

Thompson, C. (2003) Clinical experience as evidence in evidence-based practice. *Journal of Advanced Nursing*, 43(3), 230–7.

Thorne, S. (2008) *Interpretive Description*. Walnut Creek, CA: Left Coast.

Thorne, S. (2011) Toward methodological emancipation in applied health research. *Qualitative Health Research*, 21(4), 443–53.

Thorne, S. (2014) Applied interpretive approaches. In P. Leavey (ed.), *The Oxford Handbook of Qualitative Research* (pp. 99–115). New York: Oxford University Press.

Thorne, S. and Sawazky, R. (2014) Particularizing the general: Sustaining theoretical integrity in the context of an evidence-based practice agenda. *Advances in Nursing Science*, 37(1), 5–18.

Tracy, S. J. (2010) Qualitative quality: Eight 'big tent' criteria for excellent qualitative research. *Qualitative Inquiry*, 16(10), 837–51.

Traynor, M. (1999) The problem of dissemination: Evidence and ideology. *Nursing Inquiry*, 6, 187–97.

Traynor, M. (2002) The oil crisis, risk and evidence-based practice. *Nursing Inquiry*, 9(3), 162–9.

Upshur, R. E. G. (2001) The status of qualitative research as evidence. In J. M. Morse, J. M. Swanson and A. J. Kuzel (eds), *The Nature of Qualitative Evidence* (pp. 5–26). Thousand Oaks, CA: Sage.

Verhoeven, F., Steehouder, M., Hendrix, R. and van Gemert-Pijen, J. (2009) How nurses seek and evaluate clinical guidelines on the internet. *Journal of Advanced Nursing*, 666(1), 114–27.

Walker, K. (2003) Why evidence-based practice now? *Nursing Inquiry*, 10, 145–55.

Walsh, D. and Downe, S. (2006) Appraising the quality of qualitative research. *Midwifery*, 22(2), 108–19.

Wokler, R. (1995) Anthropology and conjectural history in the enlightenment. In C. Fox, R. Porter and R. Wokler (eds), *Inventing Human Science: Eighteenth-century domains* (pp. 32–52). Berkeley, CA: University of California Press.

12 Research appraisal and individual responsibility – a critique

Martin Lipscomb

The UK Nursing and Midwifery Council (NMC) requires that educators equip students so that, post registration (post licensure), 'All nurses must ... be able to understand and appraise research' (NMC, 2010: 14).[1] The NMC's rationale for this demand rests – arguably – on two overlapping assumptions. First, I presume that the NMC believes that students can be educated to appraise research at a level or depth commensurate with that appraisal productively informing practice. Second, the NMC implicitly supposes that individual involvement in research appraisal is a necessary part of ensuring that research evidence enters practice. Statements similar to those made by the NMC litter nursing's wider scholarly literature (see, for example, Laibhen-Parkes, 2014).

If, however, appraisal requires that appraisers authoritatively determine whether individual report findings are warranted then, contra NMC assumptions, students and nurses will almost always fail to adequately appraise research. To support this assertion, I note that, excepting the simplest of surveys, quantitative researchers employ statistical tests that most students/nurses do not understand and qualitative research reports label but do not generally describe the analytical processes that yield emergent codes, themes and categories. In both instances, while students/nurses may complete and pass evidence-based practice (EBP) or research educational modules at first degree level, without advanced training practitioners cannot meaningfully ascertain how findings are derived and, if substantive understanding is a necessary part of determining whether findings are defensible and warranted, appraisal fails. Conversely, if research appraisal does not include determining that findings are defensible or warranted, then the purpose and worth of appraisal must be questioned.

Synthesising and developing ideas sketched elsewhere (Lipscomb, 2012a, 2012b, 2014) this chapter explores the idea that, if appraisal involves or requires that appraisers substantively understand how findings are derived before those findings are accepted and acted upon (that is, high rather than low levels of epistemic justification should be sought by appraisers), then most students/nurses cannot meaningfully appraise research. Further, if even only some students/nurses cannot meaningfully appraise research then getting research into practice cannot rely on 'all nurses' being able to do this thing. Implications for UK nurse regulation and education regarding EBP are sketched.

'How much of this report do I need to understand?'

Individuals may read research for fun. However, students and nurses are principally influenced in their choice of professionally related reading by instrumental demands rather than the modest pleasure of unstructured serendipitous curiously. Research is therefore read purposefully and students and nurses who are not researchers predominantly read to achieve academic credit and/or acquire action guiding clinically relevant information.

Links between evidence and practice are accented in the UK by regulations, applicable to all nurses, which stipulate that care must be based on 'best evidence available and best practice' (NMC, 2015: 7) and, while evidence is a broader concept than research evidence, research and research findings are prized insofar as they ground and influence practice through the provision of an 'evidence base'. Individuals perform EBP when their actions comply with evidence-based guidelines and protocols. However, UK regulator standards for educators (NMC, 2010) stipulate, as noted, that all nurses must be prepared to 'understand and appraise research' (p. 14), and nursing students are therefore invited to access and make sense of research reports. Individual nurses are thus personally accountable for providing care grounded on best available evidence and best practice; that is, individuals are responsible for undertaking or engaging with EBP. This responsibility includes, certainly for current students and recent graduates, reading research, and this is done to assess whether report findings are robust enough to legitimately influence practice.

With this in mind, let us assume that a student or nurse has identified a patient-related problem or issue. Following recommended procedure (see, for example, Sackett *et al.*, 2000; Booth Papaioanou and Sutton, 2012; Aveyard, 2014) this problem/issue has been formulated as a potentially answerable question. A competent literature search has been conducted to find material that addresses this question and ostensibly relevant research reports are identified.

These reports now require appraisal and, put crudely, appraisal aims to determine whether results are warranted, clinically significant, acceptable and relevant to whatever situation or problem is being addressed, and affordable. If these criteria are met then practice (that is, behaviour/care) may justifiably be altered. Clinical significance, acceptability, relevance and affordability are clearly important and non-significant, unacceptable, irrelevant and unaffordable findings will not be acted upon. Yet, unless findings are in the first instance deemed warranted, other considerations are immaterial. I therefore hereafter focus on the ability of students and nurses to assess whether findings are warranted.

Numerous assessment tools and frameworks exist to guide neophyte readers through the appraisal process. Tools vary in detail and complexity. Nonetheless, they generally 'walk' appraisers formulaically through reports in a stepwise fashion. They direct appraisers' attention to the various parts of reports and they prompt appraisers to consider whether appropriate actions were taken by researchers. Some authorities suggest that only certain forms of research are worth reading and/or it is asserted that research which does not use particular methods should be passed over. However, if, following broadly reliabilist precepts, appraisers determine that each step in the research process was performed appropriately, and if no serious problems or deficiencies are apparent then, on balance, appraisers might conclude that research findings are warranted and, in consequence, they can be accepted (that is, they may provisionally be deemed correct or probably correct). Findings judged correct and probably correct can justifiably be acted upon. They can inform behaviour/care (assuming also clinical significance, acceptability, relevance and affordability). Findings not judged correct or probably correct and findings where correctness cannot be determined must be discounted. To suggest otherwise would be odd.

So far so good. However, while in some situations understanding or comprehension is simply present or absent (that is, one understands fully or not at all – a flipped coin lands heads or tails up and, following observation, no ambiguity exists), when assessors attempt to make sense of research, it is more likely that understanding is achieved in or by gradations. This is important. The level, depth or degree of understanding that appraisers must attain before research findings can reasonably or sensibly be accepted and acted upon is not adequately discussed in nursing's scholarly literature (including the literature dealing with assessment tools/frameworks), and the issue is effectively ignored by regulators. For example, NMC (2010) instructions to UK educators provide scant guidance about what 'understand' means in relation to research appraisal and this lack of clarity places educators, students and practitioners in an invidious position.

Questions of the sort 'How much of this report do I need to understand?' now attain salience because, problematically, if appraisers do not comprehend sections or elements of a research report then, potentially, they may be oblivious to significant failings or errors in that report. The danger here is that, consequent to a lack of awareness, incorrect or false findings might be accepted and applied (they may inappropriately influence behaviour/care). Alternatively, correct or robust findings could mistakenly be deemed irrelevant and overlooked. Appraisers who do not understand key sections or elements of a report do not understand that report meaningfully or substantively. By definition, the report is not understood fully and 'correctness' cannot easily be judged.

I now advance the following claim – if student and nurse appraisers need to substantively understand how individual report findings are derived before they can legitimately accept and act upon those findings then, in almost all instances, findings should not be acted upon. At face value, this statement, or at least its implications, is absurd. However, the alternatives are even more problematic. If appraisers need no understanding of how findings are derived or, if only superficial and/or partial understanding is necessary, then practice can be altered on the basis of findings that are 'understood' incompletely or merely as assertions.

For the sake of argument, to tease out the issues involved, I henceforth suggest that, with respect to quantitative research reports, while student and nurse appraisers (who are not specialists/researchers) can in principle, in theory, achieve substantive levels of understanding regards finding derivation, in practice this is not generally achieved. Alternatively and more troublingly, it is proposed that qualitative research report appraisers cannot in principle meaningfully understand how findings are derived (and critiquing tools grounded on reliabilist principles are probably inapplicable when applied to qualitative reports). These are bold statements. If carried, their acceptance would have serious ramifications for the way in which we regulate nursing practice and teach and reflect upon EBP. On the other hand, even if rejected, thinking through these issues has value, since we are thereby forced to address otherwise neglected subjects.

Quantitative research appraisal

The status and meaning that can be accorded to numerical data and the concept of generalisation are both subject to debate and contestation (see Chapter 7 in this volume). However, the nursing literature rarely engages with the problematic aspects of reduction/enumeration, event identity, causation, probability or generalisation in a sustained or detailed manner, and it is therefore unsurprising that clinicians often advance naïve statements about these topics. Putting these issues to one side, with regard to quantitative research, I here affirm a very straightforward claim, namely, most students and qualified nurses possess limited statistical knowledge *and this matters*.

Excepting the comparatively small number of people who have undertaken specialist statistical training, it is probably fair to claim that most students and nurses do not, in any real sense, understand the sorts of statistical tests that interpret data in experimental and quasi-experimental studies. That is, 'treatment comparison' research producing robust generalisable action guiding claims – loosely, studies located near or at the apex of the hierarchy of evidence. Survey findings that interpret data using basic descriptive statistics are easily comprehended. However, to reframe arguments outlined above, if – to limit error – research report appraisers (students and nurses) should substantively understand how results are obtained before they accept and act on those results, when appraisers do not substantively understand the statistical tests employed in quantitative reports, when they cannot 'follow through' how findings are derived, then regardless of the actual validity and reliability of reports (that is, regardless of what could be determined if more ability/knowledge was possessed), those findings ought not to influence the behaviour/care of appraisers who realise that their understanding of finding derivation is limited or non-existent. To argue otherwise is to argue that findings can be accepted and acted upon by appraisers who appreciate that they do not meaningfully understand how findings are derived or obtained. Appraisers may of course be mistaken, ignorant about and/or overestimate their ability to interpret statistical tests. However, I am not here interested in this sort of misunderstanding.

Further, while experienced researchers often specialise in performing studies that make use of a restricted palette of research approaches and techniques (and experienced researchers may have only a glancing awareness of alternative approaches/techniques) regulators such as the NMC, and educators more generally, place no restrictions on the types of research that students and nurses are expected to engage with (that is, locate and appraise). Indeed, 'wide reading' is (correctly) encouraged and rewarded.

However, given the diversity of research methodologies and methods that are available, and given the very different ontological and epistemological assumptions that these methodologies and methods 'carry' (to say nothing of their distinctive and often intricate nomenclatures), it is unrealistic to imagine that most student/nurse engagement will be anything other than superficial. That is, it is almost certainly optimistic to suppose that even gifted students and clinicians who are educated to first-degree level but are not themselves researchers or statisticians, can confidently and competently 'make sense' of the argumentative forms and investigative structures contained in all research forms (indeed – who can?).

Moreover, vis-à-vis quantitative studies, while statistically literate researchers will occasionally be challenged by unfamiliar tests, non-specialists cannot but, I suggest, be confounded by the diversity of approaches to data interpretation that exist. For example, a single issue of the *Journal of Advanced Nursing* (March 2015) – the sort of journal recommended to students, the sort of journal that, at my own institution, we expect to see cited in reference lists – contains or makes reference to, among others, the following statistical devices and tests: the Mantel-Haenszel test, Spearman's rho correlation coefficient, logistic regression modelling, Cronbach's alpha, *t*-tests, chi-square, standard deviations, odds ratios, and so on. Few people will understand all of these tests and devices sufficiently well to determine whether they are being used correctly. Fewer still can assess the accuracy with which findings are derived from these tests and, to restate, this short list is not exhaustive.

In summary, students and nurses read research reports to assess the use value of findings. This is not the only reason for reading research. It is however, for clinicians, the primary reason. More controversially, it is proposed that assessors should not act on research report findings that they appraise unless substantive understanding about how report findings are derived is grasped. This understanding is necessary to establish whether findings are warranted. 'Substantively' is not adequately defined. However, the term is associated with the idea that appraisers need to be able to 'follow through' how statistical tests interpret data so that assessor understandings of finding derivation are epistemically sufficient to form beliefs capable of legitimately supporting actions (that is, behaviour/care). To do otherwise, to allow appraisers to act without sufficient or substantive understanding of how findings are derived (that is, to act on the basis of low epistemic confidence) would be to sanction actions that lack good or even tolerable justification/reasons (that is, actions that, from the perspective on an appraiser, lack a known or realised evidence base). Put another way, if appraisers can accept and act on findings without understanding how findings are derived from the statistical tests that interpret data, then appraisers can accept and act on findings when they are knowingly oblivious to whether the findings being implemented are warranted or not – crudely, correct or false.

Since very few students or nurses are educated to assess statistical tests, if the above argument is accepted, in most cases quantitative studies cannot reasonably inform the behaviour/care of student and nurse appraisers.

Qualitative research appraisal

Appraisers face greater obstacles in assessing qualitative studies. For, while few students and nurses are equipped to make sense of the statistical tests that interpret quantitative research data, nothing prevents determined students or nurses from obtaining that knowledge (this knowledge is in principle attainable – anyone can enrol on a statistics training course). However, in the case of qualitative research, in almost all cases it is arguably not possible for appraisers to in principle meaningfully understand how findings are derived and – to repeat – if appraisers need to substantively understand how findings are derived before they can legitimately accept and act on findings then this destabilises the use value of qualitative research. Indeed, in an extreme formulation, it could be suggested that beliefs capable of sanctioning clinical action cannot justifiably be derived from or formed on the basis of qualitative research findings.

Risjord (2014) claims that 'Those who maintain that interpretation is a distinctive form of inquiry need to articulate how interpreters acquire knowledge of others' experiences, meanings, and values' (p. 57). If we assume that an appraiser is reading a 'typical' health-related qualitative study (that is, one involving a small number of face-to-face interviews and the subsequent interpretation of interview transcript data), then this articulation or explanation could perforce cover multiple aspects of researcher–participant interaction and subsequent data analysis. Nonetheless, a key element in this articulation presumably involves explaining how themes, codes and categories 'emerge' from qualitative data.

Students and nurses read qualitative research because, instrumentally, they anticipate that its findings may inform practice. However, the avowedly non-objective, personal and non-repeatable nature of qualitative data collection and analysis creates difficulties for report appraisers. Notably, qualitative researchers are themselves the instrument or tool by or through which codes, themes and categories are identified and, while the stages in this process can be labelled, the thinking which lies behind this labelling cannot easily be made public. Of course, research reports include purportedly illustrative participant remarks. And these remarks are attached by report writers to emergent code, theme and category descriptors with the intension of conveying to readers something of the flavour or tone of what was said and meant by study participants. Nonetheless, regardless of their affective or emotional appeal – that is, regardless of whether remarks 'seem' or 'feel' as if they support the analysis offered – plucking or highlighting comments from an interview transcript rarely if ever explains or defends the processes (psychological and logical) that lie behind code, theme and category derivation. Irrespective of the actual strength or robustness of a qualitative study, from an appraiser's perspective, the appropriateness or applicability of codes, themes and categories inevitably remain indeterminate.

Can researchers address this problem? Could they 'show their workings'? Risjord (2014) suggests that we might 'ask whether the interpreter [researcher] was aware of the ways in which the qualitative methods produced their results' (p. 64). This is an intriguing question. It spotlights the qualitative interpretive process and, as such, this move points to a particular problem for qualitative researchers – namely – in many instances they cannot, beyond post hoc rationalisation or mere assertion, explain how codes, themes or categories are derived.

Qualitative researchers will thus, following consideration, decide that a word, statement, phrase or passage should be coded, themed or categorized in some way. However, how these decisions are made generally remains obscure. The interpretation offered may or may not be sensible/defendable. Yet, while we are by definition aware of our conscious thoughts, we have little insight into the processes that lie behind those thoughts and, since the qualitative researcher is the interpretive tool, clarifying how this tool reached the conclusions that it did (that is, ascertaining how codes, themes and categories are derived) would require researcher thought processes to be explained. This is problematic. Requesting the basis of thoughts threatens a form of infinite regress and, moreover, psychological and philosophic research shows that memory, judgement and intuition are frequently unstable, irrational or systematically fallacious (Thaler and Sunstein, 2008; Kahneman, 2011; Sutherland, 2013 – see also Chapter 10 in this volume). These truths problematise many forms of research/decision making. However, since qualitative nursing research overwhelmingly relies upon participant recall and researcher judgement, psychological and philosophical challenges to these 'abilities' are especially grave (internal validity is not established).

In summary, code, theme and category choices are stated in qualitative research reports and a brief synopsis of the procedures followed in analysis is described (albeit that, often, only high-level explanatory descriptors are provided). However, merely asserting that this or that code, theme or category 'emerged' does not explain or clarify how or why this rather than that interpretation of transcript/conversation data is best or most appropriate (and, while alternative data interpretations often if not always also 'fit' the data, these alternatives are hardly ever presented to readers with an explanation as to why they were rejected). Crucially, emergent codes, themes and categories are the outcome or conclusion of processes of analysis. They carry little or no information about what occurred during analysis. They do not explain how qualitative findings are derived and, if appraisers should not accept and act on findings when they do not know how those findings were derived then, once again, appraisal stumbles.

Getting quantitative findings into practice

Nurses who lack statistical education cannot, I argue, meaningfully appraise quantitative research reports if appraisal requires that key elements in individual reports (for example, finding derivation) be substantively understood. However, this does not mean that quantitative research cannot inform practice. Instead, if we abandon the pretence that solitary students and nurses can adequately appraise research findings (to say nothing of situating 'a' set of findings within larger 'fields' of research), and if – contrary to previous assertions – we accept that actions can in some situations be deemed legitimate even when the ultimate justification for those actions remains – from the perspective of the actor – obscure, then problems evaporate. What now matters is the context of action. Thus, if we transfer responsibility for appraisal from individuals to groups and bodies with developed and possibly accredited appraisal skills, and if we require students and nurses to implement (when appropriate/applicable) evidence-based policies and guidelines generated by trusted authorities, then quantitative research findings can reasonably inform nursing actions.

In a sense, this proposal banally states current realities. It is comparatively rare for a nurse who is not undertaking an educational module or course to locate and read primary research papers (Caldwell *et al.*, 2007) and attempts to persuade or cajole nurses to do so have in some instances met with resistance (Kenny, 2005; Yoder *et al.*, 2014). For those that do, peer review arguably offers a modicum of quality control and this filtering process supplies readers with token assurance regarding the value of published research. More substantively, within the UK, the Department of Health and the National Institute for Health and Care Excellence develop and publish high-quality guidelines; Cochrane Collaboration systematic reviews are equally if not more meritorious, and few sensible clinicians knowingly overlook or ignore these commanding documents. Indeed, it must presumably be foolish for anyone who is not an 'appraisal expert' to prefer or rely upon their own location and appraisal abilities in contrast to reviews and guidelines produced by trusted bodies. To do so would, arguably, demonstrate scant regard for EBP.

However, the proposal does undercut what I take to be core assumptions implicit in current NMC instructions to UK nurse educators (assumptions mirrored by many nursing scholars). My proposal is based on the belief that not all nurses can meaningfully appraise individual reports and it likewise presumes that individual involvement in appraisal is not necessary to ensure that warranted research findings make their way into practice. Instead, my version of EBP would invite students to consider, for example, the complexity of inter- and multi-agency coordination where different ideas about evidence and evidence use may obtain (see, Chapters 2–5 in this volume), as well as the difficulty of determining whether the recommendations of 'this' guideline or 'this' systematic review apply to 'my' patients (see Chapters 7 and 13 in this volume). This later claim includes but runs ahead of acknowledging the problems inherent in generalisation. Rather, it also recognises the particular, contingent and contextual nature of practice and it emphasises the need for evidence (that is, high-quality systematic reviews and guidelines) to be integrated alongside and interpreted through what, for want of a better word, we might describe as the 'craft' of care. Students would still receive tuition on or about research forms. However, this element of EBP would take a determinedly back-seat position and questions concerning the management and coordination of change, and questions about decision making in situations of 'real world' muddle, would come to the fore.

Questions such as those thrown up when research findings, clinical experience and expressed patient preferences fail to align.

On the other hand, as a profession, nursing needs to develop and enhance its research capability and, in consequence, it could be argued that educators should treat students as putative researchers – that is, EBP education ought to focus on methodologies and methods rather than the application and 'role out' of findings deemed legitimate by others. And, moreover, the roots of EBP lie (in part) in clinical dissent – that is, EBP is 'about' individuals using research findings to challenge contemporary practice and, perhaps, requiring that students and nurses 'merely' or blindly follow guidelines developed by others might not equip them to perform this oppositional role (see Chapter 8 in this volume). Obvious dangers clearly lurk in the unthinking application of guidelines (McCartney, 2014; see also Chapters 3, 6 and 14 in this volume) and both above points have merit. However, accepting that nursing, as a profession, needs to improve its research capacity is not an argument for subjecting all students to research training of the sort required by researchers and, regards EBP's radical or disruptive potential, it is equally plausible that this would be strengthened rather than diminished if attention shifted from the consideration of abstract methods to finding implementation and the overcoming of sociocultural, organisational and political barriers to change that this involves.

Quantitative research findings can then inform the actions of students and nurses who do not substantively understand how those findings are derived – but – this is only permissible when the soundness or warrant of those findings is vouched for by trusted bodies. Bodies willing and able to explain and justify their decision making processes.

Can qualitative findings inform nursing actions?

Descriptive qualitative research may capture something of the perceptions, feelings and thoughts of study participants and this understanding, filtered through the interpretive lens of the researcher, can prompt report readers to rethink taken-for-granted assumptions and/or contemplate previously unconsidered possibilities. Qualitative findings can be interesting. They may even be important. However, it is less clear that they are 'evidence' as commonly understood (see Chapters 10 and 11 in this volume) and, if qualitative findings cannot be generalised (again, as commonly understood) then they are of limited use value to nurses in practice. We might therefore ask, from the perspective of a clinician, in what ways, if at all, can qualitative findings inform nursing actions?

Interpretive methods offer novel and 'even indispensable, ways of gathering information' (Risjord, 2014: 77). That said, practitioners confront notable problems in establishing whether or to what extent specific qualitative findings possess action guiding use value. There is nothing new or contentious in pointing towards these difficulties (Wiggins, 2011). However, the consequences and significance of well-known critiques of qualitative research are blithely disregarded by many nurse researchers and scholars and they infrequently get the attention they deserve in the sorts of EBP texts accessed by pre-registration student nurses.

Problematically, while interpretive researchers cannot but make 'general statements' (Risjord, 2014: 60) about their study objects, qualitative findings or 'knowledge can never seamlessly generalize to predict future practice' (Tracy, 2010: 845). Thus, mindful of the non-representativeness of qualitative participant selection and the subjective nature of qualitative data analysis, if we again imagine a 'standard' qualitative nursing study involving a limited number of interviews and the interpretation of transcript data, then statements in research reports concerning the meaning or implications of findings will and can logically relate only and specifically to the participants being studied.

Further, since qualitative reports are literary constructions that re-present and re-create what occurred or was said (Risjord, 2014), while qualitative findings describe 'an' interpretation of the meanings/explanations expressed by participants, this interpretation can never foretell the meanings/explanations that other similarly placed individuals would or might attribute to the same or comparable occurrences or phenomena. Moreover, because the interview event is 'nothing more than a moment in the changing, flowing narrative co-created by interviewer and subject' (Risjord, 2014: 61) the meanings and explanations that appear in qualitative study reports cannot be replicated. Thus, the same or similarly situated participants are very unlikely to make the same responses (give the same answers) to the same prompts or questions on another occasion, and the researcher, or a similarly disposed researcher, is unlikely to interpret the same data in exactly the same way on another occasion. None of this, to repeat, detracts from the interest or importance of qualitative findings. However, qualitative findings cannot be replicated or generalised and, if these 'attributes' are necessary to establish use value, then qualitative findings lack action guiding use value.

In response, some scholars have proposed that transference rather than generalisation provides use value for qualitative findings (Lincoln and Guba, 1985; Miles and Huberman, 1994). Problematically, however, transference is linked both with prolonged and 'deep' researcher emersion in or at study sites and thick or protracted descriptions of participant comments/study phenomena (Seale, 1999) and, unfortunately, not only is prolonged emersion or researcher contact with study participants rarely achieved (many qualitative nursing studies rely on single, short, transient interviews with a small number of participants) but publication restrictions on paper length allow only the briefest of conversational 'snippets' to be reproduced. If transference can substitute for generalisation, and if transference is demonstrated when report writers convey to readers significant understanding through extended descriptions of events over protracted timeframes involving 'deep' researcher emersion in the study situation, then transference is very seldom evidenced in published nursing qualitative reports.

Can analogy stand-in for generalisation? The problem here is that, for generalisation by analogy to hold, report readers would again require a lot more information than nursing qualitative report writers generally provide and, moreover, much of this information might require quantification (at which point we are no longer reading a qualitative study). For example, a student or nurse could read a qualitative report and think – these patients say things that sound like the sorts of things my patients say, and the researcher's interpretation of what this means matches my beliefs, intuitions or experience and thus, by analogy, I assume that my patients' comments can be interpreted in the same way.

However, exactly how similar are comments made by study participants to those expressed at the site/location of the appraiser? What non-similar comments (non-similar compared with the appraiser's location) were made by study participants? What non-similar comments (non-similar compared with study site participants) are made by users/patients at the appraiser's location? Were non-similar comments reproduced in the research report? What differences distinguish the appraiser's location and patients from the researcher's location and study group? Were study participants representative of those normally found at the study site? And, are they representative of patients at the appraiser's location? Clearly these sorts of question would need to be answered before generalisation by analogy could be established or deemed plausible and, equally clearly, answers to these sorts of question probably require quantification.

While research report appraisal (qualitative or quantitative) always involves elements or aspects of subjective assessment and normative evaluation, relatively objective and/or agreed appraisal criteria exist for quantitative studies and, hence, expert bodies can step in to take over the appraisal task. This option is not, however, available for qualitative work or, at least, it is not available to the same extent. Determining whether a report is interesting cannot be delegated because interest resides or is located only in the mind of the reader/appraiser. Likewise, the importance of qualitative findings – given that these findings are not generalisable – cannot be accurately fixed.

Concluding comments

Personal interest in EBP attends or stems from thirteen years' experience as a nurse lecturer in UK higher (university) education. For most of that time, I have managed a series of large pre-registration (pre-licensure) EBP-related modules and I therefore approach EBP from the perspective of an educationalist. Complacency can accompany long service. However, as anyone involved in education will testify, students have an uncanny – some say unnerving – ability to ask disturbing questions that combine rank naivety with troubling insightfulness and, for example, queries such as 'How much of this report do I need to understand?' or 'Can these findings inform my actions?' are simultaneously both artless and disquieting. Awkward inquiries can be sidestepped and stock responses such as 'Well, for the assignment you need to focus on … etcetera' generally placate students. Nevertheless, more thoughtful and nuanced solutions are required if educationalists are to prepare practitioners who can 'do' EBP (rather than simply pass modules) and, in grappling with what these answers might be, my relationship with and understanding of EBP remains distinctly unsettled.

To the extent that EBP describes a set of ideas and activities that structure and coordinate (enable) the bringing together of evidence, clinical expertise and patient/client or user preferences to productively inform and enhance decision making, EBP is simply what one would want and expect from modern healthcare providers. Alternatively, beyond platitudes, consideration of the ways in which EBP is conceptualised and implemented generate clinically apposite questions and perplexing intellectual riddles and, if taken seriously, student comments such as those described above harbour or suggest significant challenges to widely expressed assumptions concerning EBP. Further, insightful student observations disputing EBP's real world applicability, and misunderstandings that expose reasonable confusion, highlight tensions between, on the one hand, how academic and theoretical claims about EBP are presented to students and, on the other, actual clinical practice. Like others (for example, Rolfe, 2014) I see this intersection, the point at which epistemological logic/reasoning and professional aspiration confronts practice or 'how things are', as a site of considerable discord.

This chapter has explored aspects of research finding assessment and I have, as an educationalist, approached this topic mindful of student needs, capabilities and limitations. Students and nurses turn to research findings to compliment or improve clinical decision making and my role is to enable them in this task. Even talented students will, however, find it difficult to meaningfully appraise research reports and it is dishonest to suggest otherwise. Reports may be of high quality and they may contain vital action guiding information and/or important ideas and clues to facilitate service improvement. Nonetheless, if we assume that getting research into practice relies upon individual clinicians appraising these data/ideas, then this may be a misguided assumption. It is certainly one that can distort EBP education.

While Laibhen-Parkes (2014) notes that empirical demonstrations of specific beneficial consequences associated with EBP are 'limited' (p. 179) and 'Validated tools to assess EBP competence are scarce' (p. 177), let us grant that EBP has and is improving patient care (so EBP 'works'). However, it is also the case that numerous impediments hamper students and nurses in their ability to perform EBP (such as lack of time, resources, preparation, support, leadership, motivation – Gerrish *et al.*, 2008; Pravikoff, Tanner and Pierce, 2005; Yoder *et al.*, 2014). These obstructions are multi-causal and, often, organisational in character (Williams, Perillo and Brown, 2015). Nonetheless, the forms in which barriers are encountered, recognised and resolved (if indeed they are) reflect or are in part influenced by how EBP is thought about and taught (see Chapter 4 in this volume). And, if current ideas and teaching are skewed by erroneous presumptions regarding, for example, the requirement that 'All nurses must … be able to understand and appraise research' (NMC, 2010: 14) or underdeveloped beliefs concerning the use value of qualitative research, then practitioners are not best prepared to overcome the difficulties that confront them. Indeed, they are forced to take up additional and unnecessary problems.

If the arguments presented in this chapter hold, educators have, in my opinion, a key role to play in critically unwrapping EBP's assumptions so that problems associated with EBP can be fruitfully addressed and teaching and clinical care might be further improved. A significant element in this 'working through' involves clarifying educational objectives set by regulators (in the UK, the NMC). However, to avoid controversy, and despite good intentions (to make difficult material palatable), educationalists can be reticent about bringing EBP's 'prickly' or contentious features to student attention. Steered by regulatory standards, UK educationalists often employ texts and present ideas that introduce EBP to students as if students were apprentice researchers (a move that unwittingly collapses evidence to research evidence) and, regarding this later point, while we naturally need able and accomplished researchers, something is clearly amiss, insofar as so few nurses actively pursue research careers of note. Nonetheless, that said, since most nurses will not be researchers, educationalists need to present EBP to students in ways which recognise both their needs and likely career pathways.

Crucially, it is necessary to understand how knowledge claims are produced before we can decide whether those claims are warranted. Yet, importantly, clinicians operate in specific, complex, dynamic and multiagency environments and it is within these environments (rather than the classroom, library or laboratory) that the significance and potential role of evidence must be realised (Rolfe, 2014). Students and nurses need to know enough about evidence and the way in which research findings feed through into practice so that they can make sense of and, if appropriate, change behaviour/care on the basis of evidence/research. However, this capability does not perhaps require that students and nurses engage with or appraise individual reports and, instead, it may be sufficient for findings to make their impact felt through incorporation in reviews, guidelines and protocols. Further, while I would personally like to see the extent and depth of nurse scientific education/literacy greatly enhanced (my argument is not hostile to education about research), scientific knowledge is, on its own, rarely sufficient to ground practice (see Chapters 9 and 13 in this volume). Thus, unless education about research and EBP engages with the situations and decision making contexts in which nurses operate – that is, contexts in which dialogue concerning the applicability and acceptability of findings '*in this case*' and '*to meet this objective*' are as important as debates about method appropriateness – education will fail to productively assist practitioners (see Chapters 3 and 4 in this volume). Experience suggests that while UK and non-UK pre-registration curricula overemphasise individual research report appraisal, they do not always give problems associated with 'situating' or placing results in the clinical environment the attention they deserve.

Note

1   This document is, at the time of writing, being revised. Nonetheless, the full current reference is: 'All nurses must appreciate the value of evidence in practice, be able to understand and appraise research, apply relevant theory and research findings to their work, and identify areas for further investigation' (NMC, 2010: 14 – repeated pp. 23, 32 and 41).

References

Aveyard, H. (2014) *Doing A Literature Review In Health And Social Care: A Practical Guide*. 3rd edn. Maidenhead: Open University Press.

Booth, A., Papaioanou, D. and Sutton, A. (2012) *Systematic Approaches To A Successful Literature Review*. London: Sage.

Caldwell, K., Coleman, K., Copp, B., Bell, L. and Ghazi, F. (2007) Preparing for professional practice: How well does professional training equip health and social care practitioners to engage in evidence-based practice? *Nurse Education Today*. 27(6), 518–28.

Gerrish, K., Ashworth, P., Lacey, A. and Bailey, J. (2008) Developing evidence-based practice: experiences of senior and junior clinical nurses. *Journal of Advanced Nursing*. 62(1), 62–73.

Kahneman, D. (2011) *Thinking, Fast and Slow*. Harmondsworth: Penguin.

Kenny, D. J. (2005) Nurses' use of research in practice at three US Army hospitals. *Nurse Leadership (Toronto, Ont)*. 18(3), 45–67.

Laibhen-Parkes, N. (2014) Evidence-based practice competence: a concept analysis. International *Journal of Nursing Knowledge*. 25(3), 173-182.

Lincoln, Y. S. and Guba, E. G. (1985) *Naturalistic Inquiry*. London: Sage.

Lipscomb, M. (2014) Research report appraisal: how much understanding is enough? *Nursing Philosophy*. 15(3), 157–70.

Lipscomb, M. (2012a) Abductive reasoning and qualitative research. *Nursing Philosophy*. 13(4) 244–56.

Lipscomb, M. (2012b) Questioning the use value of qualitative research findings. *Nursing Philosophy*. 13(2) 112–25.

McCartney, M. (2014) *Living With Dying: Finding care and compassion at the end of life*. London: Pinter and Martin.

Miles, M. B. and Huberman, A. M. (1994) *Qualitative Data Analysis: An Expanded Sourcebook*. 2nd edn. London: Sage.

NMC (2015) *The Code: Professional Standards of Practice and Behavior for Nurses and Midwives*. London: Nursing and Midwifery Council. Available online at www.nmc-uk.org/The-revised-Code (accessed 10 March 2015).

NMC (2010) *Standards of Pre-registration Nurse Education*. London: Nursing and Midwifery Council. Available online at www.nmc-uk.org/Publications/Standards (accessed 10 March 2015).

Pravikoff, D. S., Tanner, A. B. and Pierce, S. T. (2005) Readiness of U.S. nurses for evidence-based practice. *American Journal of Nursing*. 105(9), 40–51.

Risjord, M. (2014) *Philosophy of Social Science: A contemporary introduction*. Routledge Contemporary Introductions To Philosophy. Abingdon: Routledge.

Rolfe, G. (2014) Foundations for a human science of nursing: Gadamer, Laing, and the hermeneutics of caring. *Nursing Philosophy*. doi: 10.1111/nup.12075.

Sackett, D. L., Straus, S. E., Richardson, W. S., Rosenberg, W. and Haynes, R. B. (2000) *Evidence-based Medicine: How to practice and teach EBM*. 2nd edn. Edinburgh: Churchill-Livingstone.

Seale, C. (1999) *The Quality of Qualitative Research*. London: Sage.

Sutherland, S. (2013) *Irrationality: The enemy within*. London: Pinter and Martin.

Thaler, R. H. and Sunstein, C. R. (2008) *Nudge: Improving decisions about health, wealth and happiness*. Harmondsworth: Penguin.

Tracy, S. J. (2010) Qualitative quality: eight 'big-tent' criteria for excellent qualitative research. *Qualitative Inquiry*. 16(10), 835–51.

Wiggins, B. J. (2011) Confronting the dilemma of mixed methods. *Journal of Theoretical and Philosophical Psychology.* 31(1), 44–60.

Williams, B., Perillo, S. and Brown, T. (2015) Review: What are the factors of organisational culture in health care settings that act as barriers to the implementation of evidence-based practice? A scoping review. *Nurse Education Today.* 35(2), e34–41. doi: 10.1016/j.nedt.2014.11.012.

Yoder, L. H., Kirkley, D., McFall, D. C., Kirksey, K. M., StalBaum, A. L. and Sellers, D. (2014) Staff Nurses' use of research to facilitate evidence-based practice. *American Journal of Nursing.* 114(9), 26–37.

13 Ethics and evidence-based practice

Peter Allmark

Introduction

Evidence-based practice (EBP) is roughly the use of current best evidence in making decisions about the care of patients (Sackett *et al.* 1996). At first, it seems hard to imagine how such practice could raise ethical concerns, and yet it has. These concerns are set out in the first section of this chapter. Much of the past discussion of these problems has focused on the epistemology of evidence, with critics suggesting that EBP is based on an overly narrow definition of evidence and knowledge. This chapter tacks differently, focusing instead on the epistemology of practice; in other words, what type of evidence or knowledge is needed in deciding how to act? Using the distinction drawn by Aristotle between practical and scientific knowledge, it is suggested that evidence in the form of scientific knowledge, no matter how widely defined, cannot form the basis for practice because it cannot provide the goals that action requires; for EBP, these must be provided from within practice itself, from for example, nursing or surgery. However, ultimately the goals are provided by wider personal and social goals, in particular, human flourishing. Once this is accepted, it is possible to resolve the ethical concerns that have been raised about EBP, drawing on Aristotle's account of reasoning in the practice areas of craft knowledge and of practical wisdom.

Ethical concerns

At least four ethical concerns are found in the literature on EBP:

- some types of knowledge are not included in EBP
- EBP runs counter to patient-centred care
- 'testable by randomized controlled trial' is not the same as 'most effective'
- decisions based on EBP can be unjust.

Some types of knowledge are not included in EBP

EBP downgrades or discounts types of knowledge that are used by practitioners and which are important for good practice; these include experience, intuition and anecdote (Barker 2000; Bax 2008; Milton 2007; Tonelli 1998). In health care, EBP fits best with tightly defined areas of practice, particularly pharmacology, but is ill suited for the more craft-like areas, such as surgery and nursing. In these areas, experience counts for a great deal, and a patient would be better served by an experienced practitioner rather than one well-versed in recent research evidence. The obvious riposte here is that the patient is best served by one well versed in both. However, the point is rather that experience and intuition can point in directions counter to those suggested by EBP. For example, whilst guidelines based on EBP might suggest a new treatment for all patients, a practitioner might believe that, overall, some patients who are well established on the old treatment would be best left on it (for example, those who would find it difficult to establish new routines). A surgeon during a procedure might decide to try something new on the basis of a hunch, even though little or no EBP evidence exists to support it (Stirrat 2004). Another type of example in the literature is described as a Lazarus case, in which the practitioners, despite EBP-based guidelines, decided to carry on treating a patient who unexpectedly revived and left hospital relatively well (Brant-Zawadzki 2012).

EBP runs counter to patient-centred care

The concern that EBP runs counter to patient-centred care is a continuation: the type of knowledge that is discounted by EBP is often specific to case or circumstance. By insisting that all practice is based on up-to-date research evidence where it is available, patient-centred care, which requires case-specific knowledge and intuition, is undermined. The issue arises particularly where EBP enters protocols and guidelines which are supposed to be used as the primary decision-making aid for the practitioner. There are two types of problem:

- Patients lose choice; they are constrained to have what the evidence tells them to, a phenomenon that has been described as evidence-based paternalism (Rysavy 2013; Slowther *et al.* 2004; Liberati 2004). Of course, it might be asked why patients would want a less effective treatment anyway. However, patients might have different notions of effectiveness to those measured in the research evidence. An obvious example is where the evidence-based judgement includes cost effectiveness; for example, an individual patient might prefer a treatment of only marginally superior efficacy but much greater cost. But even where cost is not an issue, patients might have factors that matter to them but which are not judged overly important in the outcome measures of EBP; for example, American guidance recommending statins for all patients with diabetes was rejected by many patients (Montori *et al.* 2013).
- Practitioners lose choice; they can no longer make choices that fit individual patients but which run counter to the guidelines of EBP (Loewy 2007; Kerridge *et al.* 1998; Gupta 2003, 2004a, 2004b, 2014). Again, it might be asked why practitioners would want less effective or unproven treatments.

However, we have already seen one case, that of allowing some patients to remain on the apparently inferior old treatment. Another might be a health visitor who senses that a new mother is under stress, struggling with breast-feeding and in need of a kind of permission to give up and switch to bottle feeding. To encourage such a switch runs counter to evidence-based guide-lines and yet in certain situations health visitors might do so. A cancer nurse might meld conventional evidence-based treatment with a patient's own unproven (or even proven not to work) treatments. A mother using ineffec-tive colic drops for their baby might be encouraged to wean the child off them rather than stop straight away, as EBP would suggest. It is almost certain that many, perhaps most, practitioners could give further examples. It is not simply that some practice has to be undertaken in the absence of good evidence, it is that practitioners' practical knowledge, based on anecdote, intuition or similar, can suggest practice that runs counter to that which is suggested by EBP.

'Testable by randomised controlled trial' is not the same as 'most effective'

EBP puts highest value on evidence from randomised controlled trials (RCTs). However, this can produce unethical results (Zwitter 2001; Vos *et al.* 2004; Vineis 2004; Rysavy 2013). Consider two treatments that are proposed to reduce rates of heart disease in an area. The first is a publicity campaign to reduce smoking; the second, a campaign focused on social determinants of heart disease, which aims to reduce poverty through welfare advice and work on financial capability. It is relatively straightforward to test the first by RCT; researchers could, for example, use a cluster randomised trial in matched areas of the country. The outcomes could be easily measured by, say, six-week quit rates. And there would be no ethi-cal concerns – the researchers would be in equipoise as to whether or not the campaign works. Equipoise is the state in which the practice community is genuinely unsure as to whether one treatment is superior to another; it is consid-ered to be an ethically necessary condition prior to any randomisation; if it does not exist then clinicians would be randomly and unethically allocating patients to a treatment they believed inferior (Ashcroft and ter Meulen 2004). By contrast, the social-determinant-orientated intervention is harder to evaluate. There would be no immediate health-related scores, such as quit rates, that could be used. It would be possible to measure other scores, such as anxiety, but the link to health improvement would be slower and less obvious. There would also be an ethical concern concerning equipoise. The researchers do not know whether or not the intervention is useful in terms of health and as such equipoise exists and a clus-ter randomised design could be used. However, it is already known that interventions like this *are* effective in terms of reducing debt problems (Allmark *et al.* 2013). In such cases, it seems unethical to randomise people into a trial knowing that one group will get a less effective treatment than another. There are two key points from the example. The first is that the EBP pyramid can lead prac-titioners to prefer treatments that are testable by RCT but which may in fact be less effective than others which are not. The second is that practitioners might be pushed towards undertaking trials that are ethically dubious, just to meet the randomisation requirement.

Decisions based on EBP can be unjust

Those funding a health system would seem well advised only to fund interventions for which there is evidence. The preference for RCT-testable interventions described in the previous paragraph easily mutates into a preference for funding such interventions (Ashcroft and ter Meulen 2004; Vos *et al.* 2004; Kerridge *et al.* 1998; Jansen 1997; Hughes 1996; Hope 1995). This can result in what seem to be unjust decisions of various types. In the first place, rare conditions are difficult to test via RCTs, as there are insufficient cases to run a trial likely to reach statistical significance. Patients with these conditions might find that promising but insufficiently tested treatments are unfunded. Other conditions are common but are such that it is difficult to find funding to run expensive RCTs of their treatment. This might be because the conditions are suffered by those with low economic power; an example might be diarrhoea in developing countries. Or it might be because the condition is such that successful treatment of it is low profit. This has been the case with the development of antibiotics for multi-resistant bacteria; the problem here is that the drugs are used on too short-term a basis for companies funding research to recoup their research costs. By contrast, conditions that are widespread in affluent populations and which require long-term treatment are likely to be supported by many treatments that are well supported by RCT evidence; depression, for example. For similar reasons, certain types of patients may be poorly supported by RCT evidence, as is the case for those with multiple pathologies, the elderly and children. Finally, certain features of patients might be ignored or insufficiently accounted in RCTs meaning that it can be unclear whether a treatment is effective for patients on the basis of, for example, ethnicity or class. In summary, rationing based on EBP is likely to be unfair across a number of axes of inequality.

Summary

EBP has the foundational belief that practice should be based on the best evidence available. This implies that some evidence is better than others; the meta-analysis of multiple well-conducted RCTs is better than the intuition of a practitioner in deciding whether, for example, one treatment is better than another. However, implementation of EBP based on a hierarchy of evidence which puts RCTs at the top has resulted in a number of ethical concerns. EBP, it is said, can result in unethical practice where: i) it overrides the decisions of practitioners borne of their knowledge gained through experience; ii) it disempowers the ability of patients to choose on the basis of their own ideas and values; iii) it results in preference given for treatments that are most easily tested by RCTs; and iv) it is used in rationing and allocation decisions which tend to favour the existence of evidence over the presence of need.

Initial responses

The critical response to these concerns has focused on epistemology as the source of problems. Some critics reject outright epistemology that prioritises RCT-style knowledge, suggesting it is unsuitable for, say, nursing, which, it is claimed, is largely based on an entirely different type of practice knowledge (Barker 2000; Bax 2008). On first examination, however, this looks implausible. The EBP pyramid is not a production of *fiat* on the part of, say, doctors over nurses or quantitative researchers over qualitative ones. It is based on recognition of the nature of scientific method as being in large part concerned with the elimination of error. The literature on sources of error in reasoning is immense and overwhelming; if a nurse is to claim that they prefer by intuition to give treatment X to this particular patient in the face of strong RCT evidence preferring the contrary, they will fall foul of this evidence (Thaler and Sunstein 2009; Glass and McAtee 2006; Sutherland 1994). Their decision will be evidently wrong because it is less likely to achieve the desired goal than a decision based on the RCT evidence.

Others have emphasised the importance of the use of other types of evidence in practice. Some accept the EBP pyramid, which puts RCT and meta-analysis as the best basis for practice but allow other evidence when the former is unavailable or unobtainable. An example is the Medical Research Council (MRC) guidance on so-called natural experiments (Craig *et al.* 2012). Such experiments are the use of environmental differences that are not in the researchers' control to assess an effect; for example, the introduction of legislation or changes in taxation on health behaviour. The MRC guidance leaves the pyramid unaltered, merely acknowledging that randomisation is either practically or politically impossible in some cases.

Other critics suggest that the pyramid itself is unsuitable for certain areas of practice. For example, Pawson (2013) and others suggest that RCTs are suitable only for research in relatively closed systems, such as drugs acting on bodies. In these closed systems, it is relatively easy to remove or reduce the effect of confounding factors. However, RCTs are not suitable for open systems, such as social interventions to change behaviour of people in society. Here, there are so many confounding factors that the attempt to impose control of them reduces the intervention to something that is nothing like what will appertain in practice. Thus, for example, you might show that an educational intervention to increase exercise works at six weeks after a stroke for under-65-year-old English speaking men attending a programme run by well-motivated researchers in Yorkshire in August 2010 but it is unlikely that the programme will be as effective (or effective at all) amongst Asian women in Lancashire in December 2014 (see Snelling's criticism, Chapter 15 in this volume, of the 'ludicrous' level of compliance required in a randomised study of intentional rounding). The realist revolution in social research currently taking place is in part based on recognition of this. However, note that this does not get the critics of EBP very far. On the realist account, there is still a hierarchy of evidence; it is just that RCTs are not always at the top; they are replaced by something like realist synthesis (Pawson 2002); but even if this were done, the four areas of ethical concern set out above would remain in some form.

The initial responses to these ethical concerns have focused on the epistemology of 'evidence'. I argue that, as well as considering the 'evidence' in EBP, it is also necessary to consider the idea of practice being 'based' on evidence. The argument draws upon Aristotle's account of practical reasoning and the various distinctions he makes. One such distinction is that between scientific and practical knowledge. I argue that EBP errs where it is uses scientific knowledge as the sole or primary basis for practical decisions. For practice, scientific knowledge is only one element (or base) of what is required. This Aristotelian approach is then brought to bear on the ethical concerns that have been set out concerning EBP. The starting point is a brief account of Aristotle's theory of action, as set out in various places, including briefly in *Nicomachean Ethics* (Aristotle 2000) and, in more depth, in *Aristotle's De Motu Animalum* (Nussbaum 1985).[1]

Knowledge-based practice

Practice of the type identified in EBP is a type of action; it is purposeful or intentional action by practitioners with goals that are generally focused on the health or wellbeing of others. Action is, for Aristotle, a movement of some kind, the origin of which lies within the thing that moves. Generally, these are living things; as such, they are able to act without being acted upon. When a tree blows in the wind it is acted upon but when it grows or sucks up nutrition from the ground, it acts. However, it does so without intention; its action is autonomic. Animals, too, can be acted upon, like trees, and they can act autonomically, as when they digest food. However, they are also able to act on the basis of their internal states of desire in combination with their perception of external stimuli; a hungry animal that perceives food will, other things being equal, move to obtain and eat the food. Humans, as a type of animal, are capable of all such motion: involuntary, as when being acted upon, autonomic, as with digestion, and voluntary, as with acting in accordance with a desire in the manner of all animals. However, humans are capable of another layer of desire: rational or reasoned desire, which gives rise to another type of action, intentional action. This is a desire that does not just arise from their animal nature, like appetite for food or sex, but which is endorsed as good or not by some process of reasoning. Thus, a person who is hungry and perceives food that is easily obtainable might nonetheless avoid it because he has a reasoned desire to lose weight (Table 13.1).

Purposeful or intentional action is, then, action which is undertaken in the light of the agent's belief that some good is to be obtained through it. This good might be instrumental, constitutive or both. For example, the activity of working as a nurse might be instrumental, say, to obtaining money to do the things the agent wants. By contrast, building model boats might be constitutive, something the agent does that he views as good in itself. Working as a nurse could also be both

Table 13.1 Types of action in inanimate and animate objects

Object⟍ Type of action	Inanimate	Plant	Animate Animal	Human/Rational animal
Involuntary: moved with origin of movement outside self	✓	✓	✓	✓
Non-voluntary: origin in self (no desire)		✓	✓	✓
Voluntary: i) origin in self (with appetite-type desire)			✓	✓
Voluntary: ii) origin in self (with rational desire) – intentional/purposive action				✓

instrumental, to get money, and constitutive, because the agent views it as worthwhile or good in itself. The simple model of reasoned action is thus,

i.   Agent has a reasoned desire for x (where x is an instrumental or constitutive good).
ii. Agent recognises the situation as one in which action φ (pronounced 'phi') is one that will achieve x without any negative effects that outweigh it.
iii. Agent decides to φ.
iv. In the absence of countervailing forces, agent φs.

Evidence in this model comes into play in the second premise; for example, the agent desires to treat an infection and knows that RCTs have shown treatment A to be most effective. However, note that no decision will form and no action take place without the first premise, the goal and desire. This point is important: evidence of itself does not have and cannot provide a goal. No action, be it practice or other, can be based on evidence alone. 'Mere thought, however, moves nothing; it must be goal-directed and practical' (Aristotle 2000, 1139a).

Action requires, first, some kind of evidence such that the agent recognises the situation as one where a desire can be fulfilled plus, second, the desire. Thus, in judging the reasonableness or otherwise of an action, we need to consider at least two sets of evidence: first, the evidence by which the agent recognises the situation that requires φ in order to achieve x and, second, the evidence (or other considerations) by which the agent forms the reasoned desire for x at the outset.

The evidence referred to and discussed in relation to EBP belongs primarily in the first category; that is, it is evidence for φ as the most likely means of achieving x. Where does the evidence of the second type originate; that is, the evidence for the goal itself? Here, it is useful to draw upon a distinction that Aristotle makes between two categories of practical activity: production or craft (*techne*) and praxis. (The latter term is transliterated as it is awkward to translate; it will, however, be defined by explanation.)[2]

Production/craft is practical activity best shown by examples, such as playing a musical instrument, constructing a boat, performing surgery and nursing a patient. Here, the goal is provided from within the craft, to play a tune, build a boat, repair an aneurysm or return a patient to reasonable living. The goal will typically be broken down into stages, although this is more obvious in examples like building a boat than in playing a tune. To do the production/craft well, the agent will need a variety of attributes or, broadly, what Aristotle terms (craft-specific) 'virtues'. For playing a tune, these might be specific technical abilities but also the discipline to practice and apply them. For nursing, the range of virtues required will be different, including knowledge of up-to-date research evidence; but, as well as knowing this, the nurse will need the ability to apply it to specific situations. Finally, note that the goals of production/craft do not have to be good for the agent or for the wider world. Assassination could be termed a craft; a good assassin would require a range of skills and knowledge but being an assassin seems unlikely to be something that serves the individual or the world well in general.

Praxis is practical activity of which there is also a huge variety but (unlike crafts) in broad terms only one goal, that of living well. It is the activity undertaken by people as either constitutive of or instrumental to doing or living well (*eupraxia* and *eudaimonia*). As such, it might be thought that everything the agent does is praxis, including all production/craft activities. The assassin has goals and skills internal to their craft but also presumably undertakes it in the belief it is instrumental to living well overall. However, for Aristotle, such a person may be a good assassin but be mistaken about living well, hence mistaken in their praxis. It might be better to say that everything the person chooses to do is done in part as praxis but that it is not necessarily good praxis. To achieve good praxis, certain specific virtues and skills are required. These can be broadly divided into ethical and intellectual virtues.

Ethical virtues relate to desire. In order to act, a person must desire; we noted the example earlier of the hungry dieter who forgoes available food. Ethical virtue is possessed by someone whose desires are in line with good reasoning, with the choices that will constitute good praxis. But, for good reasoning itself, the person needs intellectual virtues of various types. The overall one is practical wisdom (*phronesis*) but this has many elements, key amongst which are:

- *Nous*, a word that has come down directly into English (usually pronounced 'nowse') to mean a kind of worldly wise attitude, perhaps a slightly cynical one. In right action, it has three roles: i) to read current circumstances correctly as, for example, something that requires urgent action; ii) to recognise the features of the situation that are relevant prior to deliberating; and iii) to recognise that deliberation is complete and an action settled upon.

- Good-end deliberation (*euboulia*); that is, reasoning well about living well, correctly reasoning about what goes into making a happy, flourishing life.
- Cleverness (*deinotes*), which is the ability to work out the particular means to particular goals. Aristotle recognises that this third element can be damaging if it is possessed by someone with bad goals.

These ideas can be summarised and developed as shown in Table 13.2. As illustrated by the assassin, production/craft does not require ethical virtue; for similar reasons, neither does it require good-end deliberation. However, the craft-person does require types of nous and cleverness that are specific to the production. The nurse referred to earlier requires not just research evidence but also the nous-like ability to know that this is a situation in which it is pertinent. She also requires the ability to work out specific steps in particular situations to achieve a goal, an ability termed quasi-cleverness in Table 13.2. With this account of practical knowledge in hand, it is now possible to return to the puzzles with which this chapter began and to attempt to resolve them.

Practical knowledge and the ethics of EBP

The 'evidence' referred to in EBP relates largely to scientific knowledge; to what is, or is probably on current evidence, the case. In terms of its relation to action, it is neutral because it is not tied to any particular ends. To take a simple example, the Romans and Ancient Greeks were aware that human effluent poisoned a water supply. One action that resulted from this scientific knowledge was building settlements such that effluent was disposed of downstream. However, another was the earliest known example of chemical warfare, when troops would deliberately poison the water supplies of cities under siege (Roffey *et al*. 2002). Here, the same knowledge forms the basis for completely opposed actions. Thus, one form of knowledge that EBP cannot supply is that of the right ends. Where does this knowledge come from and what evidence relates to it?

Table 13.2 Two types of productive activity and their related features

Productive activity	End	Virtue	Knowledge/evidence required
Praxis	Living or doing well	Ethical virtue Nous Good-end deliberation Cleverness	Knowledge of the good
Production/craft	Craft-specific	Craft-specific	Craft-specific, sometimes including research evidence

The ends of action can be provided from within a practice, such as nursing, surgery and assassin-craft (for want of a better word). The scientific knowledge of causes of infection will fuel different choices of action within each practice; surgeons and nurses avoiding it and assassins, perhaps, deliberately causing it. In this process, they are likely to use other types of knowledge. The executive knowledge of cleverness results in their knowing how to develop a plan for achieving the end; the how-to knowledge of experience results in their knowing how to, for example, do things aseptically. With such practical knowledge, scientific type knowledge of the RCT type seems tangential at best. Aseptic technique is learnt largely by doing, not by learning the results of experiments.

This gives purchase to some of the concerns about EBP; a nurse or surgeon making executive decisions of skill will use knowledge that is not of the EBP type, based as it rather is in the experience of the practitioner. However, this has not yet taken us to the heart of the problem. Proponents of EBP should have no difficulty acknowledging that skill-type and executive-type knowledge will be required, as well as the scientific knowledge that they champion. What they would not acknowledge would be the possibility of conflict between them; roughly, if you want to achieve ends within a practice, they would claim, then you should use the best scientific knowledge available; surgery requires practical skill but the surgeon should not use procedures, however skilfully, that have been shown to be less then best in terms of health outcomes.

It is then to outcomes and ends that we should look to resolve the concerns detailed at the beginning of the chapter. Table 13.2 shows that the ends of a practice are set by that practice such that different practices might use the same knowledge for contrary ends, such as saving lives and ending them. One way in which EBP might run counter to good practice would be where its proponents were advising the wrong ends. A number of examples where this might be claimed were given earlier: the nurse who advised some of their patients to stick with their old, apparently inferior, medication; the health visitor who did not advise breastfeeding; the nurse who combines evidence-based medication with the patient's own preferred non-evidence based ones. If the goal of practice in this case was to provide evidence-based care then such practitioners would indeed be wrong. However, it is not.

To take the health visitor example, the actual goal is, something like, to take the steps most likely to lead to a happy and healthy parenting of the child. Despite the health visitor knowing that breastfeeding is in general associated with healthier children, in this case she can see, on the basis of knowledge from beyond health research, that it might well go wrong and that not pushing breastfeeding is a better option. Much of this is down to nous, particularly here the ability of the health visitor to discern the relevant particulars (Sherman 1989). EBP-style evidence will be of great import but is defeasible by local particular factors. Thus, the EBP evidence shows that babies who are breastfed generally do better on a large number of indicators that are important in this specific case; as such, the health visitor will be inclined to recommend it. However, she discerns specific differences here; the mother's awkward relationship with her own body; her family's lack of support; her signs of emotional distress – and these cause the health visitor to choose a different action.

That this is a tricky and hazardous argument can be illustrated in the Lazarus-type cases. In these cases, practitioners make a decision to carry on treating apparently hopeless cases and then find themselves vindicated by successful outcomes. Might not such practitioners also point to nous, to discerning there was something about this case that made them feel they should press on? Such *post hoc* reasoning is notoriously unreliable. How can a distinction be made between the implausible magical-type nous claimed in some Lazarus cases from the more plausible examples, such as that of the health visitor?

Broadie's discussion of practical wisdom and the present author's own example provides a possible answer (Broadie 1991; Allmark 2005). An old master painting is for auction and an art expert is sent at short notice to bid for it on behalf of a client. He arrives late and bidding is apparently near its end. He has been told to bid above the present level but when he looks at the painting he instantly decides not to bid; he believes it to be a fake. The painting is sold and a legal dispute subsequently arises between the successful bidder and the auction house as to the painting's authenticity. In this case, the art expert could reasonably point to nous; he could sense something wrong about the painting. However, were he asked to set out in detail his concerns, he could do so: the brush strokes were too broad; the colours were of a type this painter never used; and so on. He did not go through this step by step but, rather, he instantaneously used a chain of reasoning that he could provide if called upon. The same must apply in these cases of particular judgement. The health visitor can provide such a chain; the Lazarus practitioner cannot. This is an important caveat to notions such as reflection-in-action (see Chapter 8 in this book); reflexivity of itself is of little practical use unless it is in-principle visible and analysable. This gives sufficient detail to tackle the problems set out at the beginning of this chapter:

- Some types of knowledge are not included in EBP.
- EBP runs counter to patient-centred care.

Some types of knowledge are indeed not included in EBP, of which skill-type knowledge (know-how) and nous (knowing what to do and when to act) are particularly relevant to practice. However, these will only lead to apparent disputes with EBP where there are specific details in the particular situation which are relevant and which are not accounted for in the evidence base, such as the mother's awkwardness. Practitioners calling upon such knowledge need to be cautious and need to provide a credible account of why such particulars are relevant in any particular case.

- 'Testable by RCT' is not the same as 'most effective'.

This concern was largely dealt with in the section 'Initial response' above. As it stands, this is a problem not of EBP but of the inappropriate placing of RCTs at the top of the pyramid of evidence types. As stated earlier, recent developments in realist methodology have shown that alternative methods might sit atop the pyramid in relation to research in open systems. It remains the case that EBP, even of this type, may yet be what practitioners choose not to apply in particular cases for the reasons just given and with the same caveats.

- Decisions based on EBP can be unjust.

Consider a nurse facing a patient with a pressure sore and another having a cardiac arrest; she would clearly prioritise the latter even though the evidence base for the treatment of the former might be stronger. Although this example is clear, in practice such decisions can go wrong in ways that are easily masked. Thus, community practitioners might decide that there is insufficient evidence to attempt a health-screening intervention in an under-researched community, such as the Roma, even though it is used successfully in the majority community. For the individual healthcare practitioner, the message is that the availability of evidence should not guide decisions about priorities of treatment; these priorities must be decided on the basis of the ends of the practice itself.

On a larger scale, funding decisions might be made by health commissioners, managers and, ultimately, politicians; decisions about what to research will be made by research funding bodies, drug companies and the like. It is worth recalling that, for all practitioners, their practice choices will also constitute praxis; that, as well as meeting the goals of their practice, they attempt to meet their overall goal of doing or living well. Some practices are such that their goals are likely to run foul of the goal of living well. Successful criminals, terrorists and assassins are not, *pace* relativists, living well. But most practices, including those outlined here relating to health care and management, are compatible with living well; a good nurse will also be someone who, barring ill luck, lives well. Hence, as practitioners, they will be concerned that there is an insufficient evidence base in some areas of practice or that there is injustice in resource allocation. This concern is seen in numerous ways, such as government reports. The response to the injustice that relates to EBP should be to encourage research in those areas, not to turn away from EBP itself.

Conclusion

The practice of EBP is largely exonerated in this account; it does not of itself give rise to ethical concerns, whereas failure to practice based on evidence often would. However, right action requires more than good evidence; it requires also the right ends, the right desires and the ability to apply all this as a package in any particular situation. This latter ability is practical wisdom and it combines various abilities, including the nous ability to discern the relevant particulars. And it is in the particular situations where EBP might appear to diverge from ethical best practice where the relevant particulars may diverge from those measured as important outcomes in the original research. There is a second way in which EBP might appear unethical. This is when strength of evidence is used as a method of prioritisation of health care; this seems obviously wrong once it is noticed but can slip through as apparently rational or 'scientific' if it is not. By providing the tools for practitioners and researchers to note the difference between epistemic wisdom and practical wisdom, Aristotle helps to resolve one area of concern relating to evidence-based practice.

Notes

1   The appendix to this chapter sets out some of the Aristotelian terms used in this chapter and compares them with alternatives found in translation, as well as with the original Greek.
2   Lipscomb (Chapter 12 in this book) addresses the specific issue of how much and what research evidence a particular practitioner needs or could be expected to have. This is an important issue not specifically addressed in the current chapter.

References

Allmark, P., Baxter, S., Goyder, E., Guillaume, L. and Crofton-Martin, G. (2013) Assessing the health benefits of advice services: using research evidence and logic model methods to explore complex pathways. *Health and Social Care in the Community*, 21(1), 59–68.

Allmark, P. (2005) Health, happiness and health promotion. *Journal of Applied Philosophy*, 22(1), 1–15.

Aristotle (2000) *Nicomachean Ethics* (trans. and ed.) R. Crisp, Cambridge: Cambridge University Press.

Ashcroft, R. and ter Meulen, R. (2004) Ethics, philosophy, and evidence based medicine. *Journal of Medical Ethics*, 30(2), 119.

Barker, P. (2000) Reflections on caring as a virtue ethic within an evidence-based culture. *International Journal of Nursing Studies*, 37(4), 329–36.

Bax, A. (2008) Evidence-based practice: ethical questions for nursing. *Nursing Science Quarterly*, 21(2), 183.

Brant-Zawadzki, M. (2012) The Lazarus syndrome: The ethics of evidence-based versus experience-based medicine. *Radiology*, 263(3), 629–32.

Broadie, S. (1991) *Ethics with Aristotle*, New York: Oxford University Press.

Craig, P., Cooper, C., Gunnell, D., Haw, S., Lawson, K., MacIntyre, S., Ogilvy, D., Petticrew, M., Reeves, B., Sutton, M. and Thompson, S. (2012) Using natural experiments to evaluate population health interventions: new Medical Research Council guidance. *Journal of Epidemiology and Community Health*, 66(12), 1182–6.

Glass, T. A. and McAtee, M. J. (2006) Behavioral science at the crossroads in public health: extending horizons, envisioning the future. *Social Science and Medicine*, 62(7), 1650–71.

Gupta, M. (2003) A critical appraisal of evidence-based medicine: Some ethical considerations. *Journal of Evaluation in Clinical Practice*, 9(2), 111–21.

Gupta, M. (2004a) Evidence-based medicine: Ethically obligatory or ethically suspect? *Evidence-Based Mental Health*, 7(4), 96–7.

Gupta, M. (2004b) Reconsidering rationality and ethics in the evidence-based medicine debate: A reply to commentators. *Journal of Evaluation in Clinical Practice*, 10(2), 143–6.

Gupta, M. (2014) *Is Evidence Based Psychiatry Ethical?* Oxford: Oxford University Press.

Hope, T. (1995) Evidence based medicine and ethics. *Journal of Medical Ethics*, 21(5), 259–60.

Hughes, J. C. (1996) Evidence based medicine and ethics. *Journal of Medical Ethics*, 22(1), 55–6.

Jansen, R. P. S. (1997) Evidence-based ethics and the regulation of reproduction. *Human Reproduction*, 12(9), 2068–75.

Kerridge, I., Lowe, M. and Henry, D. (1998) Personal paper. Ethics and evidence based medicine. *BMJ*, 316(7138), 1151–3.

Liberati, A. (2004) Introduction to the symposium: what evidence based medicine is and what it is not. *Journal of Medical Ethics*, 30(2), 120–1.

Loewy, E. H. (2007) Ethics and evidence-based medicine: Is there a conflict? *MedGenMed Medscape General Medicine*, 9(3), 30.

Milton, C. L. (2007) Evidence-based practice: Ethical questions for nursing. *Nursing Science Quarterly*, 20(2), 123–6.

Montori, V., Brito, J. and Murad, M. (2013) The optimal practice of evidence-based medicine incorporating patient preferences in practice guidelines. *Journal of the American Medical Association*, 310(23), 2503–4.

Nussbaum, M. (1985) *Aristotle's De Motu Animalium*, Princeton, NJ: Princeton University Press.

Pawson, R. (2002) Evidence-based policy: the promise of 'realist synthesis'. *Evaluation*, 8(3), 340.

Pawson, R. (2013) *The Science of Evaluation*, London: Sage.

Roffey, R., Tegnell, A. and Elgh, F. (2002) Biological warfare in a historical perspective. *Clinical Microbiology and Infection*, 8(8), 450–4.

Rysavy, M. (2013) Evidence-based medicine: a science of uncertainty and an art of probability. *Virtual Mentor*, 15(1), 4–8.

Sackett, D. L., Rosenberg, W. M. C., Gray, J. A. M., Haynes, R. B. and Richardson, W. S. (1996) Evidence based medicine: what it is and what it isn't. *BMJ*, 312, 71–2.

Sherman, N. (1989) *The Fabric of Character: Aristotle's theory of virtue*, Oxford: Oxford University Press.

Slowther, A.-M., Ford, S. and Schofield, T. (2004) Ethics of evidence based medicine in the primary care setting. *Journal of Medical Ethics*, 30(2), 151–5.

Stirrat, G.M. (2004) Ethics and evidence based surgery. *Journal of Medical Ethics*, 30(2), 160–5.

Sutherland, N. (1994) *Irrationality*, New Brunswick, NJ: Rutgers University Press.

Thaler, R. and Sunstein, C. (2009) *Nudge: Improving Decisions about Health, Wealth and Happiness*, Harmondsworth: Penguin.

Tonelli, R. (1998) The philosophical limits of evidence-based medicine. *Academic Medicine*, 73(12), 1234–40.

Vineis, P. (2004) Evidence-based medicine and ethics: A practical approach. *Journal of Medical Ethics*, 30(2), 126–30.

Vos, R., Willems, D. and Houtepen, R. (2004) Coordinating the norms and values of medical research, medical practice and patient worlds: The ethics of evidence based medicine in orphaned fields of medicine. *Journal of Medical Ethics*, 30(2), 166–70.

Zwitter, M. (2001) A personal critique: Evidence-based medicine, methodology, and ethics of randomised clinical trials. *Critical Reviews in Oncology/Hematology*, 40(2), 125–30.

Appendix: Terminology used in this chapter alongside Greek and alternative translations

Term used in this chapter	Greek Transliteration	Greek	Other translations Crisp	Irwin	Important alternatives
Scientific knowledge	Episteme	'επιστήμη	Scientific knowledge	Scientific knowledge	
Good deliberation	Euboulia	'ευβουλια	Noble deliberation	Fine deliberation	
Practical knowledge	Dianoia Praktiken	διάνοια πράκτικην	Practical thought	Practical thought	
Practical wisdom	Phronesis	φρονήσις	Practical wisdom	Intelligence	
Cleverness	Deinotes	δεινότητα	Cleverness	Cleverness	
Voluntary	Hekousion	'εκουσιον	Voluntary	Voluntary, willing	Intentional
Involuntary	Akousion	'ακουσιον	Involuntary	Involuntary, unwilling	Unintentional
Desire	Orexis	'ορέξις	Desire	Desire	
Desire of appetite	Epithumia	'επιθύμια	Appetite	Appetite	
Rational choice	Prohairesis	προ'αιρεσίς	Rational choice	Decision	Choice

14 Ethical competence and evidence based practice

Derek Sellman

One problem of evidence lies in its relationship with belief. Despite the secularization successes of the Enlightenment project and the undoubted triumph of science in many areas of human endeavour, there remains scepticism about claims that laws can be determined to explain and predict human actions and reactions. Even if laws in the social world could be identified, it is unlikely they would be afforded a value equivalent to that of currently accepted laws of nature. Yet, even the laws of nature remain contestable, at least theoretically, and in relation to the ideals of scientific integrity. Nevertheless, it seems that, in general terms, experience of the natural world provides sufficient evidence to warrant strong beliefs about the laws of nature. In contrast, experience of the social world can only provide evidence for relatively weak beliefs regarding 'laws' of human behaviour. Of course, unlike theories of the natural world, there are many and varied theories of human behaviour competing for attention and the appeal of each differs among individuals. For some, the appeal of a particular theory provides grounds for a set of more or less firmly held beliefs but the evidential credentials to support strong beliefs in the social realm struggle to approximate those of established natural world theories such as those that give rise to, for example, the laws of physics or the laws of chemistry. Strong beliefs drawn from or aligned with theories of the social world might then be said to give rise to controversy and uncertainty regarding evidential claims, particularly where those claims relate to how or when evidence is to inform action in practice-based activities within social practices such as nursing.

In concert with the general position taken in the book, this chapter accepts the notion that evidence-based practice is, on balance, a good thing. The issue of concern in this chapter is in relation to the epistemic responsibilities that accompany claims of evidence based practice. Regardless of the nature or status of the evidence, epistemic responsibilities stem from the integrity that is said to be a *prima face* requirement of the scientific method and for this no apology is offered. As several authors in this volume indicate, and to misquote Winston Churchill, no one pretends that the scientific method is perfect. Indeed, it might be said that the scientific method is the worst form of discovery, except for all the others that have been tried. For what the scientific method offers that other approaches cannot is a genuine attempt to account for and avoid bias, wishful thinking, and capriciousness – or as Paley (2005) might put it, the scientific method and all its accoutrements offer opportunities for evaluation against the 'error criterion' test. But, as Bluhm points out (Chapter 7 in this volume), even if a research study does pass this test, it may not generate evidence of the value often assumed by those who wish to use it to guide practice. For the purposes of this chapter, however, the debates about what should and should not count as evidence are of only tangential relevance. What is under consideration here is the transfer of the requirements of scientific integrity from the producer to the consumer of evidence as part of the process of attempting to put evidence to use in the pursuit of effective, safe, competent and compassionate nursing practice.

As Thorne (Chapter 11 in this volume) reminds us, it is not unknown for nurses to demonstrate tendencies of ambivalence towards evidence: championing evidence in the decision-making process when it aligns with existing beliefs regarding, for example, how resources are allocated within healthcare systems; while being, if not antagonistic, then less accepting of evidence that challenges firmly held normative beliefs about cherished nursing practices. This tendency to be more receptive to evidence that supports rather than that which refutes firmly held beliefs is not a phenomenon restricted to nurses – politicians demonstrate this tendency perhaps more publically than most – but what it points to is a neglect by evidence consumers of the very epistemic responsibilities that are expected of the evidence producers. For it would seem, if not necessary then at least desirable, that those who aim to use evidence as a basis for practice should apply the same rigorous intellectual standards to their evaluation of the evidence as is expected of those who produce the evidence. This is no small matter for it requires a demanding set of intellectual habits that approximate what Williams (2002) refers to as 'truth acquiring processes'. What both Thorne and Williams are talking about here is the idea of integrity or, more accurately, the scientific integrity of the kind that research ethics committees expect researchers to display. As Macrina puts it: 'Integrity is expected, because science is built upon a foundation of trust and honesty. Long before federal agencies published definitions of scientific misconduct, it was obvious that lying, cheating, and stealing in the conduct of research were wrong' (Macrina, 2005: 1).

Researchers are expected to exhibit ethical conduct no less than are registered nurses; ethical conduct is, after all, a requirement of professional nursing as identified in nursing codes throughout the world and, further, nurses who are researchers are bound by their professional nursing codes in the same way as are nurse academics and nurse practitioners. In terms of being consumers or users of evidence, the requirements of ethical practice as outlined in nursing codes apply as equally as they do to all other aspects of nursing practice. In other words, scientific integrity in the form of the application of rigorous intellectual standards is a requirement of ethical practice for nursing and, if this true, then nurses need to discharge appropriately the demands of epistemic responsibility before any claims of ethical competence can be made.

Ethical competence

For the purposes of this chapter, ethical competence is defined as the demonstration of those skills of intellect necessary to provide an accurate assessment of both the value of evidence and the value of evidence in terms of its application to a given set of circumstances. While the focus of this definition remains located in the intellectual domain there is an assumption that it provides impetus for action such that wherever a practitioner, by virtue of ethical competence, has come to the belief that evidence x should be used to inform and guide practice in situation y then that belief must by necessity obligate that particular practitioner to practice in a way that is consistent with their evidential belief.

This formulation of the idea of ethical competence in relation to evidence based practice might appear to indicate no more than that the registered nurse must know what they are doing and know why they are doing it. Something that is seen as a basic requirement of safe and effective nursing practice. Yet, while this simple interpretation may capture the essential elements of ethical competence there is a more to say and the remainder of this chapter is devoted to outlining some of the implications of ethical competence for evidence based practice.

From critical thinking to intellectual integrity, epistemic responsibility and ethical competence

Critical thinking is regarded as a fundamental requirement for nursing practice in the twenty-first century. The nine intellectual skills of clarity, accuracy, precision, relevance, depth, breadth, logic, significance and fairness are considered by Paul and Elder (2006) as 'universal intellectual standards' that provide the cornerstone of critical thinking necessary to avoid thinking that would otherwise be 'biased, distorted, partial, uniformed or down-right prejudiced' (Paul and Elder, 2006: 4). For a practice-based activity such as nursing, the application of a set of thinking skills such as Paul and Elder's universal intellectual standards is utilitarian insofar as it has as a core purpose the development of habits of mind conducive to ensure best practice in critical thinking and beyond.

This much is relatively uncontroversial, as sentiments consistent with this position appear explicitly and implicitly within the clauses of nursing's codes. But beyond any easy acceptance of these sentiments lies a moral obligation to bring such habits of mind to bear on all relevant evidence; that is, to examine critically the evidence that supports current practice as well as the evidence that contests current practice. Each of the standards identified by Paul and Elder are implicated in this apparently simple task. A practitioner has every right to anticipate these standards are met by those who produce evidence but also needs to recognise the obligation to adopt those same standards in order seek answers to questions that will give confidence in the value of the evidence, and of the value of the evidence as it relates to a particular set of circumstances. If not Paul and Elder's standards, then some similar set of intellectual standards can provide the wherewithal for an appraiser to asses the integrity of the evidence for without an understanding of the requirements of such standards it seems unlikely that a useful appraisal can be made of anything claiming to be evidence. It is not clear that checklist approaches to research appraisal can encourage the habits of mind necessary for effective evaluation of evidence.

Underpinning the idea of intellectual standards are a number of anticipated commitments; commitments that might emerge from a requirement to take the appraisal of evidence seriously. High among these commitments are a commitment to honesty, a commitment to fairness, a commitment to open-mindedness and a commitment to act on the findings of evidence. In other words, a commitment to intellectual integrity, epistemic responsibility and ethical competence, which at a very basic level includes a willingness to accept that one might be wrong about any one firmly held belief or wrong about beliefs in the effectiveness of any one practice behaviour. One implication of this might be formulated thus: ethical competence requires a nurse not only to recognise they may be wrong about what they believe in addition to what they do but also to acknowledge the necessity to amend beliefs and change practice in the light of evidence sufficient to warrant such changes. The rational logic of this would seem inescapable but so often, as those charged with effecting change will surely testify, rationality alone is rarely sufficient to motivate individuals to change their beliefs or their behaviours.

Belief is related to identity. To the extent that we generally expect people to behave in a way consistent with their beliefs then it is reasonable to suppose that, in some sense at least, individuals are defined according to their beliefs. When those who we understand to hold strong beliefs regarding the value of honesty act in dishonest ways we are surprised because we expect them to behave in honest ways; when those who we understand to believe in fairness when dealing with others demonstrate uncharacteristic prejudice we wonder why their usual concern with justice has evaded them on this occasion. This view assumes that beliefs are closely associated with identity and consequently implicates challenges to beliefs, particularly challenges to strongly held beliefs, as threats to personal identity. If true, then the challenge that the very idea of evidence-based practice poses to personal identity is underestimated at the cost of its rejection whenever and wherever evidence threatens the strongly held beliefs of an individual practitioner. It also points to one possible explanation of why individuals are wont to demonstrate ambivalence towards the value of evidence; illustrated by those who readily entertain evidence supportive of their strongly held beliefs while minimising or dismissing the value of evidence that contests those strong beliefs.

It also suggests a reactionary rather than a revolutionary tendency when it comes to belief formation and maintenance which in turn aligns with Kuhn's (1970) view of scientific progress. For, following this logic, evidence that requires only minor changes in beliefs – changes in beliefs that can be incorporated into existing sets of beliefs without a radical challenge to the core beliefs implicated in identity – can be accommodated within the existing framework of beliefs of an individual. As such, evidence indicating changes in beliefs and practices can continue to be accommodated just so long as those changes do not threaten the edifice of beliefs upon which a practice rests. In this way, it would seem possible to introduce change incrementally and with some confidence of success – and in this scenario it is relatively easy to remain open minded. It is when the evidence begins to suggest more radical changes in belief are necessary or when evidence begins to point to the unsustainability of existing sets of beliefs – sets of beliefs that sustain existing organisational, professional or political structures – that resistance to changes in beliefs are likely precisely because of the threat such evidence poses to those whose position relies on maintaining the primacy of existing sets of beliefs. In this scenario, the possibilities for maintaining scientific integrity, discharging epistemic responsibilities, or retaining ethical competence are limited not only by threats to personal identity but also by pragmatics and political power. It is where evidence comes up against the power of belief.

Open mindedness

Collectively the intellectual standards that Paul and Elder (2006) consider essential as habits of mind for those wishing to be or to become critical thinkers would seem a necessary condition of ethical competence as conceived here. It is difficult to imagine that a claim of intellectual integrity could be sustained in the absence of any one of the standards. As Paul and Elder note, each standard can be viewed as a stand alone skill and each can be learned separately but the synergy of combining all allows a comprehensive perspective not available to any one standard alone. In terms of evidence-based practice, intellectual integrity is thus served when the habits of mind allow for a review of evidence taking account of each of the intellectual standards necessary to determine the value of that evidence. And herein lies the idea of epistemic responsibility. If a nurse is to lay claim to evidence-based practice then it would seem that she or he must be prepared to pay attention, and give a fair hearing, to any evidence that impacts the phenomenon under consideration. Being selective will only compound charges of bias.

The use of intellectual standards such as those endorsed by Paul and Elder (2006) also provides a platform for the formation, revision, and maintenance of both strongly and weakly held beliefs. If nurses are to pursue evidence-based practice then the epistemic responsibilities that follow include a responsibility to take seriously the appraisal, without bias, of everything that claims to be relevant evidence. And to do this requires adoption of a set of justifiable intellectual standards that among other things approximates an unbiased review of the evidence. While one conclusion would indicate the necessary suspension of existing beliefs (for how else can an unbiased appraisal take place?), such a demand is unrealistic because appraisal must by definition involve belief – even it is only belief of a minimal kind such as belief in the validity of the criteria against which evaluation is to be made. A more realistic proposal is that an unbiased review of evidence is one in which the appraiser adopts a disposition that suspends judgement on the value of a particular piece of evidence – and of the value of that evidence in relation to a particular situation – until such time as the appraisal has been completed. And this requires the appraiser to have an open mind in the sense that they are open to the possibility that they may be wrong about one or more of their existing beliefs and willing to change those beliefs in the light of compelling evidence. As noted, beliefs can be held in a weak or strong (or anywhere in between) sense and, presumably, the weaker the belief the easier the task of being open to the possibility of error in that belief. The implications of this insight for evidence-based nursing practice would seem manifested in a need for autonomous practitioners to be proactive in seeking evidence both *for and against* existing beliefs and current practices in the attempt to discharge the epistemic responsibilities evidence based practice entails. Being proactive in seeking evidence requires nothing less than being open minded about what counts as evidence and open minded about what the evidence might require in terms of revising existing beliefs including beliefs about what practice actions are supported by the evidence. The heady demands of the requirements of open mindedness might turn out to demonstrate that one is less open minded than one would like to believe, for a belief in one's own open mindedness may yet to turn out to be a false belief. As Hare (2003) puts it 'To be open-minded is, after all, to be critically receptive to alternative possibilities, to be willing to think again despite having formulated a view, and to be concerned to defuse any factors that constrain one's thinking in predetermined ways' (Hare, 2003: 4–5), which indicates that the open-minded person will recognise a need to ensure their strongly held beliefs do not interfere with genuine attempts to remain true to the ideals of scientific integrity while undertaking appraisal of evidence. As Hare (1979) claims elsewhere 'open-mindedness appears to be written into the notion of having a scientific outlook, inasmuch as this involves being willing to revise and/or reject the views one has in the light of fresh evidence' (Hare, 1979: 30).

Yet, this desire, consistent with the scientific ideal of following the evidence to wherever it leads and adapting practice accordingly places unreasonable demands on individual practitioners. As intimated earlier in this chapter, being open minded is relatively easy when all that is at stake is a change in beliefs that do not threaten those core beliefs implicated in personal identity but even here, the pace of practice leaves little time for individual nurses to attend to all of the requirements of epistemic responsibilities and so the rise of guidelines, protocols, and organisations such as the UK National Institute for Health and Care Excellence (NICE) to assist in the pursuit of evidence based practices are understandably welcomed by busy practitioners. But such protocols as developed do not abrogate individual nurses from their epistemic responsibilities for as I have argued elsewhere (Sellman, 2003, 2011) there is a professional obligation to not only ensure that a protocol reflects current best evidence but also to ensure that protocol applies to any given patient situation. To do otherwise is the equivalent of blindly following orders and one of the justifications for evidence-based practice is precisely to avoid such myopic practice. Yet the authority vested in protocols and guidelines is rapidly becoming (in some places may have already become) such that to act against protocol is to invite censure even if an individual practitioner has followed the epistemic responsibilities required of evidence-based practice. The idea that protocols and guidelines should remain under constant review is a given but inevitably the decision to change protocols must wait until those with the authority to change the content of the protocol decide that the evidence is sufficient to warrant a change. This poses something of a conundrum for while there may be protocols in place to assist the process of review and revision of policy and protocols, that process ultimately relies on the effective discharge of epistemic responsibilities of a group of individuals who may have differing views not only about the collective weight of evidence required to necessitate a change in the protocol but also differences of opinion about the value of individual pieces of evidence. While the practitioner awaits the outcomes of the deliberations of whichever committee ultimately decides and, while under the threat of censure for acting outside of protocol, the practitioner would seem obligated to follow current guidelines even if the those guidelines might change tomorrow or the next day; even if, according to the ideals of scientific integrity, the protocol should have already been changed in the light of evidence sufficient to warrant a change.

In addition, it is possible that the vested interests of those in the positions of power afforded by being selected to serve on committees that make decisions regarding when protocols and policies should be amended in the light of new evidence presupposes expertise of a kind that leaves them vulnerable to charges of having the most to lose should the evidence contradict existing beliefs in general and the strongly held beliefs of those individuals in particular. Furthermore, given the political patronage required for membership of many of these types of committees then the precarious (nay, capricious) nature of continued membership can distort the outcomes of deliberations if members acknowledge a need for recommendations to remain consistent with the organisational, economic or even ideological imperatives of those with the power to change the membership of the committee, or the power to dissolve the committee altogether. Pressure can also be brought to bear in less subtle ways as the case of Professor Bengtsson amply demonstrates. Professor Bengtsson resigned only weeks after being appointed to the Global Warming Policy Foundation Academic Advisory Council following what was described as 'the disgraceful intolerance within the climate science community which ... prompted his resignation' (Peiser, 2014). In response to Bengtsson's letter of resignation, David Henderson (Chairman of the Advisory Council) noted that 'The reactions that you speak of, and which have forced you to reconsider the decision to join us, reveal a degree of intolerance, and a *rejection of the principle of open scientific inquiry*, which are truly shocking' (Global Warming Policy Foundation, 2014; emphasis added). The disturbing aspect of this incident (of which there are likely many less reportable occurrences) is that it points to a failure of scientific integrity when its pursuit shows signs of disrupting the firmly held beliefs of those with powerful vested interests; be those interests reputational, political, economic, or ideological. The scientific community is, it seems, not above attempting to silence evidence that does not conform to the cherished assumptions on which a given scientific community relies for its authority and influence – and it does this in subtle as well as not so subtle ways. The peer review process, for example, requires the discharge of the very epistemic responsibilities as have been outlined in this chapter precisely because the alternative is a cartel of self-proclaimed experts acting as gatekeepers to the dissemination of evidence. There is, of course, a need for a gatekeeping function for the sake of scientific credibility but there is a fine line to be drawn between the promotion of disseminating evidence that deserves a hearing and the prevention of the publication of material that challenges existing dogma. Again, while the scientific integrity that underpins the peer review process is not perfect, it at least has the support of the scientific community and moves to make the process transparent by opening up to scrutiny the comments of reviewers and author responses along with publication of articles would seem one further step in acting in ways consistent with the ideals of scientific integrity in the publication process.

In nursing it is no different. Nursing has its own epistemic communities or what Fox Keller (2010) would call, its own *'epistemological cultures* – i.e., the collectivity of shared assumptions about what counts as an explanation, and about what suffices for understanding' (Fox Keller, 2010: 133; original emphasis). I think that Fox Keller would anticipate a single epistemological culture for nursing but judging by the continuing debates even within this volume about what does and does not count as evidence for nursing it would seem nursing cannot yet claim a single epistemological culture. Indeed, it is not clear that a single epistemological culture would serve nursing well, if for no other reason than the wide and varied nature of nursing practice. Nevertheless, there are personal and/or professional vested interests within nursing and it is reasonable to assume that wherever the pursuit of scientific integrity leads to conclusions unpalatable to the strongly held beliefs of those with vested interests, then the ideals of epistemic responsibility come up against the pragmatics of practice. In this sense, ethical competence in terms of the discharge of epistemic responsibilities seemingly required by scientific integrity would seem beyond the reach of ordinary practitioners.

Given these conditions, being open-minded and discharging one's epistemic responsibilities seems far from straightforward. But as with so much human activity, the recognition that the logical ideal might not be possible should not prevent efforts to minimise the effects of the limitations identified. The scientific method is not perfect but without it the current state of knowledge would be so much the poorer. Similarly, evidence-based practice might not be the panacea that some would have us believe but the genuine pursuit of the epistemic responsibilities that come with it provide the elements of ethical competence that can assist in the discharge of ethical nursing practice.

References

Fox Keller, E. (2010) Evelyn Fox Keller. In R. Rosenberger (ed.), *Philosophy of Science: 5 Questions*. Copenhagen: Automatic Press/VIP.

Hare, W. (1979) *Open-mindedness and Education*. Montreal: McGill-Queen's University Press.

Hare, W. (2003) The ideal of open-mindedness and its place in education. *Journal of Thought*, 38(2), 3–10.

Henderson, D. (2014, May 14) Your letter of resignation. In Global Warming Policy Foundation, Lennart Bengtsson resigns: GWPF voices shock and concern at the extent of intolerance within the climate science community [Press release]. Available online at www.thegwpf.org/lennart-bengtsson-resigns-gwpf-voices-shock-and-concern-at-the-extent-of-intolerance-within-the-climate-science-community (accessed 13 March 2015).

Kuhn, T. S. (1970) *The Structure of Scientific Revolutions* (2nd ed.). Chicago, IL: University of Chicago Press.

Macrina, F. L. (2005) *Scientific Integrity: Text and cases in responsible conduct of research* (3rd ed.). Washington, DC: ASM Press.

Paley, J. (2006) Evidence and expertise. *Nursing Inquiry*, 13, 82–93.

Paul, R. and Elder, L. (2006) *The Miniature Guide to Critical Thinking: Concepts and tools*. Dillon Beach, CA: Foundation for Critical Thinking.

Peiser, B. (2014, 14 May) It is with great regret, and profound shock, that we have received Professor Lennart Bengtsson's letter of resignation from his membership of the GWPF's Academic Advisory Council. In Global Warming Policy Foundation, Lennart Bengtsson resigns: GWPF voices shock and concern at the extent of intolerance within the climate science community [Press release]. Available online at www.thegwpf.org/lennart-bengtsson-resigns-gwpf-voices-shock-and-concern-at-the-extent-of-intolerance-within-the-climate-science-community (accessed 13 March 2015).

Sellman, D. (2003) Open-mindedness: A virtue for professional practice. *Nursing Philosophy*, 4, 17–24.

Sellman, D. (2011) *What Makes a Good Nurse: Why the virtues are important for nurses*. London, England: Jessica Kingsley.

Williams, B. (2002) *Truth and Truthfulness: An essay in genealogy*. Princeton, NJ: Princeton University Press.

15 Rounding on the smokers

The myth of evidence based (nursing) policy

Paul Snelling

Introduction

The enterprise of evidence-based practice is undertaken at many levels, from the funding and performance of international multicentre trials and their incorporation into evidence-based guidelines, to individual nurses driven by professionalism or curiosity, or by the requirements of an academic programme, accessing and appraising evidence to inform practice in line with what their regulatory body requires of them. As the chapters in this book make clear, conceptual and practical problems make this process far more complex than it might at first appear. However, at minimum, it could be argued that if nurses follow properly constructed evidence-based guidelines they can point to them, if they needed to, as justification for a claim that their care is based on 'the best available evidence and best practice' (Nursing and Midwifery Council, 2015: 7). There cannot be a guideline for every eventuality, of course, and nurses 'must be able to respond autonomously and confidently to planned and uncertain situations' (Nursing and Midwifery Council, 2010: 7). Autonomous practice is one of the defining features of professional practice but it clearly does not amount to practising exactly as each nurse sees fit, independent of all external considerations.

The Nursing and Midwifery Council (NMC) *Standards for Competence* document (Nursing and Midwifery Council, 2010: 6) also requires that nurses 'must show professionalism and integrity and work within recognised professional, ethical and legal frameworks'. These sorts of regulatory and explanatory documents are candidates for analysis of almost infinite regress. What, for example, does 'recognised' mean in this context, and recognised by whom? This is an analysis for another day and of more immediate concern is a framework omitted from the list: a framework of employment. The large majority of nurses work for an employer under a contract which stipulates terms of employment, and these terms will include the expectation or requirement that employers' policies will be followed in the course of employment. These policies cover many aspects of work, governing behaviour by both employer and employee. They set out working arrangements like shift patterns and leave entitlement as well as the working environment to which employees are entitled. For example, safety is assured (or at least it should be) by health and safety policies which apply to all employees, capable of separation from professional considerations. However, some policies also cover aspects of professional practice and it is often claimed that these are formulated on the basis of evidence. If these claims are not credible, there may be tensions between a requirement for nurses to follow reasonable instructions and policies required of her by her employer, and the professional requirement articulated in standards documents, for autonomous and evidence-based practice, within ethical frameworks. This chapter explores these tensions offering critical and occasionally polemic analysis in relation to two developing areas of policy: the introduction of intentional rounding and hospital smoking bans. I argue that policies concerning intentional rounding are defended by reference to evidence but its quality and application are so poor that a claim that it is evidence-based policy is simply not credible; and, although supported by authoritative bodies like the National Institute of Health and Care Excellence (NICE), authoritarian policies that seek to prevent smoking at hospitals are based not on factual evidence but on normative values. Before considering these practical nursing applications, the chapter proceeds with a brief discussion of the many levels of policy, how it differs from guidance and the claim that it is based on evidence.

The nature of policy

The word 'policy' is used freely but its frequency of use belies a complexity uncaptured by simplistic definitions, such as 'something like "a formal course of action proposed or adopted"' (Traynor, 2013: 126). In a standard textbook, Ham (2009) was tempted, following Cunningham, to suggest that 'policy is rather like the elephant – you recognise it when you use it but you can't easily define it' (Ham, 2009: 131). In relation to public health policy, Coggon's (2012) discussion demonstrates that the notion of policy can be taken to mean both the aims of 'considered decision making by an agent or agency' (Coggon, 2012: 75) and the means by which they are procured. Policies can be seen at many different levels. At the highest level, statements of intent are articulated by governments and in some cases these are implemented by detailed procedures, for example in contractual arrangements in the National Health Service which must be followed by all commissioners of services. In other cases, high-level policy aims are implemented at local level, and discretion is sometimes allowed to account for local circumstances and preferences.

These conceptual details, although of great interest to policy makers and managers, need not necessarily concern the practising nurse caring for her patients, although the NMC standards can be read otherwise. The competence standards cited earlier go on to require that all nurses must 'contribute to the collection of local and national data and formulation of policy on risks, hazards and adverse outcomes' (Nursing and Midwifery Council, 2010: 8). In a sense, this requirement typifies the sorts of tensions that the chapters in this book explore, as regulatory requirements of practice, expressed in standards documentation, appear to leave little room for manoeuvre in what nurses are (theoretically) required to do, rather than what they are advised or exhorted or allowed to do, or what they actually do. In this particular clause, it is not the collection of data but the contribution to the formulation of policy that is problematic; something that all nurses might be encouraged to do but hardly required to do. The recent revision of the revalidation process and professional code was the subject of wide consultation undertaken by the NMC but received only 1649 individual responses (Nursing and Midwifery Council, 2014), meaning that fewer than one in about 300 nurses contributed to the formulation of these policies, that is if they can be regarded as policies at all.[1]

Of more immediate concern to the practising nurse, seeking to follow the injunctions of the NMC by practising autonomously according to the best available evidence, is the extent to which they must follow the policies and guidelines of their employing organisation. Whether something can be properly regarded as a policy or a guideline is likely to be settled, for the nurse at least, by its title. There are clearly overlaps between them and the words are sometimes used interchangeably. However, there are also a number of differences between guideline and policy, but the discussion here focuses on two: justification and force.

Policies and guidelines

The first distinction between policies and guidelines is in their justification. I do not claim that guidelines are always and only based on evidence but, in the context of evidence-based practice, their primary purpose is to locate and evaluate evidence and synthesise it so that it can usefully inform practice. Evidence-based policy is, in contrast, a much more diffuse concept. It is far from clear about what counts as evidence and how causal links between policy and its claimed consequences can be demonstrated (Greenhalgh and Russell, 2009), yet these causal claims are made in many different areas of government activity. As I write this, in December 2014, a decision to reduce night-time street lighting has been criticised because it has led to an increase in accidents (BBC, 2014; Automobile Association, 2014). Here, the policy debate requires both a view about the veracity of the causal claims and, following this, a weighing up of the different options. The claimed increased number of road accidents and deaths is pitted against savings of energy and cost.

It is well recognised that there are a number of different drivers of policy making in addition to evidence, including ideology, values, public opinion and lobbying (Smith and Joyce, 2012) and, in one sense, the multiple drivers of policy might be seen as diminishing the need for evidential justification. But this is not how it is presented. Government ministers and others frequently make claims that policy is based on evidence, and yet, even allowing for the difficulty in deciding what would count as good evidence, these claims sometimes lack credibility, and there is a reasonable suspicion that despite the rhetoric concerning the value of evidence, that policy is being directed for political reasons, including ideology and short term political advantage. Core values are emphasised in the most recent white paper on public health in England which claims to take a radical new approach to public health by setting out how the approach will 'reflect the

Government's core values of freedom, fairness and responsibility by strengthening self-esteem confidence and personal responsibility; positively promoting healthy behaviours and lifestyles; and adapting the environment to make healthy choices easier' (Department of Health, 2010: 6).

In the same document, a claim to evidential justification is clear:

> the Government will balance the freedoms of individuals and organisations with the need to avoid serious harm to others. We will look carefully at the strength of the case before deciding to intervene and to what extent. This must be based on a rigorous assessment of the evidence about health and wider harms, with the potential benefits balanced against the social and economic costs to individuals, organisations and wider society.
>
> (Department of Health, 2010: 28)

Is this a credible claim for the coalition government? The Liberal Democrat minister in the Home Office, Norman Baker, resigned following the publication of a report (Home Office, 2014), which detailed evidence about drugs policy in other countries. In his resignation letter (Baker, 2014), he expressed pleasure in what he had been able to achieve: 'not least to have been the first minister with responsibility for drugs to have put prejudice aside and published an evidence-based approach to this important issue, despite repeated Conservative efforts to block release'. Despite his claims, this is not primarily a party political manner. The previous Labour government also became embroiled in controversy about how evidence informs drug policy.

What evidence that exists suggests that alcohol and tobacco, both legally available, are more harmful than cannabis and LSD, both of which are prohibited (Nutt *et al.*, 2007). According to an editorial in the *Lancet* (MacDonald and Das, 2006), the lack of appreciation of evidence by politicians has resulted in a classification system that 'almost defies belief' (p. 559). It is perhaps unsurprising that the principal author of the study into comparative harms, Professor David Nutt, was dismissed by Home Secretary Alan Johnson in 2009 from his position as Chair of the Advisory Council on the Misuse of Drugs after claiming that alcohol (Nutt, 2009a) and horse riding (Nutt, 2009b) were more dangerous than some proscribed drugs. A year earlier, he had criticised the reclassification of cannabis from class C to class B, reversing a decision taken five years previously. This decision, in effect increasing the penalties for cannabis use, was justified, politically, on the ground that evidence was strengthening that cannabis causes schizophrenia (see, for example BBC, 2009), although it has been estimated that, even for heavy users, over 1000 people would need to be prevented from using cannabis to prevent a single case (Hickman *et al.*, 2009).

A similar lack of evidence has been claimed in relation to organisational changes which have increased competition in the NHS, introduced by successive governments. A review published by the independent think tank New Economics Foundation (Coote and Penny, 2014) argues that there is no sound evidence to support the claim that increased competition can improve efficiency and quality of care. Yet successive governments, most recently David Cameron's coalition government have insisted not only that the reforms will improve care but also that they have improved care. Coote and Penny (2014) cite a speech given to NHS staff in June 2011 in which the Prime Minister claimed that a study 'found hospitals in areas with more choice had lower death rates'. He referred to a paper by Cooper *et al.* (2011), which found that mortality fell fastest in areas where there was greater competition. This paper has been critiqued on several grounds, not least for failing to show a causal relationship (Pollock *et al.*, 2011) and, in a review, Bevan and Skellern (2011) concluded that most studies found that competition has been ineffective.

This is not the place in which to attempt an evaluation of these studies but it could be done. Rigorous assessment of evidence of the sort that precedes guideline production would take account of contradictions within the body of evidence. Despite the claims made in the White Paper, there has not been a 'rigorous assessment' of the evidence in relation to drugs and competition policy. Instead, there has been an attempt at *post hoc* evidential justification by the use of selected evidence to defend policy that has been decided upon for other reasons. In evidence-based practice, evaluation of research comes prior to the production of guidelines. In much of evidence-based policy, evaluation of research evidence is a secondary and retrospective concern.

The second difference between guidance and policy is in their directive power. Properly formulated guidance assesses evidence and, where necessary, also takes into account cost effectiveness. Thereafter, it is offered to the clinician as advice and, while justification may be required if the advice is disregarded, clinicians take other factors into consideration, not least patient preference and their own clinical experience and expertise. Guidance guides. In contrast, policy can be clearly directive, and this can cause problems for individual practitioners who wish to act outside policy in pursuit of their own professional (evidence-based) judgement and patients' wishes.

The implementation of intentional rounding

The widespread implementation of intentional rounding is an interesting and illustrative case study, which demonstrates the way that spurious evidential claims are used to defend what are easily capable of being seen as politically motivated nursing interventions. Levenson defines intentional rounding as:

> the timed planned intervention of health care staff in order to address common elements of nursing care, typically by means of a regular bedside ward round that proactively seeks to identify and meet patients' fundamental care needs and psychological safety.
>
> (Levenson, 2013: 5)

The key features are that all patients are visited at set frequencies and that a standardised approach to care is used. In the UK, Castledine (2002) proposed them as 'a new idea' in nursing in 2002, and intentional rounding has been popular in the United States for some time.

In the wake of high-profile failures in care, the idea of regular and universal checking was promoted by the Prime Minister, who said in January 2012 during a visit to Salford Hospital, that 'in place of non-essential paperwork and other unnecessary activities, nurses will be able to undertake regular nursing rounds which will ensure that every hour, they will be able to check that every patient is comfortable' (Department of Health, 2012a). Intentional rounding was noted with approval in the Francis (2013) report and, although open to some interpretation, it was recognised in recommendation 238 (Francis, 2013: 1610): 'Regular interaction and engagement between nurses and patients and those close to them should be systematised through regular ward rounds.' In its initial response to the Francis report, the government gave rounding as an example of a 'comply or explain' approach to be used in hospital inspections: 'Inspectors will expect to see these being used across hospitals, or a valid explanation given if this is not the case' (Department of Health, 2013: 17). It is not clear what would constitute a 'valid' explanation.

At the same time as the Prime Minister was setting out his expectations, claims about the effect of intentional rounding were released in the form of a press release from the NHS trust, supported by the Chief Nurse's newsletter (Department of Health, 2012b), which stated that quality improvement initiatives have led to:

- 92 per cent of patients harm free as measured by the safety thermometer
- 78 per cent reduction in *Clostridium difficile*
- 71 per cent reduction in cardiac arrests
- 56 per cent reduction in pressure ulcers
- 17 per cent reduction in falls.

It should be noted that these figures were not claimed to be the result of intentional rounding alone. Intentional rounding was also being promoted by the King's Fund, an influential independent think tank. A PowerPoint presentation available on their website presents the evidence base for intentional rounding as being from a study undertaken in the United States by the Studer Group (Meade *et al*., 2006), which found the following in a 'controlled trial (Bartley, 2011):

- 38 per cent reduction in call lights
- 12 point mean increase in patient satisfaction
- 50 per cent reduction in patient falls
- 14 per cent reduction in pressure ulcers.

These evidential claims are repeatedly given as rationale for local policies. Even more impressive results, including a 56 per cent reduction in pressure ulcers have been claimed in a further Studer Group publication (Studer Group, 2007).

Also in response to concerns about the quality of nursing care, notably at Mid Staffordshire NHS Foundation Trust, the Prime Minister established the Nursing and Care Quality Forum (NCQF), an 'independent group of nursing and care experts [which] aims to spread best practice in all care settings and make recommendations about tackling barriers to high quality, safe and effective care' (Department of Health, 2012b). It is interesting to note that the word 'evidence' is absent from their mission statement, which instead includes, as an aim to: 'achieve their ambition of providing the very highest quality of care through supporting the adoption of best practice and promoting innovation' (Department of Health, 2012c). In its initial recommendations to the Prime Minister, the NCQF (Nursing and Care Quality Forum, 2012a) indicated its desire to accelerate the implementation of rounding and a further report, in September 2012 (Nursing and Care Quality Forum, 2012b), noted that demonstrator sites had been established. The report on the implementation of the demonstrator sites for the NCQF was published in August 2013 (Levenson, 2013).

The report is clearly concerned with the implementation of intentional rounding rather than its effectiveness and has involved a good deal of work with observations and interviews. In a sense, the report, and those like it, can be regarded as a form of qualitative enquiry. It has some significance, but despite its 39 pages, it cannot be properly regarded as academically presented qualitative research which can be properly evaluated. There was scant reference to the literature: 'while a systematic literature review was beyond the scope of the report, it was useful to look at recent key articles' (Levenson, 2013: 35), a cursory examination that would be unacceptable to any peer reviewer. The report uncritically notes the extraordinary claims made by the Studer Group about the effectiveness of rounding, simply noting that some see the evidence base as flawed and some are less than enthusiastic. The future of the NCQF is unsure and it was reported, in March 2014, that its members feared that it has been disbanded (Stephenson, 2014). It seems odd that this body, established with an authoritative prime ministerial fanfare and an ambitious remit two years previously simply did not know whether or not it existed. What can be said with some confidence is that it was influential in ensuring that intentional rounding has become established. However, not only were recommendations, including by Robert Francis, made without referral to evidence but an evaluation report also cited supporting evidence without evaluating it and simply noted that some people disagreed. So much for best practice.

Fuller evaluations of the evidence and process are available elsewhere (Snelling, 2013a, 2013b). There are a number of worrying issues concerning the quality of the evidence cited and the use to which it has been put. Nearly all evidential trails about intentional rounding lead to Meade *et al.* (2006). This was a multicentre trial carried out by the Studer Group, which found significant reductions in falls and increases in patient satisfaction following the introduction of hourly and two-hourly rounding regimes. Some of the shortcomings of the study design were acknowledged by the researchers: the groups were not matched and individual units self-assigned to specific groups, which may have been for self-interest. Data were provided by the hospitals themselves. Design and statistical concerns are reported by Vest and Gamm (2009). Data were discarded from 19 of the original 46 units because the rounding logs had more than five per cent of data elements missing, suggesting that 'nursing staff members hadn't consistently performed the rounding' (Meade *et al.*, 2006: 62). The hourly rounding regime consisted of a visit every hour between 0600 and 2200 with two-hourly visits overnight; that is, 20 visits per 24 hours, and so a single daily missed or unrecorded visit constitutes the cut-off point of 95 per cent of data. This means that the results are generalisable (if they are at all) only to areas where this ludicrous level of compliance is maintained. For comparison, a more academically rigorous study (Tucker *et al.*, 2012) also undertaken in the United States, which did not support Meade *et al.*'s findings, documented compliance to be 22–60 per cent. A cursory read of Meade *et al.*'s (2006) paper will suffice to show that it is not a disinterested and open-minded study. A nested box within the text describes the conversion of a ward manager from sceptic to evangelist and another follows up hospital units one year later referencing further Studer Group publications. A video training package for intentional rounding based on the impressive results in the study is for sale for US$995 via its website (Studer Group, no date).

The second Studer Group publication (2007) takes the form of a best practice supplement, largely detailing implementation processes and documents. The first two pages simply state the results, which were also cited uncritically by Levenson (2013). There is neither methodological detail nor data analysis; the reader is simply told, via bar charts, that five months after implementing intentional rounding, patient satisfaction increased by 71 percentage points, falls reduced by 33 per cent and hospital-acquired pressure ulcers fell from 16 to 7, a reduction of 56 per cent. These completely unsubstantiated and, as they are presented, meaningless claims published in what amounts to an advertising brochure for a management consultancy selling to US hospitals, have been cited by Levenson (2013) and elsewhere (for example, Forde-Johnston, 2014) as evidential support for intentional rounding in the UK. Even more worrying is the claim that Meade *et al.*'s (2006) study reduced pressure ulcers by 14 per cent, which has been cited in a number of publications (for example, Fitzsimons *et al.*, 2011). This finding is simply not in the paper and presumably indicates that those citing it have not read it. A review of the literature (Forde-Johnston, 2014) promulgated this error and also failed to locate a paper (Snelling, 2013a) which pointed it out. A systematic review completed in 2013 and published in 2014 (Mitchell *et al.*, 2014) found only one study (Saleh *et al.*, 2011), since retracted, which used pressure ulcers as an outcome measure. The claim that intentional rounding reduces pressure ulcers has become accepted within 'evidence-based' policies without the support of a single study that can be properly evaluated.

As well as uncritically reporting and serially misreporting findings of very poor quality research, there has been a complete failure to consider the wider concepts underpinning intentional rounding. The intervention has been claimed to increase patient satisfaction but it is far from clear that this is a valid indicator of quality of care, particularly in a different healthcare environment from that where most studies have been undertaken. In the UK, NICE (2012: 10) states that 'the concept of satisfaction has been explored in various formats over the last two decades within the NHS; it is now widely acknowledged that it is a poor indicator for evaluating quality from a patient experience perspective'.

Of course patient satisfaction is important but the oversimplification represented by the conflation of quality and perception of care can obscure a detailed analysis of what interventions improve quality. Additionally, the frequency of call-bell usage has been used as an indicator to assess the effectiveness of rounding in a number of studies, including Meade *et al.* (2006), but this is not supported by evidence or argument. Tzeng and Yin (2009) found that increased number of call bells correlated with less fall related harm and their recommendation was that wards encourage call-bell usage. In a further study, Tzeng *et al.* (2012) confirmed this finding and also found that, after correlating for covariates, both the number of falls and number of injurious falls were associated with lower call-bell response time rather than usage, something barely considered in the literature on intentional rounding.

Primary research on intentional rounding is of a very poor standard and what little there is has not been properly evaluated before being given as justification for widespread intervention. In the UK, the National Institute for Health Research (NIHR) has awarded a grant approaching £450,000 to investigate further the implementation of intentional rounding. The grant application notes that:

> Ideally a randomized experimental study would be used to assess the effectiveness of a new intervention. However the use of this approach is not possible as the implementation of intentional rounding has been strongly advocated and promoted by the current government and very few trusts are reported not to have implemented it.
>
> (Harris *et al.*, 2014: 5)

Instead, realist evaluation methodology will be used, with the aim of investigating trends in patient outcomes rather than seeking to demonstrate cause and effect.

It is clear through the many poor-quality local reports published largely in professional journals that there is some appetite within the nursing profession to undertake intentional rounding and that some studies also report some benefit. It has become *de facto* national policy and this is recognised locally, as the vague recommendations have been operationalised in line with local experience. It should be clear that the preceding analysis does not suggest that there is anything necessarily wrong with intentional rounding. There is every possibility that it is effective in promoting increased quality of care. From the perspective of evidence-based practice, the rapid and widespread implementation is a case study of a top-down political intervention which allowed the government to move debate away from institutional failings and lack of resources as an explanation for the poor care experienced by many at Mid Staffordshire and beyond (Paley, 2014). The *Daily Telegraph* reported the Prime Minister's visit to Salford Hospital under the headline 'David Cameron: There is a real problem with nursing in our hospitals' (Kirkup and Holehouse, 2012) and, while the Prime Minister's words were a little more circumspect, the effect of focusing, at this time, on simple measures to change nursing practice rather than addressing resource and organisational issues was a deliberately chosen political act.

There is at the heart of the implementation a simple logical conundrum. If intentional rounding is performed on all patients as the Prime Minister says that it should be, then it will be performed on many patients who do not need it and they are as likely to be annoyed as reassured by the constant intrusion by nurses who, in these circumstances, are likely to see the intervention as an exercise in ticking boxes, taking them away from more important work. Conversely, if regular checks are made only on patients who require them on the basis of sound nursing assessment, then it is not intentional rounding at all and cannot be presented as a political and managerial response to poor care. It is just, well, individualised nursing. There is some evidence that some local policies are adapting the Prime Minister's injunction by assessing patient needs and performing regular checks only if required (for example, Royal Cornwall Hospitals NHS Trust, 2013a, 2013b) and this is to be welcomed. Until this is the norm (and Professor Harris's research will throw some light on this), intentional rounding cannot be regarded as evidence-based policy. The evidence base, what little there is of it, is tainted by commercial self-interest and poor quality and this has been exacerbated by serial misreporting and a complete failure to evaluate the quality and transferability of primary sources. It is a clear example of politically based policy implementation and the nursing profession has done a disservice to itself and its patients by acquiescing in its implementation, all the while claiming that it is underpinned by evidence. It is not.

Hospital smoking bans

The history of implementation of hospital smoking bans is a case study of the interplay between facts and values. Hume famously observed that you cannot derive an ought from an is. Evidence is, mostly, factual, although values guide its production, but it is helpful for analysis to attempt to keep facts and values apart as far as possible. If treatment A produces the best results in treating disease X (which leads to early death), it does not follow logically that treatment A should be offered. Factual and normative premises link something like this:

Factual premise (research):	Disease X causes early death.
Normative premise (policy):	Early death (caused by X) should be avoided.
Normative conclusion (policy):	Disease X should be treated.

Normative premise (policy):	The most effective treatment should be used.
Factual premise (research):	Drug A is the most effective treatment.
Normative conclusion (action):	Drug A should be used.

The normative conclusion would form the basis of a guideline. Of course, it is not quite so simple. In a publically funded health service, which places an opportunity cost on each treatment, it is not so much effectiveness as cost effectiveness that decides treatment. Funding allocation by use of quality adjusted life years (QALYs) is an attempt to get the most benefit for each healthcare pound spent, even though serious concerns are raised in relation to its fairness in regard to particular illnesses. See, for example, Garau *et al.* (2011), in relation to the difficulties in using QALYs in cancer. This could change the premises to 'cost effective' instead of 'effective' and this would increase the evidence required (NICE, 2012b). Patient consent is also required before a treatment is administered so that the normative conclusion could be recast as 'Drug A should be *offered*' instead of used. In the context of evidence-based practice, as in all forms of professional practice, consent is morally very important (as well as legally required) because it is the practical manifestation, albeit an imperfect one, of the bioethical principle of respect for autonomy (Beauchamp and Childress, 2013), seen by many (Gillon, 2003) as the predominant principle, based on the ultimate value. In these heuristic syllogisms for evidence-based practice, facts derived from research and values from elsewhere are kept apart, so far as is possible, but what is offered depends on available evidence. In the ordinary run of events in evidence-based practice, much time and effort is spent on investigating the effects and costs of drugs and other treatments. In most cases, although not all, the values that drive empirical investigations are largely uncontested.

The development of policies to reduce smoking similarly involves facts and values, though here the emphasis is different. Some treatments, for example nicotine replacement therapy offered to individuals follow the standard 'treatment' evidence cascade. Other public health measures to reduce smoking at the group level are also based on evidence; for example, policies of enforcing plain packaging of cigarettes are based on evidence, derived from experience from other countries (Freeman *et al.*, 2008), that they would reduce smoking. Unsurprisingly, manufacturers are opposed but the provision does not directly restrict liberty and threatens autonomous decision making barely at the margins or not at all.

Some smoking policies are, however, more directly liberty threatening. The Health Act 2006 introduced a number of changes into the NHS but it will be best remembered for changing forever the experiences of smokers in England and Wales. From 1 July 2007, smoking was no longer permitted in public places and in certain places of work. The given justification for the ban was other-regarding; for example, by the House of Commons Health Committee (2005), para 41: 'The justification for the principle of a ban is straightforward: workers have a right to be protected from SHS (second hand smoke)'. Unlike care homes and hospices, which were excluded from the legislation, mental health units were given a temporary exemption order for one year, which, upon expiry, meant that, where smokers could not be permitted to go outside, they were forced to stop smoking. The ban was unsuccessfully challenged by patients at Rampton and Carstairs hospitals using the European Convention on Human Rights (ECHR) in the English and Scottish courts where Lord Stewart, presiding in the Scottish Court noted that: 'Article 8(2) ECHR authorizes interventions which are 'necessary in a democratic society ... for the protection of health or morals: it is not a warrant for lifestyle fascism'.[2]

Despite his observations here, Lord Stewart found for the appellants only reluctantly.[3] His judgement also included: 'It is a perfectly reasonable proposition, given contemporary understanding about the effects of tobacco smoking, that patients in a hospital should not be permitted to smoke'.[4] His judgement was subsequently overturned on appeal.

In these political and judicial comments, a move can be seen from prevention of harm to others towards prevention of harm to the smoker. Similar justification can be found in NICE guidance: *Smoking Cessation in Secondary Care: Acute, maternity and mental health services* (NICE, 2013a). There is an extensive evidence base given in support of a wide range of guidance, including recommendation number 11: 'Develop smokefree policies', including the removal of shelters or other designated outdoor areas, and ensuring policies are in place to 'facilitate compliance with, and resolve immediately, any breaches of smokefree policies' (p. 16). There is a large amount of, often weak, evidence detailed in the accompanying evidence statement document (NICE, 2013b), mainly drawn from the United States, about impacts on patients; for example, frequency of violent episodes and use of restraint in mental health units. But there cannot be direct evidence for the important policy provision that smoking ought to be prohibited in hospital grounds, because it is a normative question. It does not follow from a fact that smoking bans can be implemented effectively that they should be implemented.

The guidance is directed not at clinicians but at employing organisations, many of which have policies of the sort recommended. The NICE guidelines recommended 'no exceptions for particular groups' (p. 6) but this is clearly incorporated into some local policies formulated before the NICE guidance was released (see, for example, the policies of West London Mental Health NHST, 2012, and Manchester Mental Health and Social Care Trust, 2012). Tameside Hospitals NHS Trust's policy, revised after the guidance, has no exceptions and includes the forthright clauses:

> Staff will not be permitted to assist patients who wish to smoke. Staff must not accompany patients who wish to smoke, and any member of staff who does so will be subject to disciplinary action in line with Trust policy. All staff should receive the support of senior colleagues and Security Officers if patients or visitors place staff under pressure to violate the Trust's No Smoking status.
>
> (Tameside Hospitals NHS Trust, 2014, para 7.8)

> If a patient leaves a Ward without permission from Ward staff, the patient will be wholly responsible for anything that may occur as a result of their action.
>
> (para 7.9)

The significant point for consideration for this chapter is that, despite the evidential legitimacy offered by inclusion in NICE guidelines, sitting as they do at the very top rung of the evidence-based practice ladder, these guidelines and the policies that follow are not based upon evidence but upon values. These values are in tension with both the professional requirement for autonomous practice and the patient's right to make decisions for himself in what he perceives to be his best interest.

Conclusion

Policy is legitimately influenced by many considerations and yet, as I have argued, evidential justification is frequently sought and claimed. Intentional rounding has been widely implemented in the interest of a political need for action, supported by appeasing managers in the absence of credible evidence. Authoritarian and paternalistic smoking policies are given evidential gloss by NICE guidelines but are driven by imposed values. Despite claims made to the contrary, evidence-based policy is often a myth and it exposes important tensions for practicing nurses and perhaps more importantly, nurse managers.

The NMC requires nurses to practise autonomously based on the best available evidence. Both of these injunctions are significantly compromised by the policies I have discussed. It is plausible that nurses are forced to choose between following these professional requirements, acting as advocates for their patients, and following a policy that requires them to do neither of these things. Clarity about what regulatory injunctions amount to may prevent them from having to argue the case for their autonomous evidence-based practice before a disciplinary panel or employment tribunal.

Notes

1   As a matter of logic, it might be suggested that even if consultation on a new professional code is regarded as 'formulation of policy', it might not be regarded as policy on 'risks, hazards and adverse outcomes', but I suggest that few of the 299 (of 300) nurses failing to respond to the consultation would offer this in justification.
2   *C M v The State Hospitals Board for Scotland*. 2013 WL 4411375. Paragraph 52.
3   There was a dissenting judgement (Keene LJ) in the English Court of Appeal. *R(N) v The Secretary of State for Health*. [2009] EWCA Civ 795.
4   *C M v The State Hospitals Board for Scotland*. 2013 WL 4411375. Paragraph 5.

References

Automobile Association (2014) Turning off street lights: inquests reveal pattern of death on councils' blacked out roads. *theaa.com*, 4 July. Available online at www.theaa.com/newsroom/news-2014/streetlights-ignoring-inquest-findings.html (accessed 14 March 2015).

Baker, N. (2014) A statement from Norman Baker MP [blog post]. Available online at http://normanbaker.org.uk/2014/11/04/a-statement-from-norman-baker-mp (accessed 14 March 2015).

Bartley, A. (2011) *Making It Happen: Intentional rounding*. London: King's Fund.

BBC (2009) Debate over cannabis classification. *BBC News*, 31 October. Available online at http://news.bbc.co.uk/1/hi/uk/7845023.stm (accessed 14 March 2015).

BBC (2014) Labour attacks street light cuts. *BBC News*, 22 December. Available online at www.bbc.co.uk/news/uk-politics-30569215 (accessed 14 March 2015).

Beauchamp, T. L. and Childress, J. F. (2013) *Principles of Biomedical Ethics*, 7th edn. Oxford: Oxford University Press.

Bevan, G. and Skellern, M. (2011) Does competition between hospitals improve clinical quality? A review of evidence from two eras of competition in the English NHS. *BMJ*, 343(10), d6470.

Castledine, G. (2002) Patient comfort rounds: a new initiative in nursing. *British Journal of Nursing* 11(6), 407.

Coggon, J. (2012) *What Makes Health Public?* Cambridge: Cambridge University Press.

Cooper, Z., Gibbons, S., Jones, S. and McGuire, A. (2011) Does hospital competition save lives? evidence from the English NHS patient choice reforms. *Economic Journal*, 121(554), F228–60.

Coote, A. and Penny, J. (2104) *The Wrong Medicine: A review of the impacts of NHS reforms in England*. London: New Economics Foundation.

Department of Health (2010) *Healthy Lives, Healthy People. Our strategy for public health in England*. London: Department of Health.

Department of Health (2012a) PM announces new focus on quality and nursing care [press release]. *gov.uk*, 6 January. Available online at www.gov.uk/government/news/pm-announces-new-focus-on-quality-and-nursing-care (accessed 14 March 2015).

Department of Health (2012b) A commitment to quality – Salford Royal NHS Foundation Trust welcomes Prime Minister and Secretary of state. *Chief Nursing Officer Bulletin*, 31 January. Available online at http://cno.dh.gov.uk/2012/01/31/a-commitment-to-quality (accessed 14 March 2015).

Department of Health (2012c) Nursing and Care Quality Forum, Mission Statement. Available online at www.gov.uk/government/uploads/system/uploads/attachment_data/file/216805/Nursing-and-Care-Quality-Forum-Mission-Statement.pdf (accessed 14 March 2015).

Department of Health (2013) *Patients First and Foremost. The Initial Government Response to the Report of The Mid Staffordshire NHS Foundation Trust Public Inquiry, Presented to Parliament by the Secretary of State for Health by Command of Her Majesty*. Cm 8576. London: TSO.

Fitzsimons, B., Bartley, A. and Cornwell, J. (2011) Intentional rounding: its role in supporting essential care. *Nursing Times*, 107(27), 18–21.

Forde-Johnston, C. (2014) Intentional rounding: a review of the literature. *Nursing Standard*, 28(32), 37–42.

Francis, R. (2013) *Report of the Mid Staffordshire NHS Foundation Trust Public Inquiry, Chaired by Robert Francis QC. Presented to Parliament pursuant to Section 26 of the Inquiries Act 2005*. HC947. London: TSO.

Freeman, B., Chapman, S. and Rimmer, M. (2008) The case for the plain packaging of tobacco products. *Addiction*, 103(4), 580–90.

Garau, M., Shah, K. K., Mason, A. R., Wang, Q., Towse, A. and Drummond, M. F. (2011) Using QALYs in cancer, *Pharmacoeconomics*, 29(8), 673–85.

Gillon, R. (2003) Ethics needs principles – four can encompass the rest – and respect for autonomy should be 'first among equals', *Journal of Medical Ethics*, 29, 309–12.

Greenhalgh, T. and Russell, J. (2009) Evidence-based policymaking: a critique. *Perspectives in Biology and Medicine*, 52(2), 304–18.

Ham, C. (2009) *Health Policy in Britain*, 6th edn. Basingstoke: Palgrave MacMillan.

Hickman, M., Vickerman, P., Macleod, J., Lewis, G., Zammit, S., Kirkbride, J. and Jones,

P. (2009) If cannabis caused schizophrenia-how many cannabis users may need to be prevented in order to prevent one case of schizophrenia? England and Wales calculations. *Addiction*, 104, 1856–61.

Harris, R., Gourlay, S., Ross, F., Sims, S. and Levenson, R. (2014) HSandDR-13/07/87: Intentional rounding in hospital wards: what works, for whom and in what circumstances? [project portfolio]. National Institute for Health Research. Available online at www.nets.nihr.ac.uk/projects/hsdr/130787 (accessed 14 March 2015).

Home Office (2014) *Drugs: International Comparators*. London: Home Office.

House of Commons Health Committee (2005) *Smoking in Public Places: First report of session 2005–2006*. London: TSO.

Kirkup, J. and Holehouse, M. (2012) David Cameron: There is a real problem with nursing in our hospitals. *Daily Telegraph*, 6 January. Available online at www.telegraph.co.uk/health/healthnews/8996771/David-Cameron-There-is-a-real-problem-with-nursing-in-our-hospitals.html (accessed 14 March 2015).

Levenson, R. (2013) *A Report on the Implementation of Intentional Rounding at Demonstrator Sites for the Nursing and Care Quality Forum*. London: NHS England. Available online at www.6cs.england.nhs.uk/pg/cv_content/content/view/81294/76110?cindex=0andcview=81295andctype=allandcflag=createdandcdvault=76117and container=76110# (accessed 14 March 2015).

MacDonald, R. and Das, A. (2006) UK classification of drugs of abuse: an un-evidence-based mess. *Lancet*, 368(9535), 559–61.

Manchester Mental Health and Social Care Trust (2012) Directorate of Nursing and Therapies Smokefree Policy. Available online at http://mentalhealthforum.org.uk/uploads/file/Manchester%20Smoke%20Free%20Policy.pdf (accessed 14 March 2015).

Meade, C. M., Bursell, A. L. and Ketelsen, L. (2006) Effects of nursing rounds on patients' call light use, satisfaction and safety. *American Journal of Nursing*, 106(9), 58–70.

Mitchell, M. D., Lavenberg, J. G., Trotta, R. L. and Umscheid, C. A. (2014) Hourly rounding to improve nursing responsiveness: a systematic review. *Journal of Nursing Administration*, 44(9), 462–72.

NICE (2012a) *Patient Experience in Adult NHS Services: Improving the experience of care for people using adult NHS services; patient experience in generic terms*. Clinical guidance, methods, evidence and recommendations. London: National Institute for Health and Clinical Excellence.

NICE (2012b) *The Guidelines Manual: 7 – Assessing Cost Effectiveness*. London: National Institute of Health and Care Excellence. Available online at www.nice.org.uk/article/pmg6/chapter/7-assessing-cost-effectiveness (accessed 14 March 2015).

NICE (2013a) *Smoking Cessation in Secondary Care: Acute, maternity and mental health services*. Public Health Guidance 48. London: National Institute of Health and Care Excellence.

NICE (2013b) *Smoking Cessation in Secondary Care: Acute, maternity and mental health services*. The evidence statements. London: National Institute of Health and Care Excellence.

Nursing and Care Quality Forum (2012a) Letter to the Prime Minister, 18 May. Available online at http://webarchive.nationalarchives.gov.uk/20130123162410/www.wp.dh.gov.uk/ncqf/files/2012/07/NCQF-letter-to-PM-_Final_.pdf (accessed 14 March 2015).

Nursing and Care Quality Forum (2012b) Letter to the Prime Minister, 30 September. Available online at http://webarchive.nationalarchives.gov.uk/20130123162410/

www.wp.dh.gov.uk/ncqf/files/2012/10/NCQF-letter-to-the-PM-Sept-2012.pdf (accessed 14 March 2015).

Nursing and Midwifery Council (2010) *Standards of Competence for Registered Nurses*. London: Nursing and Midwifery Council.

Nursing and Midwifery Council (2014) *Revalidation Evidence Report*. London: Nursing and Midwifery Council.

Nursing and Midwifery Council (2015) *The Code: Professional standards of practice and behaviour for nurses and midwives*. London: Nursing and Midwifery Council.

Nutt, D., King, L.A., Saulsbury, W. and Blakemore, C. (2007) Development of a rational scale to assess the harm of drugs of potential misuse. *Lancet*, 369, 1047–53.

Nutt, D. (2009a) Estimating drug harms: a risky business. *Centre for Crime and Justice Studies Briefing*, 10. Available online at www.crimeandjustice.org.uk/publications/ estimating-drug-harms-risky-business (accessed 14 March 2015).

Nutt, D. (2009b) Equasy: An overlooked addiction. *Journal of Psychopharmacology*, 23(1), 3–5.

Paley, J. (2014) Cognition and the compassion deficit: the social psychology of helping behaviour in nursing. *Nursing Philosophy*, 15(4), 274–87.

Pollock, A., Macfarlane, A., Kirkwood, G., Majeed, F. A., Greener, I., Morelli, C., *et al.* (2011) No evidence that patient choice in the NHS saves lives. *Lancet*, 378(9809), 2057–60.

Royal Cornwall Hospitals NHS Trust (2013a) Policy for the Management and Reduction of Risk of Falls in Hospital Care and the Safe Use of Bedrails with Adult Patients, v3.2. Available online at www.rcht.nhs.uk/DocumentsLibrary/RoyalCornwallHospitals Trust/Clinical/General/FallsPolicy.pdf (accessed 14 March 2015).

Royal Cornwall hospitals NHS Trust (2013b) Safe and Supportive Observation Policy, v2.1 Available online at www.rcht.nhs.uk/DocumentsLibrary/RoyalCornwallHospitals Trust/Clinical/SafeguardingAdults/PolicyAndProceduresForTheSafeAndSupportiveO bservat.pdf (accessed 14 March 2015).

Saleh, B. S., Nusair, H., Al Zubadi, N., Al Shloul, S. and Saleh, U. (2011) Retracted: The nursing rounds system: Effect of patient's call light use, bed sores, fall and satisfaction level. *International Journal of Nursing Practice*, 17(3), 299–303.

Smith, K. E. and Joyce, K. E (2012) Capturing complex realities: understanding efforts to achieve evidence-based policy and practice in public health. *Evidence and Policy*, 8(1), 57–78.

Snelling, P. C. (2013a) Ethical and professional concerns in research utilisation: Intentional rounding in the United Kingdom. *Nursing Ethics*, 20(7), 784–97.

Snelling, P. C. (2013b) Intentional rounding: A critique of the evidence, *Nursing Times*, 109(20), 19–21.

Stephenson, J. (2014) PM's expert nursing forum fears it has been scrapped. *Nursing Times*, 19 March. Available online at www.nursingtimes.net/nursing-practice/clinical-zones/management/pms-expert-nursing-forum-fears-it-has-been-scrapped/5068967.art icle (accessed 14 March 2015).

Studer Group (no date) Hourly rounding improving nursing and patient care excellence DVD [advertising webpage]. Available online at www.firestarterpublishing.com/ videos/sample-category/hourly-rounding-br-em-improving-nursing-and-pa-(1)#. VJcN8l4h7A (accessed 14 March 2015).

Studer Group (2007) *Hourly Rounding Supplement. Best practice: Sacred Heart Hospital Pensacola, Florida*. Available online at www.mc.vanderbilt.edu/root/pdfs/nursing/ hourly_rounding_supplement-studer_group.pdf (accessed 14 March 2015).

Tameside Hospitals NHS Foundation Trust (2014) No smoking policy. Available online at www.tamesidehospital.nhs.uk/documents/NoSmokingPolicy.pdf (accessed 14 March 2015).

Traynor, M. (2013) *Nursing in Context: Policy, politics profession*. Basingstoke: Palgrave Macmillan.

Tucker, S. J., Bieber, P. L., Attlesey-Pries, J. M., Olson, M. E. and Dierkhising, R. A. (2012) Outcomes and challenges in implementing hourly rounds to reduce falls in orthopedic units. *Worldviews on Evidence-Based Nursing*, 9(1), 18–29.

Tzeng, H. M. and Yin C.-Y. (2009) Relationship between call light use and response time and inpatient falls in acute care settings. Journal of Clinical Nursing, 18, 3333–3341.

Tzeng, H. M., Titler, M. G., Ronis, D. L. and Yin, C. Y. (2012) The contribution of staff call light response time to fall and injurious fall rates: an exploratory study in four US hospitals using archived hospital data. *BMC Health Services Research*, 12(1), 84. doi:10.1186/1472-6963-12-84.

Vest, J. R. and Gamm, L. D. (2009) A critical review of the research literature on Six Sigma, Lean and StuderGroup's Hardwiring Excellence in the United States: the need to demonstrate and communicate the effectiveness of transformational strategies in healthcare. *Implementation Science*; 4, 35. doi:10.1186/1748-5908-4-35.

West London Mental Health NHS Trust (2012) Policy: S5. Smoke Free Policy. Available online at www.wlmht.nhs.uk/wp-content/uploads/2014/10/S5-Smoke-Free-Policy.pdf (accessed 14 March 2015).

Index

CPSIA information can be obtained
at www.ICGtesting.com
Printed in the USA
LVOW01*1317200716

497082LV00007B/30/P